This book is dedicated to the men and women around the world who, in large measure and small, give of themselves to heal others.

The companies below generously provided 100 world-class photojournalists with the necessary funding and support to travel throughout the world on this extraordinary assignment. We are grateful to these companies for giving us the opportunity to tell the story of humanity's growing ability to heal.

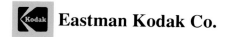 Eastman Kodak Co.

PARKE-DAVIS

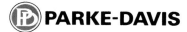 United States Surgical Corporation

Empire Blue Cross Blue Shield

PAN AM.

Apple Computer, Inc.

Nikon

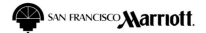 SAN FRANCISCO Marriott.

THE
POWER TO HEAL
Ancient Arts & Modern Medicine

Rick Smolan
Phillip Moffitt
Matthew Naythons, M.D.

Designed by Thomas K. Walker

PRENTICE
HALL
PRESS

New York   London   Toronto   Sydney   Tokyo   Singapore

in association with
THE RxMEDIA GROUP

Created and Produced by
Rick Smolan
Phillip W. Moffitt
Matthew Naythons, M.D.

Project Administration
Jennifer Erwitt
Project Director
Chris Noble
Production Coordinator

Office Administration
Kate Warne
Office Manager

Medical Advisor
Robert Rabkin, M.D.

Legal Advisor
Douglas P. Ferguson
Ferguson, Hoffman,
& Finney, Inc.

With special support from
Lukas Bonnier
Raymond H. DeMoulin
John Sculley
Joseph E. Smith

Design
Thomas K. Walker
Creative Director
Amy Schmitt
Senior Designer
Alex G. Sorger
Junior Designer

Picture Editing
Guy Cooper
Newsweek Magazine
Mike Davis
Albuquerque Tribune
Dennis R. Dimick
National Geographic Society
Sandra Eisert
San Jose, CA
Alfonso Gutierrez
A.G.E. Fotostock
Bill Kuykendall
University of Missouri
School of Journalism
Michelle McNally
Fortune Magazine
Eric Meskauskas
New York Daily News
Maddy Miller
People Magazine
George Olson
San Francisco, CA
Dieter Steiner
Stern Magazine
Anne Stovell
Time Magazine

Editorial
Bernard Ohanian
Editor and Caption Author
Dawn Sheggeby
Assistant Editor

Assignment &
Research Editors
Belle Adler
Laura Fraser
Elizabeth W. Heckscher
Robert Ivry
O. David Spitzler
Rob Waters

Leslie S. Feldman
Assistant

Copy Editors
Ruth Henrich
Jonathan A. Schwartz

Marketing and Sales
Preston C. Williams
Consulting Director
Peter Goggin
Coordinator

Public Relations
Kristin Joyce
Director
Patti Richards
Consultant

Business Consultants
Ira O. Glick
Cheryl MacLachlan
Dan O'Shea
Marvin M. Smolan

Accounting
Carla C. Levdar
Black Oak Services

Prentice Hall Press
15 Columbus Circle
New York, NY 10023

Copyright © 1990 by The RxMedia Group

Library of Congress Cataloging-in-Publication Data

Smolan, Rick
      The power to heal/ by Rick Smolan, Phillip Moffitt, and Matthew Naythons
      p. cm.
      ISBN 0-13-684549-5
      1. Medicine--Miscellanea--Pictorial works. 1. Moffitt, Phillip
II. Naythons, Matthew. III. Title.
R706.S56 1990
610--dc20   89-71017
                                                        CIP

Designed by Thomas K. Walker, GRAF/x

Manufactured in Japan

10   9   8   7   6   5   4   3   2   1

First Edition

Contents

Humanity's First Quest

When we began *The Power to Heal,* the original idea was to create a photography book of health, healing, and medicine around the world. We wanted it to reflect our belief that in the 1990s, wellness and longevity would be a central consideration in how people made decisions about their lives.

As it turned out, the book you now hold in your hands is about a much larger story, of which our original premise became only one small part. Almost on its own, the project was transformed into an exploration of the whole concept of healing. We found ourselves on a quest to understand the connection between the ancient arts of healing and the modern science of medicine. We were forced to answer questions such as, "What does it mean to be healed? What is the difference between physical healing and psychological healing? What is the nature of healing if one is not going to recover physically? How is our understanding of disease itself changing as we face the new millennium? Does this mean that medicine too must be redefined?"

We began to examine the role of the doctor, both as the primary healer and as a scientific fighter against ever more complex diseases. The rationality of the doctor and biomedicine brought up, in turn, the "softer" healing techniques of the mind, of attitude, and of the possibility of a spiritual component in healing. Our quest brought us to the conclusion that health and wellness are not an end goal, but are rather an ongoing process—a state of constant change and development that is in fact the process of life itself.

With *The Power to Heal,* then, we dedicated ourselves to telling the stories of the wondrous progress in medicine over the last century, and modern medicine's connections to older, traditional healing arts. We wanted to show, through visual images and word pictures, the compassion and humanity that transcend—and link—all varieties of medicine and healing.

It is this last point, we hope, that makes *The Power to Heal* noteworthy, in that it shows how all people everywhere are connected in the struggle to heal and be healthy and yet how their personal experiences of the process differ radically. This is a book filled with stories of heroes and individual acts of courage by both healers and patients.

Most of all, *The Power to Heal* captures time and again the beautiful and mysterious power that one human being can have on another through the mere act of caring. Our strongest wish is that this book carries forward this great truth—that the act of caring is the first true step in the power to heal.

—Phillip Moffitt

Health worker Wingti Mininbi examines sixty-five-year-old Tona Kowil at Aviamp Aide Post in the Pacific island nation of Papua New Guinea. *Photo by Sarah Leen*

Ancient Arts to Modern Medicine

*Long before the growth of modern medicine,
before the wizardry of pharmaceutical drugs and the
miraculous dexterity of surgery, men and
women were seeking the source of illness and the elixir of
good health. Stone Age cave dwellers dug for
medicinal plants, and the healing repertoire of the Egyptians
included herbal remedies for crocodile bites.*
—Wade Davis, Ph.D.

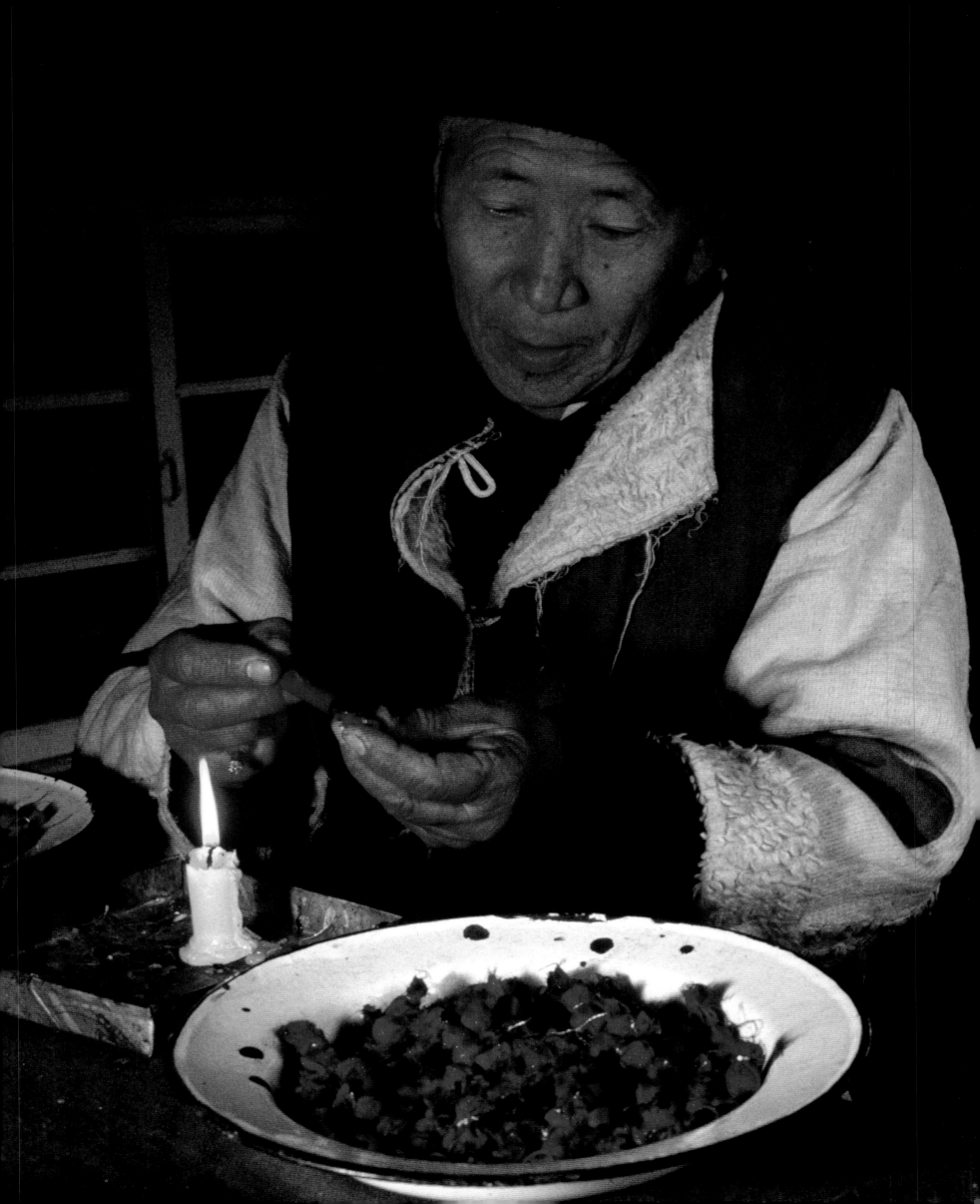

The Many Paths
of a Healer

WADE DAVIS, PH.D.

THE DEVELOPMENT WITHIN THE PAST 100 YEARS OF A MODERN, SCIENTIFIC system of medicine represents one of the greatest episodes of human endeavor. The achievements are astonishing: the elimination of countless diseases through immunology, parasitology, and the discovery of antibiotic drugs and vitamins; the advances in surgery made possible by antiseptics and anesthesia; and the discovery of insulin and human growth hormones.

But long before the growth of modern medicine, before the wizardry of pharmaceutical drugs and the miraculous dexterity of surgery, men and women were seeking the source of illness and the elixir of good health. Stone Age cave dwellers dug for medicinal plants, and the healing repertoire of the Egyptians included herbal remedies for crocodile bites. The Ayurvedic texts of ancient India are replete with magical treatments, botanical drugs, and charms designed to vanquish demons. The Chinese, who discovered smallpox immunization a thousand years before Europeans did, saw man as a mirror of the universe, infused with *qi*, vital energy that courses through channels in the body. Surgery began in prehistoric times: ancient Peruvians cut holes in the skulls of the living to provide disease with an avenue of escape.

Now, as we approach the year 2000, Western medicine views the body essentially as a machine, an exceedingly complex mechanism that can be understood and, as appropriate, modified and repaired. Specificity is the tradition's greatest asset: our physicians work best when they can identify and eliminate a known cause of disease that comes from outside the body, and our surgeons are unsurpassed in dealing with acute trauma.

But the narrow focus of modern medicine is both a strength and a weakness. In much of the world, Western medicine is too expensive, is unavailable, or is presented in a way that is inconsistent with traditional beliefs. What's more, there is an increasing sense that certain ancient and esoteric healing practices, long ignored by Western science, may in fact represent profound insights into the very nature of well-being.

In Western society, health is defined in strictly clinical terms by physicians, with the fate of the spirit being relegated to religious specialists who, significantly, have little to say about the physical well-being of the living. But for early humanity and for most societies around the world today, priest and physician are one, for the condition of the spirit determines the physical state of the body. Sickness is disruption, imbalance, and the manifestation of malev-

◄ **Tibetans say that "precious pills," often made of crushed minerals, can effectively treat cancer, high blood pressure,** and nerve paralysis, in addition to prolonging life. Lobsang Tsewang puts the finishing touches on a pill by sealing it in a small silk wrapper at the Tibetan Medical and Astrological Institute in Dharamsala, India. Dozens of varieties of precious pills are manufactured at the institute, which serves as the world center of Tibetan medicine. The most complex of the pills contains 165 different ingredients, including gold, silver, diamonds, and rubies. *Photo by Galen Rowell*

olent forces in the flesh. Health is a state of balance, of harmony, and for most societies it is something holy.

As a result, traditional medicine acts on two quite different levels. Ailments may be treated by herbal baths and massage, the administration of medicinal plants, physical isolation of the patient in a sacred place and, in certain traditions, an animal sacrifice so that the patient may return to the earth a gift of life's vital energy. But almost invariably it is intervention on the spiritual plane that ultimately determines a patient's fate, and for this the healers must often sail away on the wings of trance to distant realms where they may work their deeds of magical rescue.

For the Native American shaman the vehicle to the gods is the sweat lodge, the rhythm of drums, the pain of ordeal, and the arrows of the magic plants. The Huichol ingest peyote, the tracks of the little deer. Tibetan healers mediate the fate of their patients by ritually transforming themselves into Tantric deities capable of influencing the passage of time. African priests also become gods, often demonstrating their omnipotence by handling burning embers. In the high Andes of Peru traditional healers divine the future and diagnose ailments by reading the coca leaves, a sacred practice reserved only for those who have survived a lightning strike. In such traditions there is no rigid separation between the sacred and the secular, and thus every act of the healer becomes a prayer for the entire community, every ritual a form of collective preventive medicine.

Issues that lie at the very heart of traditional medicine—ideas concerning the spiritual realm, mind/body interactions, notions of the interplay among humanity, the environment and the cosmos—are summarily dismissed by Western medicine because they don't fit into its scientific model, even though some of these themes echo in the roots of our own tradition and remain profound existential questions.

Science will continue to give much to modern medicine, but there is a growing recognition that the mysteries of health and healing cannot be readily extracted from the totality of the human experience. In the future, people throughout the world will continue to benefit from the wonders of modern medicine. But increasingly, medicine will draw into its fold new possibilities, lessons derived from other types of healers who, lacking the technical ability to dissect the human body, chose instead long ago to embrace the human being as a whole.

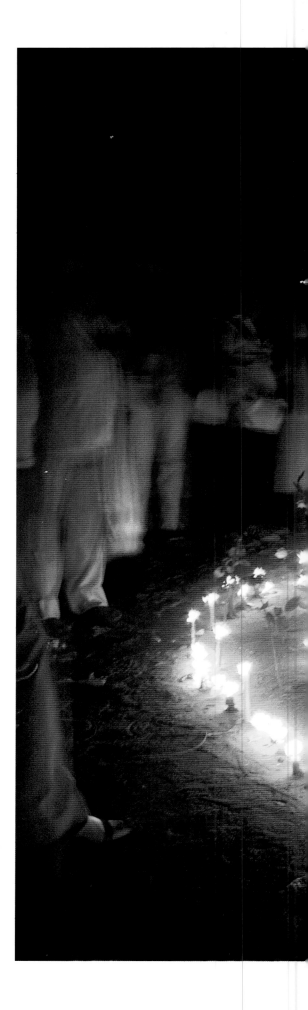

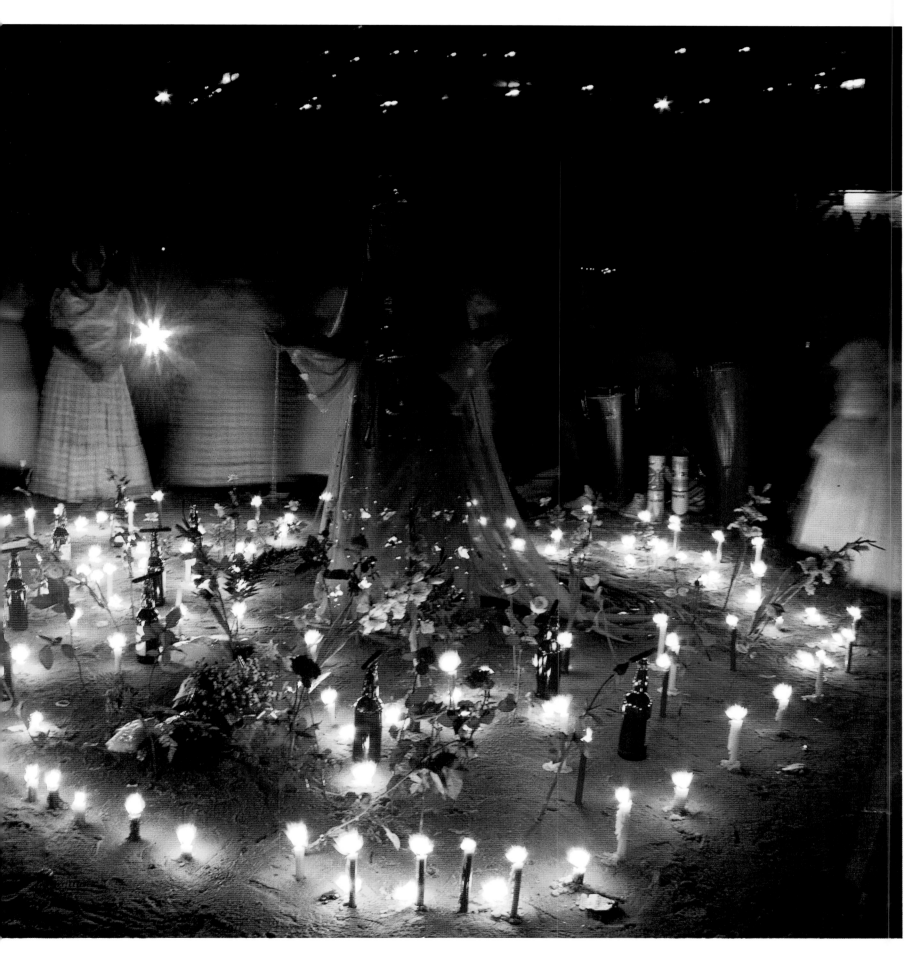

▲ **Looking to the spirit world as a source of healing,** a Brazilian woman stands transfixed by the spirit of Iemanjá, the goddess of water in several Afro-Brazilian religions. By becoming possessed by Iemanjá on New Year's Eve, the woman hopes to bring good fortune and well-being to herself and her community, many members of which have gathered to share in the spirit's blessing for the year to come. On other occasions, followers of the Macumba, Candomblé, and Umbanda religions may seek out the goddess to help with financial difficulties, community complaints, and love problems. For these rural residents of Latin America's largest country, as for many traditional peoples around the world, the Western distinction between physical and spiritual health does not exist. Most Brazilians are Catholic, but a sizable minority also follow religions brought to South America by slaves in the sixteenth and seventeenth centuries. *Photo by Wade Davis, Ph.D.*

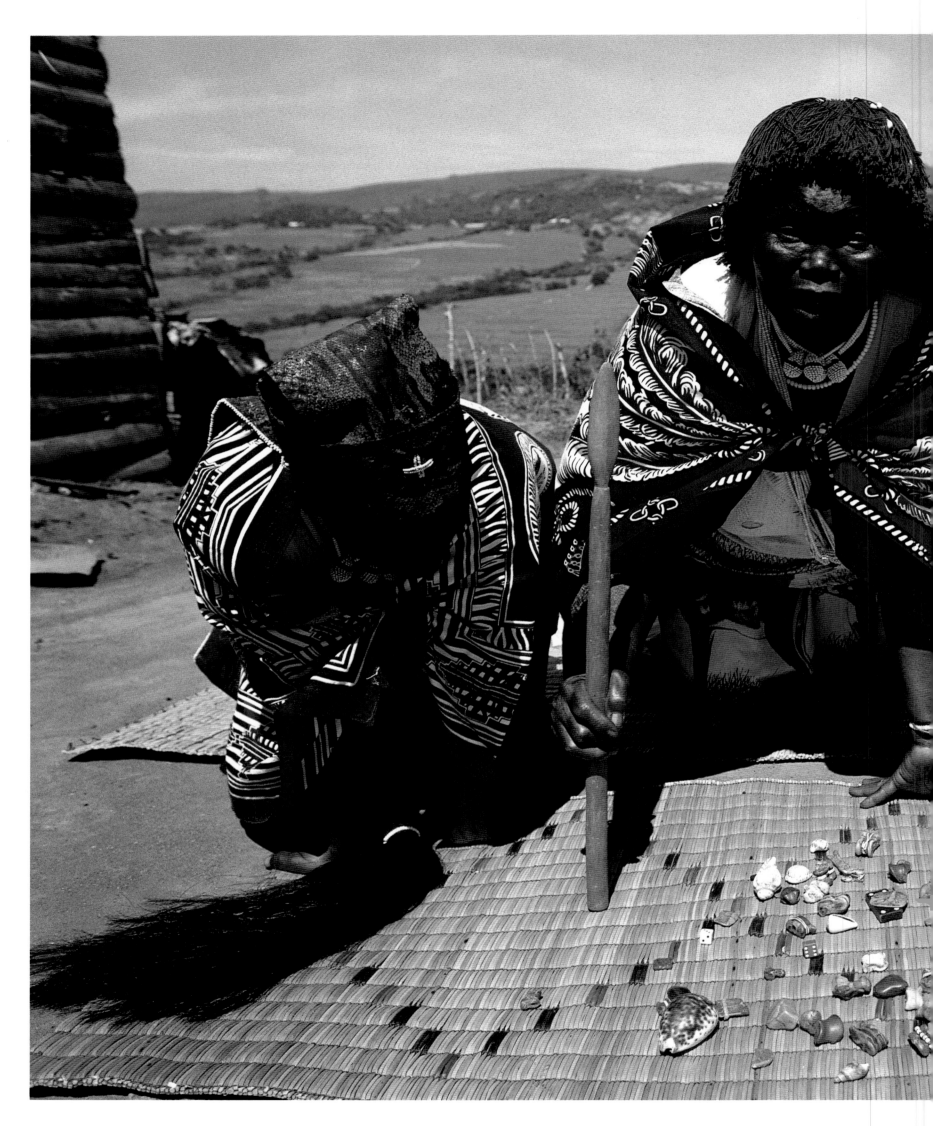

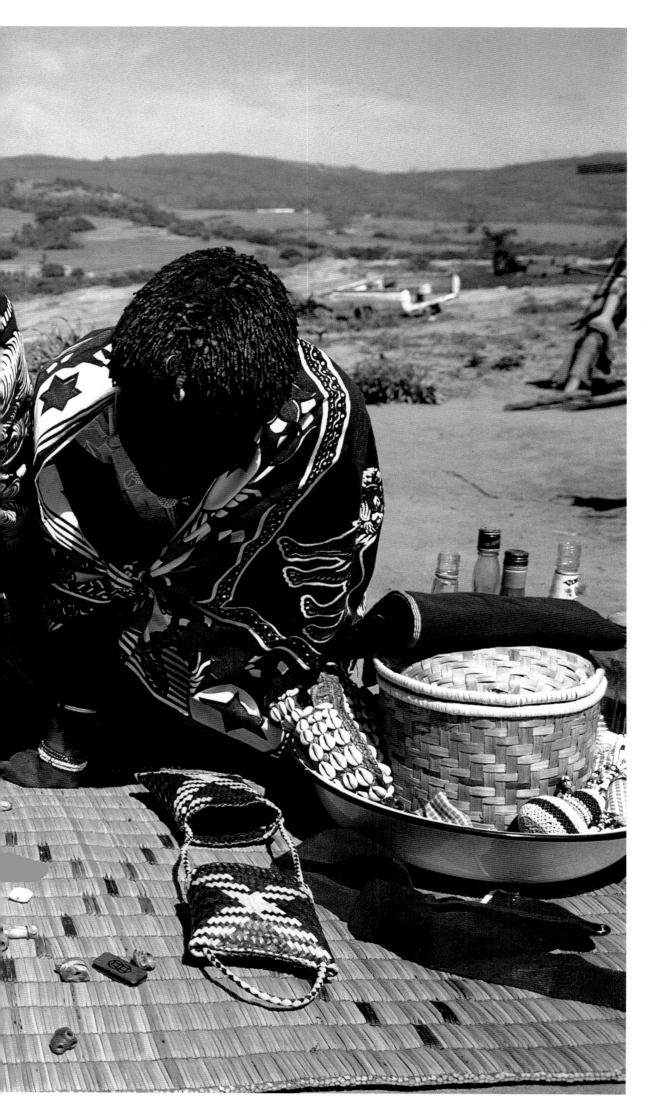

◄ **A *sangoma* and her two trainees study a series of objects to diagnose a patient's illness** in the southern African nation of Swaziland. She will use the spear in her right hand to point to the objects, which were thrown onto the mat from a small bag, and may prescribe any number of treatments, ranging from a special bath to the slaughter of a goat. The patient hopes that the objects — a mah-jongg tile, dice, a snail shell, polished stones, seashells, bones, beads, and a domino — face upward after they're thrown; objects facing downward are bad omens and may mean death. The horse's mane in front of the *sangoma*-in-training on the left is a key weapon in the arsenal of a traditional healer in southern Africa; to ward off evil, the *sangoma* will dip the mane in liquid and twirl it.
Photo by Mark Peters

▶ **The faithful ask for miracles at the graves of two Moslem saints in Badaun, India,** one of Islam's holiest cities. Pilgrims from other religions, most notably Hindus and Sikhs, also travel to the graves. As many as 2,000 people can be found visiting the graves at any one time, many of them staying several months at nearby camp-grounds or in small rental huts. "Miracles happen every day here," says Jabbar Hussein, whose family has been the caretaker of the graves for almost 700 years. "The blind see and the lame walk. I myself was cured of throat cancer after one of the saints, Bare Sarkar, appeared to me in a dream." *Photo by Bhawan Singh*

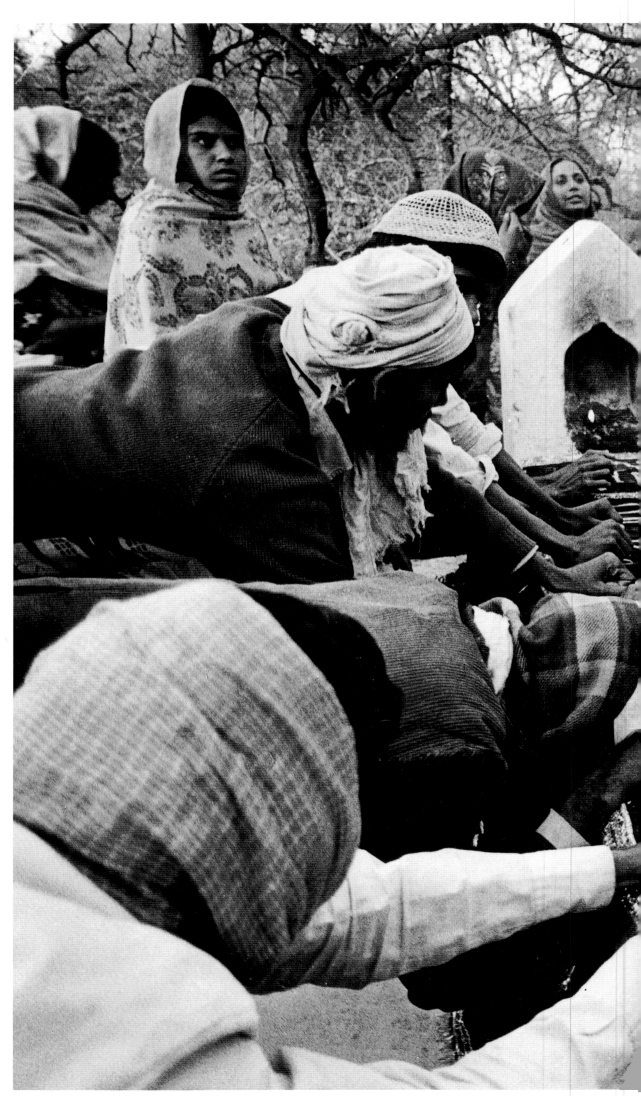

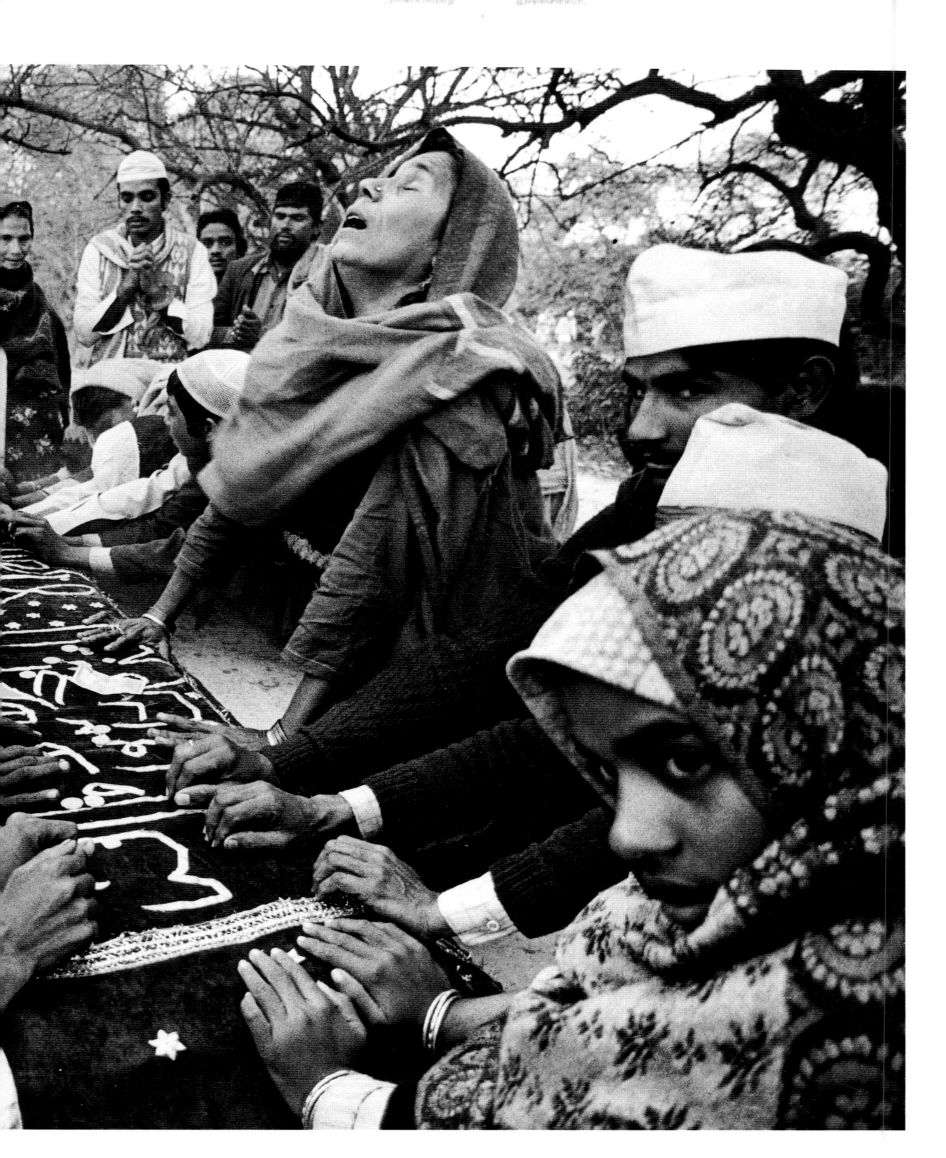

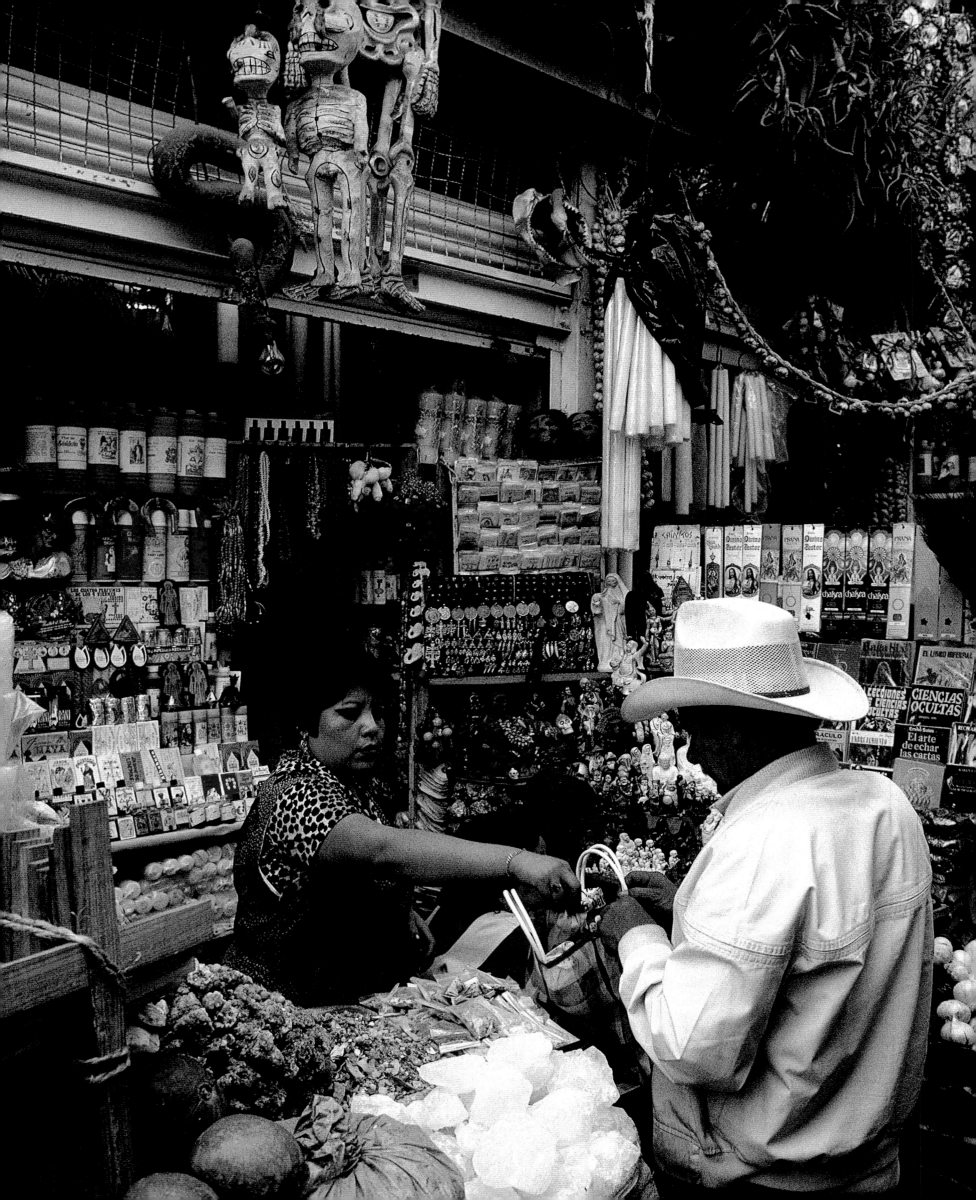

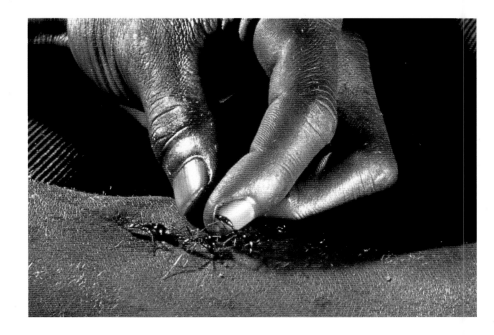

▲ Using soldier ants to stitch a cut is a tradition in central Africa, where it is still observed but slowly disappearing with the proliferation of hospitals and clinics on the continent. Holding the edges of a cut together, a healer places the ants, of the genus *Dorylus*, on the wound. Instinctively, the ants bite down and lock their jaws, sealing the cut. The healer then cuts off the thoraxes and tails of the ants, leaving the jaws in place for several days until the flesh is healed. *Photos by Geneviève Renson*

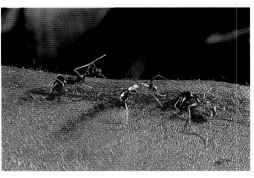

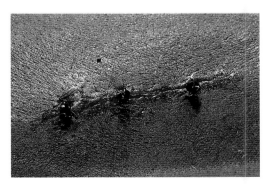

◄ Candles, shark jaws, Buddhas, dried flowers, magic powders, and incense highlight the merchandise at a *botánica*, or herbal stall, in Mexico City. *Botánicas* are a common sight throughout Latin America, with most of the herbs, potions, and charms intended to help the users improve their health, financial standing, or love life. *Photo by Eric Lars Bakke*

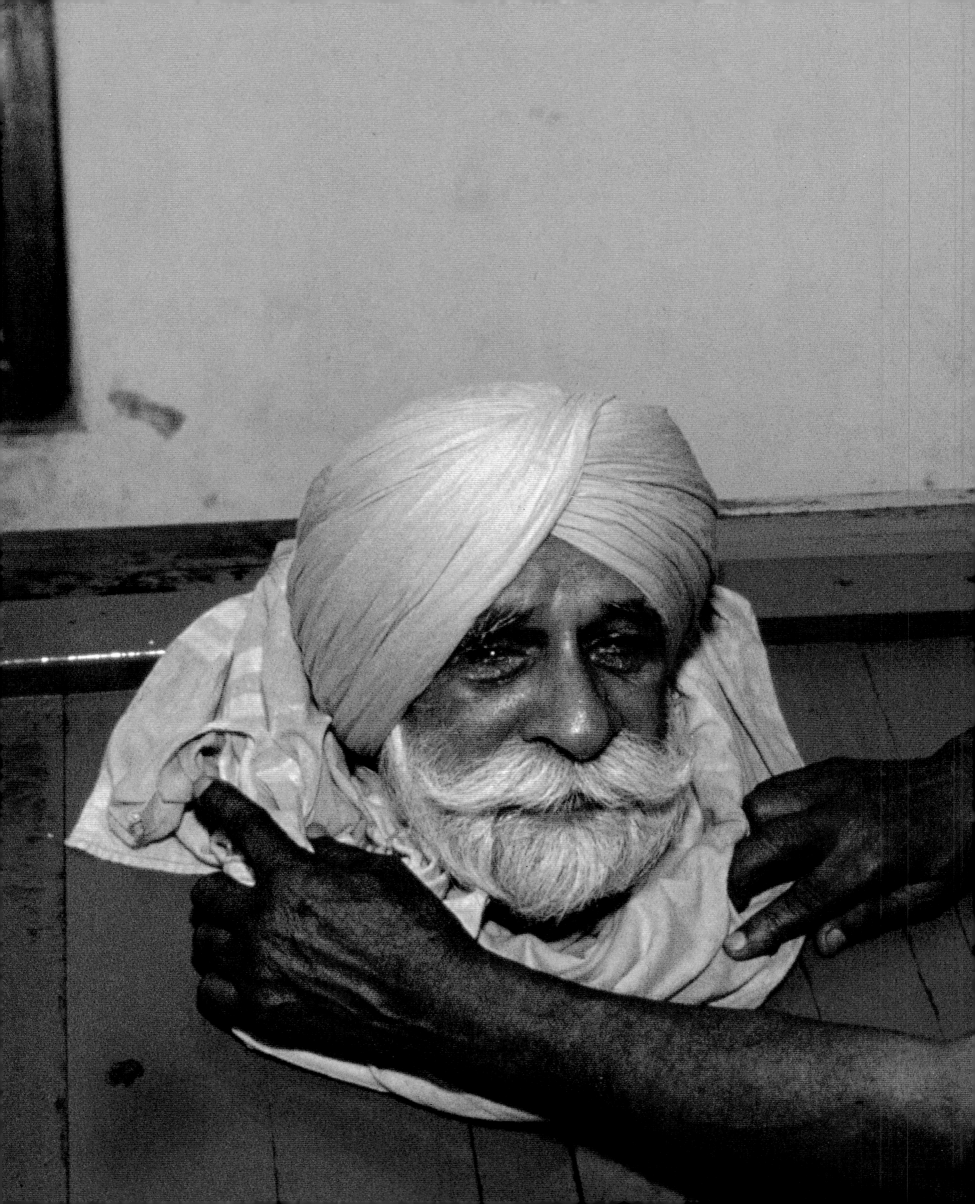

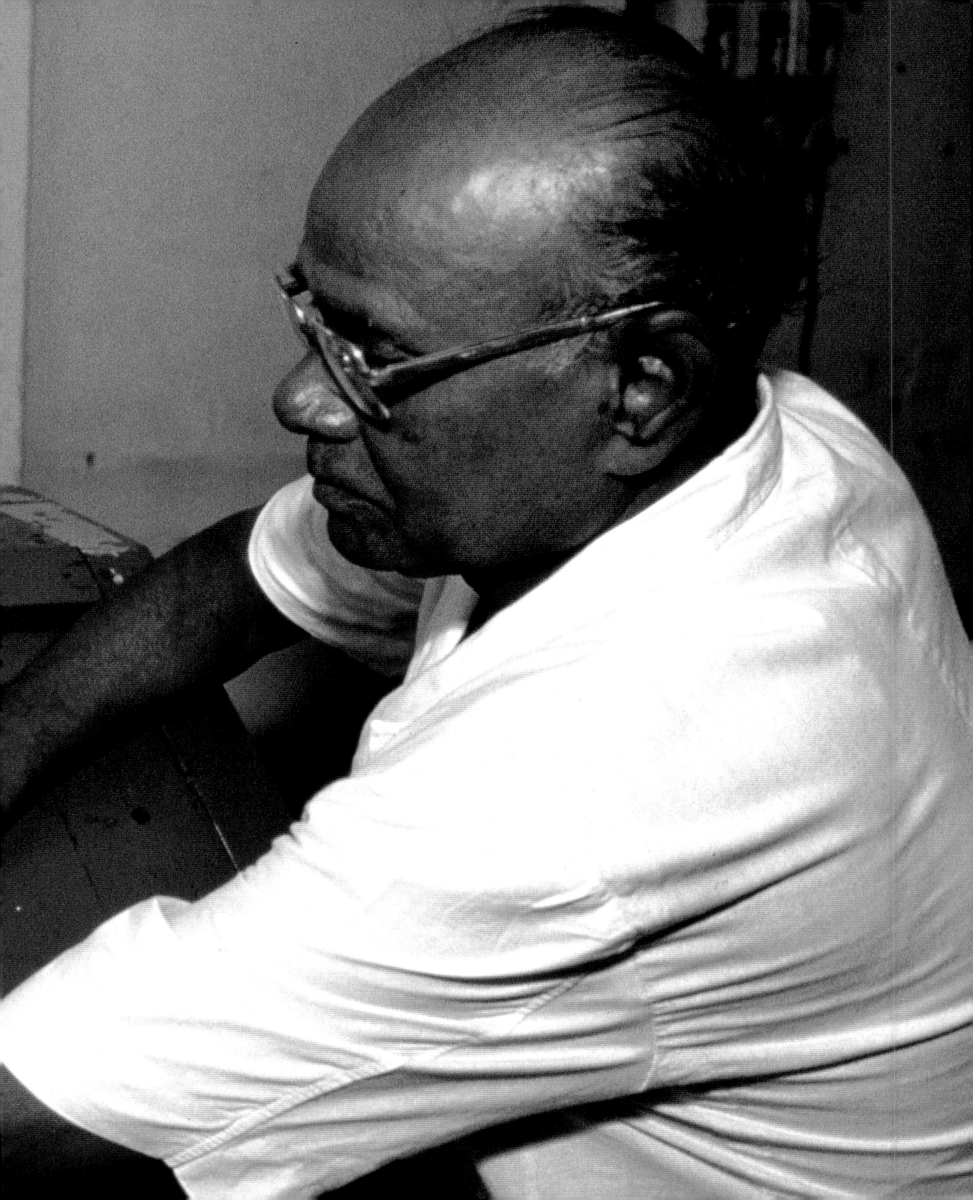

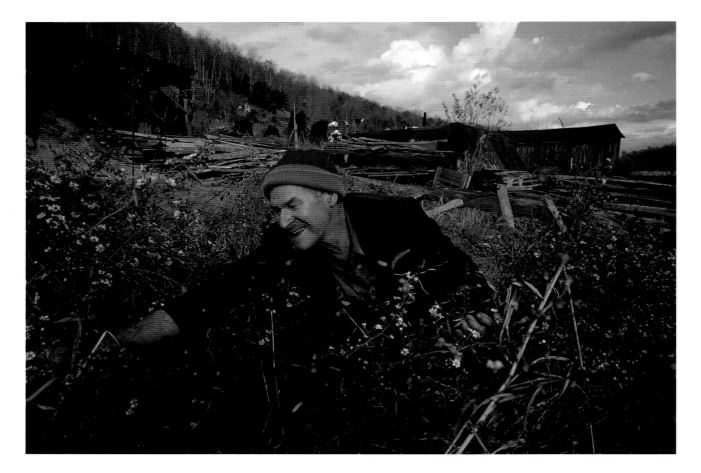

◄ **Cleansing the body, a key element of ayurvedic medicine,** is the goal of this session in a steam-filled sweatbox at Podar Hospital in Bombay, India. Ayurvedic medicine teaches that patients become ill when their bodies and spirits are not in harmony; the prescription usually features some combination of diet, yoga, medicine, and cleansing sessions like this one.
Photo by Dilip Mehta

▲ **Catfish, Man of the Woods, searches for the plants** that people from all over the United States order from him by mail. Says Anne Garcelon of the West Virginia Department of Health about the Appalachian herbalist, whose real name is Clarence Gray: "He's someone we want to promote and encourage. He's part of our heritage."

Catfish claims that his "bitters," as he calls them, can cure arthritis, impotence, gallstones — even cancer and black lung. The trick, he says, is to combine taking the bitters, which he sells for fifty cents a bag, with clean Christian living

and a special diet. According to mailings he sends out from his home in Glenwood, West Virginia — the walls of which are lined with letters from satisfied customers *(right)* — foods to avoid include eggplant, tomatoes, pork, oranges, potatoes, salt, saccharin, and "fish that don't wear scales." On the plus side, he says, dill pickles, olives, olive oil, ginseng tea, carrots, head lettuce, lemonade, sassafras tea, and a host of wild roots are the keys to good health — and, he adds with a twinkle, a good sex life.
Photos by Lynn Johnson

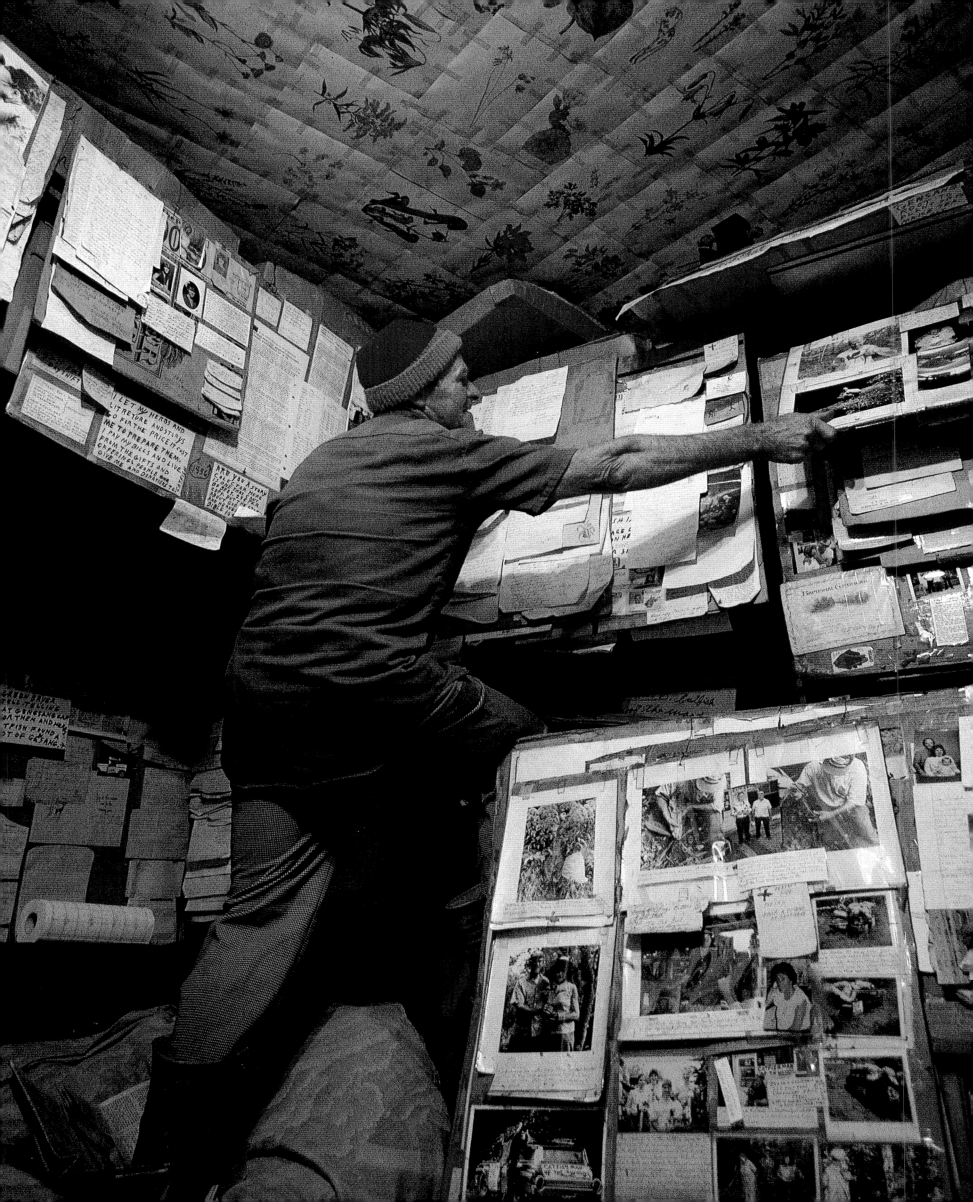

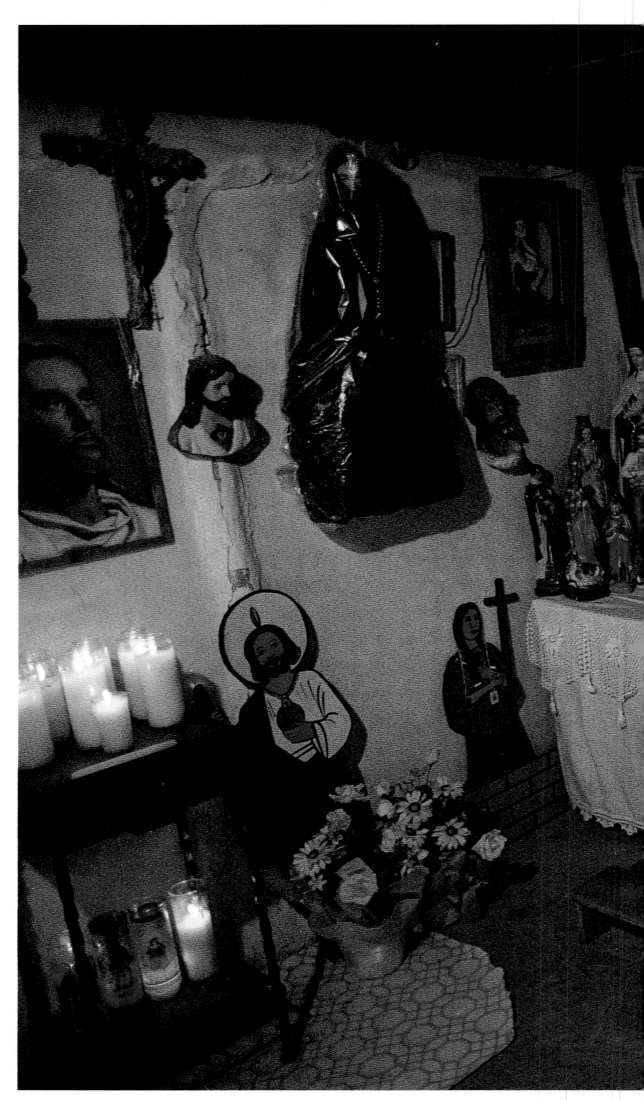

▶ **Frances Chavez offers a prayer before the holy dirt of Chimayo,** the New Mexico shrine visited annually by 250,000 people seeking a cure for rheumatism, cancer, paralysis, arthritis, blindness, and a host of other maladies. The faithful come to the shrine — a little church built in 1813 on the site where a crucifix was found three times in the early 1800s — to eat the dirt, mix it with water and drink it, rub it on their bodies, or take it home to stash in places of symbolic importance.
Photo by Jim Richardson

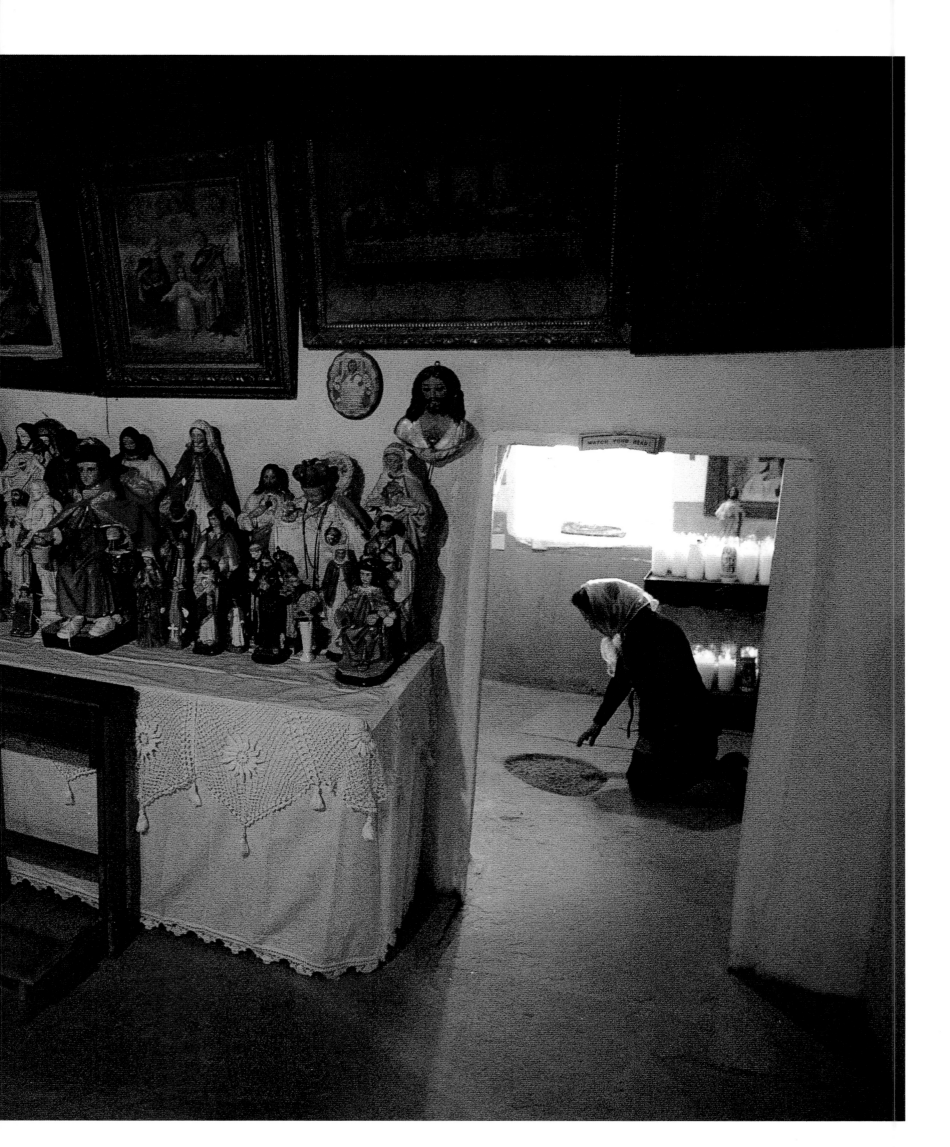

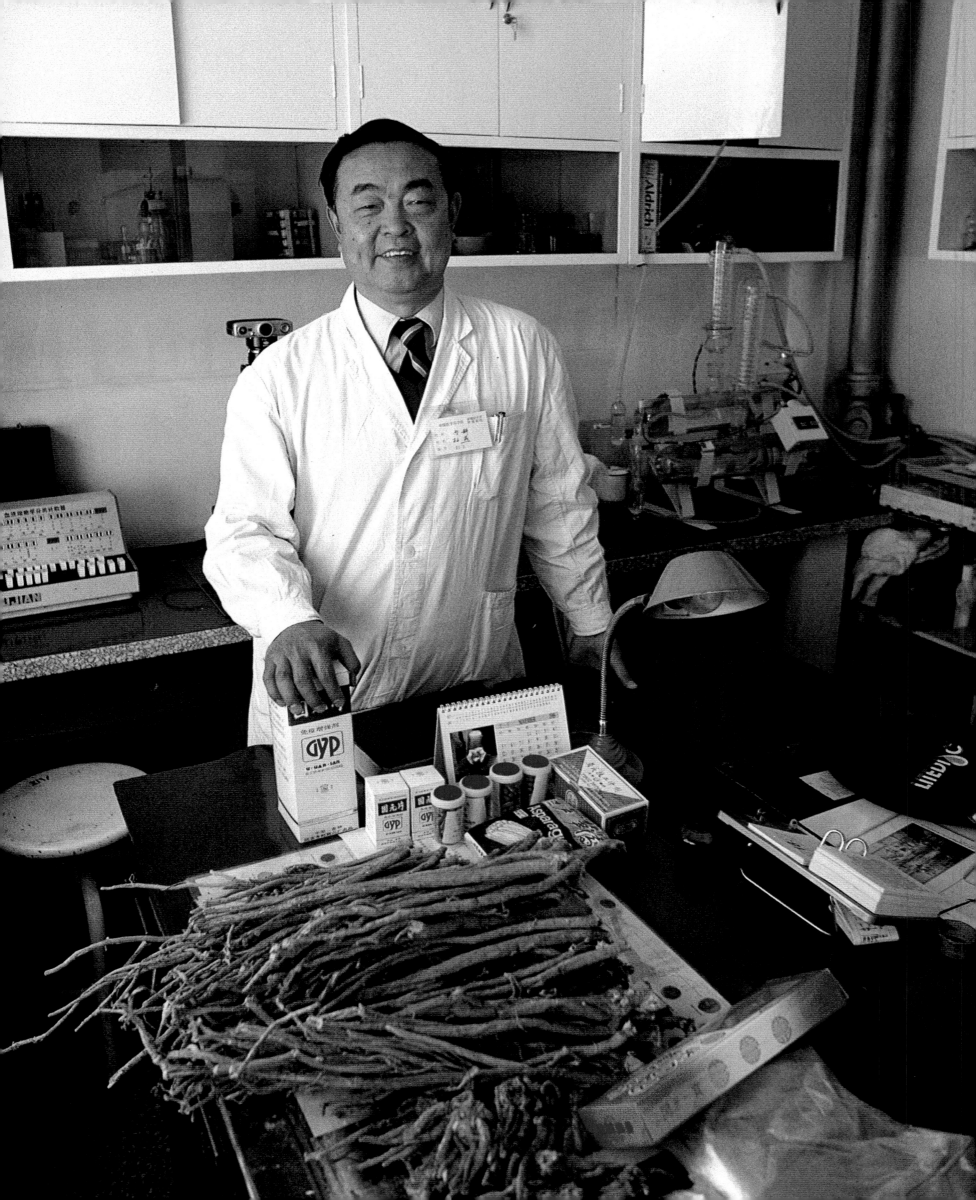

A Chinese Doctor
in America

MAXINE HONG KINGSTON

I WAS A SICKLY CHILD AND AM NOW AN AGGRESSIVELY HEALTHY ADULT, which may be the result of being raised by a doctoring mother. In 1934, my mother graduated from the To Keung School of Midwifery in Canton, China. The school had been founded in 1904 by European doctors, whose mission was to train Chinese women in Western medicine.

My mother's diploma certified that she "completed a period of two-years course of instruction of Midwifery, Gynecology, Pediatrics, Medicine, Surgary [sic], Therapeutics, Physiology, Anatomy, Embryology, Ophthalmology, Bacteriology, Dermatology, Nursing, Hygiene, [and] Bandage." Upon graduation, my mother returned to her village.

She and a fellow graduate were the only doctors in the Sun Hui countryside. I imagine them as two scientifically trained girls among villagers who demanded "the herbal brew mixed by the rabbit-on-the-moon." Faced with people who wouldn't be cured unless the doctor gave them medicine they believed would heal them, my mother went native.

After five years of practice, my mother came to California, where she has been dispensing strange information for half a century. She did not bring to this country the Western scientific knowledge that her teachers had brought from Europe to China; only scraps of her To Keung education remained, such as her denouncement of acupuncture as quackery.

She was not allowed to practice medicine in the United States, but as a child I provided her with a willing patient. She taught me that cause-and-effect is most often invisible—whether bacteria, microbes, energies, yin and yang. She made me drink elixirs; she spanked the tiredness out of my joints, so that it broke out on the skin as black and red dots. She tweaked my ears to pull the spirit back into the body. What she used on me was folk medicine she had picked up from the people she healed.

She called in a regular American doctor to give me pills, X rays, shots, urine tests, and blood tests. But this regular doctor was extraordinary—a Chinese-American woman not much younger than my mother, with a degree in psychiatry. (She had become a general practitioner when no one in our community would admit to needing psychotherapy.)

My mother brought from China her diploma, her stethoscope, a microscope, and seeds from which she raised generations of bok choy, cilantro and other herbs, melons, squashes, peaches, tangerines, almonds. We also raised ducks, turkeys, rabbits, and chickens. After almost fifty years of eating at

◄ **Complementing modern cancer treatments with traditional herbs in China,** Dr. Sun Yan prescribes *Radix Astragali* roots along with the shorter *Radix Angelicae Sinensis* roots to combat the side effects of chemotherapy. He and his colleagues at the Chinese Academy of Medical Sciences Cancer Institute and Hospital in Beijing also say that the herbs can strengthen a cancer patient's immune system.
Photo by Robin Moyer

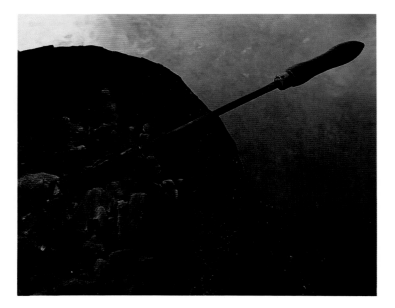

my doctor mother's table, I understand that every food is a medicine, everything in the universe connecting with everything else. Spirit is made up of two winds that blow in us and through us. Everything we eat and do bestirs the yin wind and the yang wind. When the winds inside of the body are in balance, one is in harmony with the world.

My mother made us eat yin food to balance the yang. Melon soups, vegetables, ginger, chicken seem to strengthen yin, which is cool, feminine, and dark. Chocolate, nuts, french fries, potato chips, liquor, and duck seem to stoke yang, which is hot, masculine, and bright. By eating *jai*, monks' food, on holidays, we ate ethics and morals. And even today, she keeps trying to serve me a soup that has made quite a few ladies pregnant.

She taught me that some foods are puns—"long noodles" sounds like and looks like and is eaten on birthdays for "long life"; "lettuce" sounds like and is eaten for "aliveness." I got much of my ability at words from eating puns. And I got my ability to stay healthy because we fed our animals and plants good food and water, no artificial hormones and pesticides. I know where my food comes from, and how animals and plants are born, live, and are killed. Knowing the connectedness of all things, I am healthy in body and spirit.

My mother says she refuses to doctor people who are too far gone. I suppose she ran her clinic in China like the well-baby clinics of today, with the emphasis on growing a healthy body rather than trying to repair a sick one. She learned from her patients the medicine of staying well, and she lost what she had been taught at the To Keung School, the medicine of illness.

My mother will live to be 100, and I expect to live at least that long. Our family's talent for longevity comes from our having ideas, visions, plans, and work that take time to carry out. When I've pushed myself too hard in wrong directions and get sick, and impatiently want a quick fix, I go to a doctor who injects an antibiotic or acupuncture needles. But in my heart I understand that the body is a manifestation of the spirit, and that Eastern or Western, the doctor is best who helps me find right directions for continuing my life long-term.

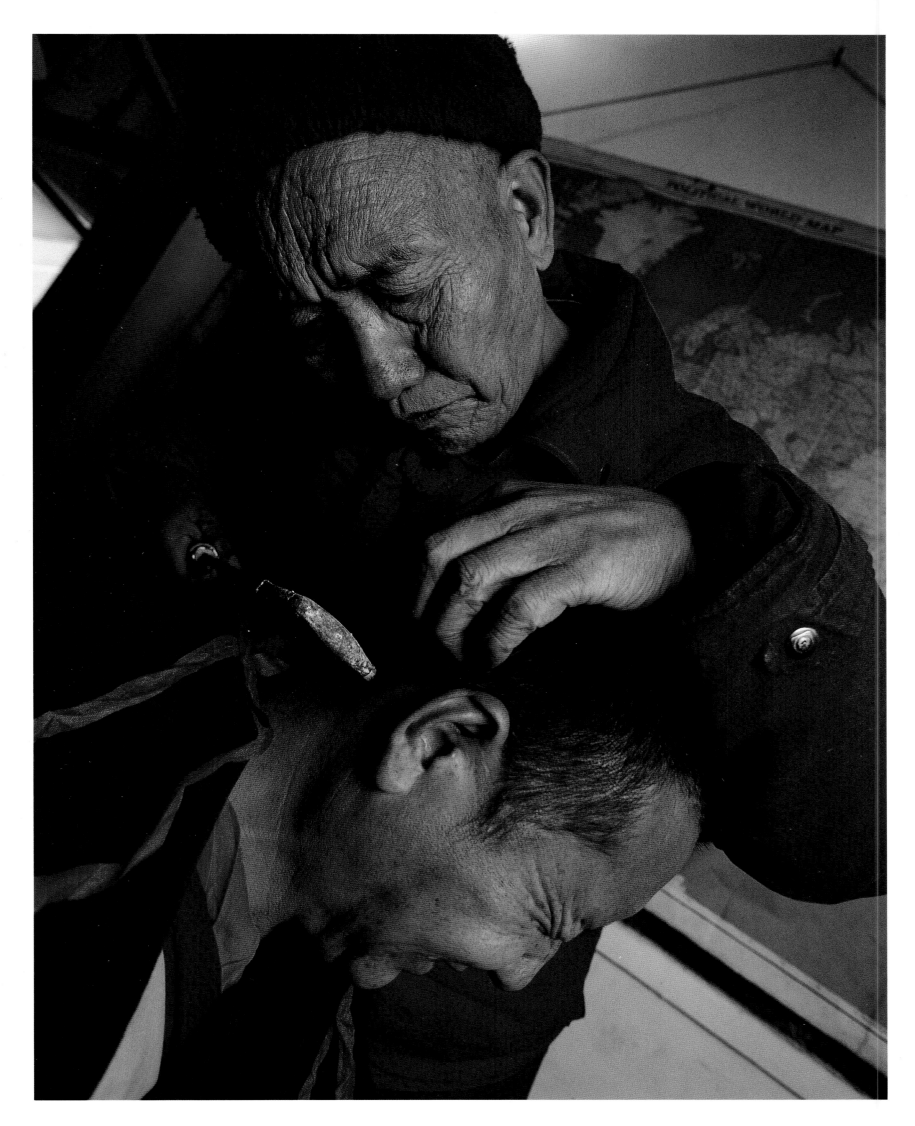

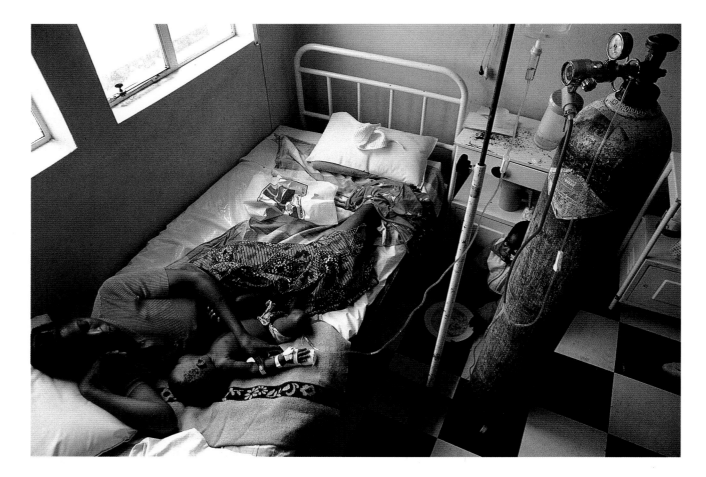

▲ **Struggling to avoid joining the 40,000 children who die each day** in the developing world — most of them from dehydration and starvation — one of Mozambique's one million war refugees suckles at his mother's breast while hooked up to an intravenous feeding tube at the José Mocamo Hospital in Maputo. An older brother eats solid food behind an unused oxygen tank in their room on the "malnourished pediatrics ward."
Photo by Larry C. Price

▶ **Underneath a poster warning of the dangers of adult anemia and child dehydration,** Eftu Handse and her young son wait outside an Ethiopian health center to see a doctor. The poster, with drawings to aid the illiterate, offers instructions for parents whose children suffer from diarrhea, a major cause of fatal dehydration among Third World children. Dehydration can be treated with oral rehydration solution, which was hailed two decades ago by the British medical journal *The Lancet* as "potentially the most important medical advance of the century." The solution consists of a carefully balanced formula of glucose, sodium chloride, potassium chloride, and sodium bicarbonate.
Photo by Rick Rickman

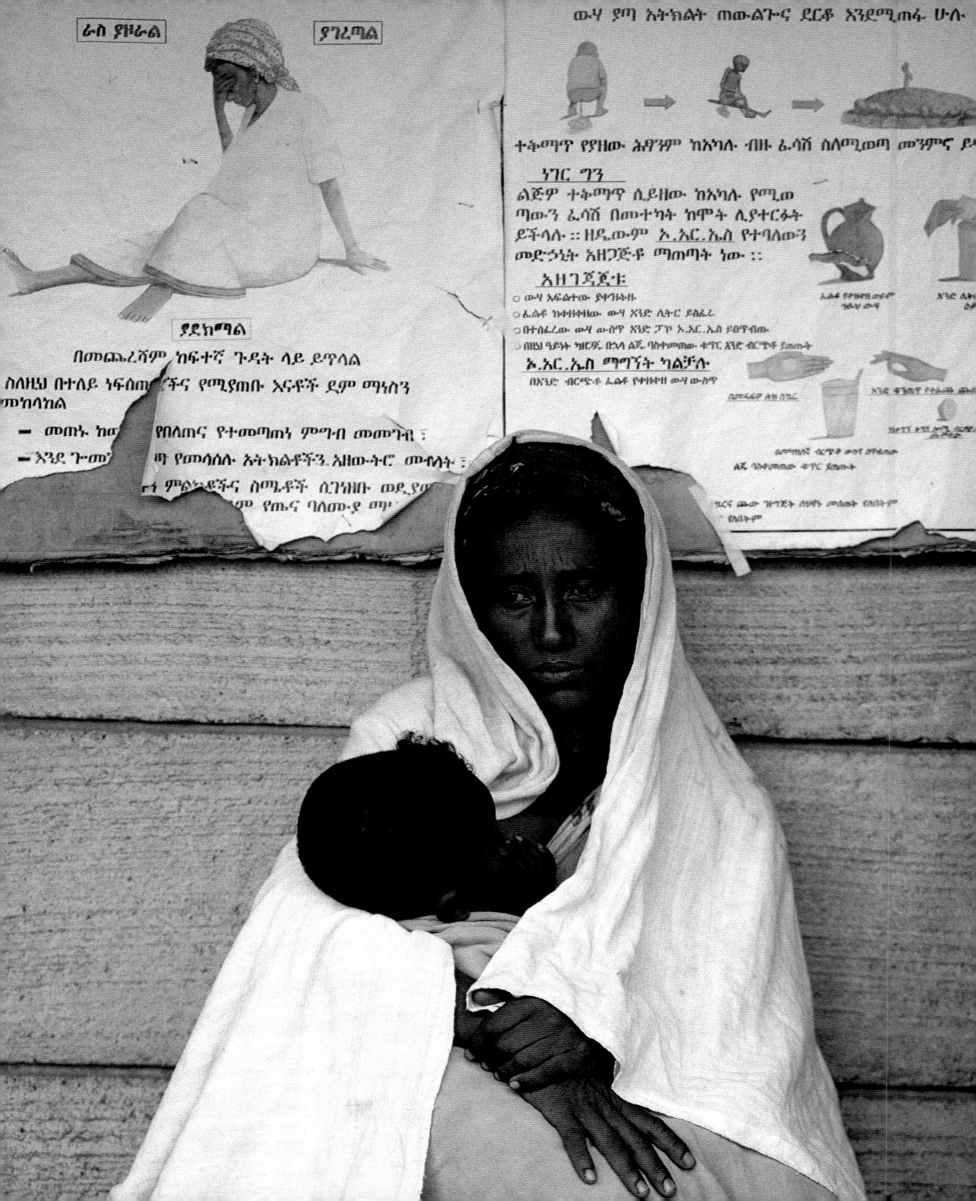

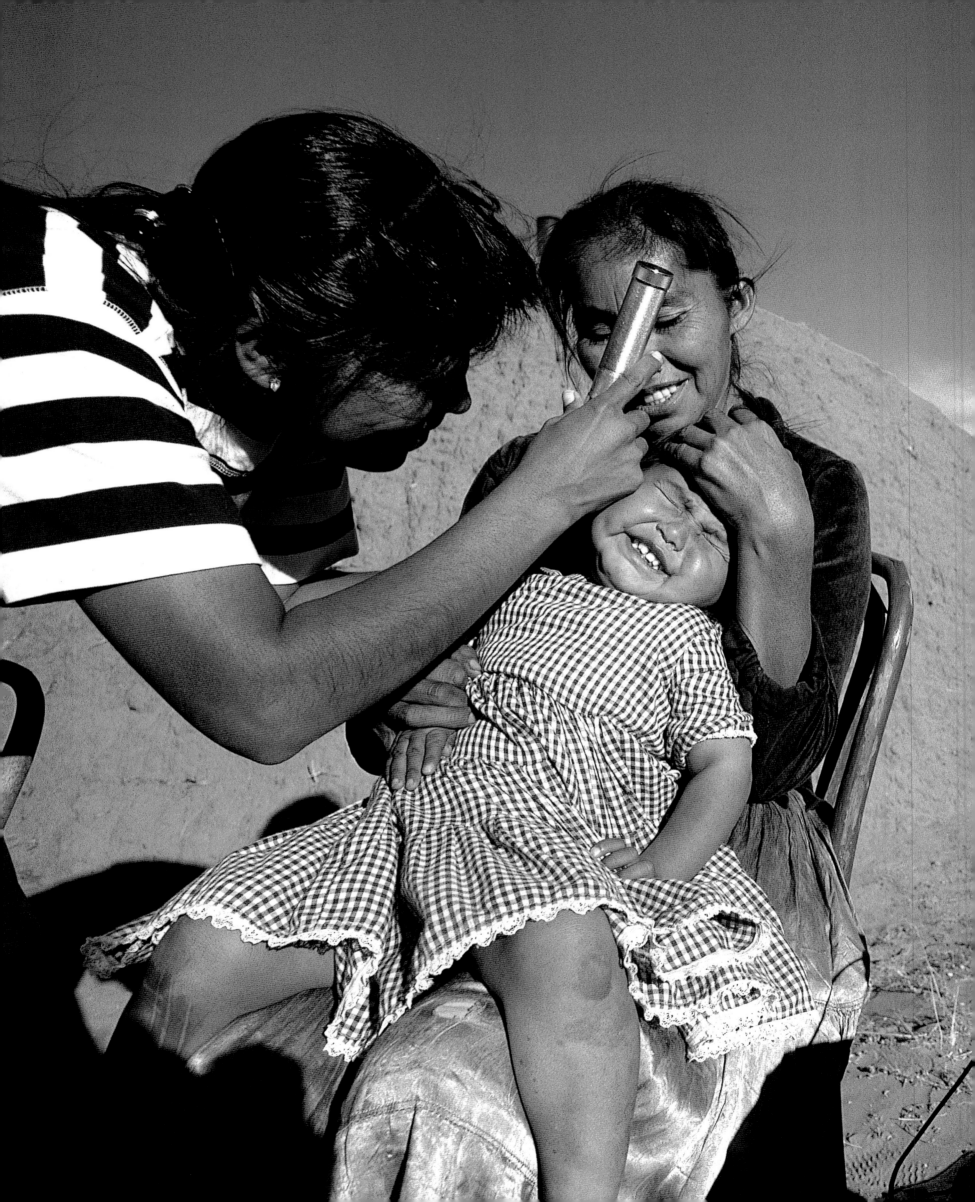

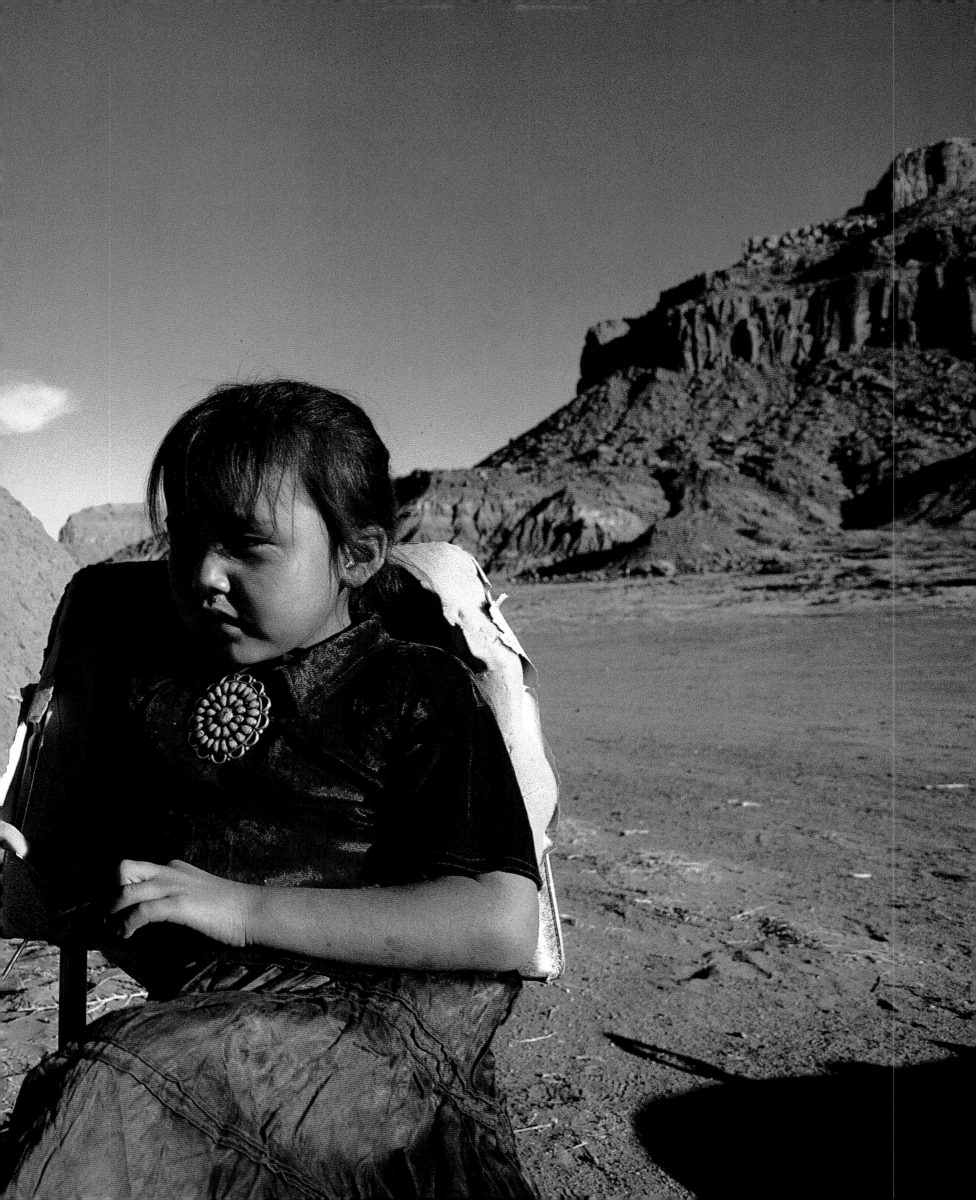

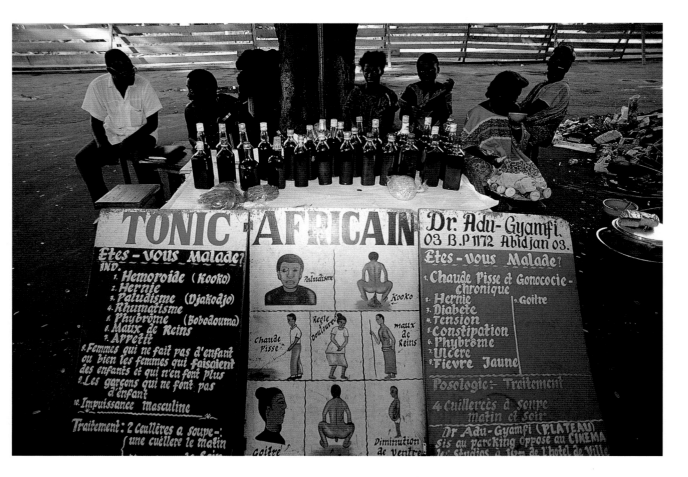

The image shows a street vendor's stall with rows of bottles and hand-painted signs reading "TONIC AFRICAIN" and "Dr. Adu-Gyamfi, 03 B.P 1172 Abidjan 03." with illustrations and French text listing ailments.

◀ **On her daily rounds through the Navajo reservation** in northern Arizona, health worker Linda Duane checks up on a squirming Tanya Grass. Duane carries a stethoscope, a blood pressure kit, first aid equipment, and splints as she travels the reservation; she's not allowed to distribute any medicine stronger than an aspirin substitute, so she takes a nurse with her if there's a medical emergency. High blood pressure and diabetes remain major problems on the reservation. But "the general health of the Navajos has gotten much better," says Indian Health Service nurse Carol Goldsmith — thanks to immunizations, early detection of diseases, better water and sanitation, and increased community awareness.
Photo by Ethan Hoffman

▲ **A few tablespoons of an African herbal remedy** can cure hemorrhoids, hernias, infertility, and impotence — or so says Dr. Adu-Gyamfi, far left, who sells the herbal potion each day on the streets of Abidjan, the capital of the Ivory Coast. Adu-Gyamfi's sign promises that "African Tonic," which sells for about eight dollars a bottle, will also successfully treat diabetes, constipation, and yellow fever.
Photo by Roland Neveu

▶ **On a busy Bangkok street,** Pratuang Yodkam fits a drop-in patient for dentures. Yodkam learned his trade from his brother-in-law, who operates a similar booth less than a block away. Neither man will perform sophisticated dental work, preferring to send patients to trained dentists instead.
Photo by Doug Hulcher

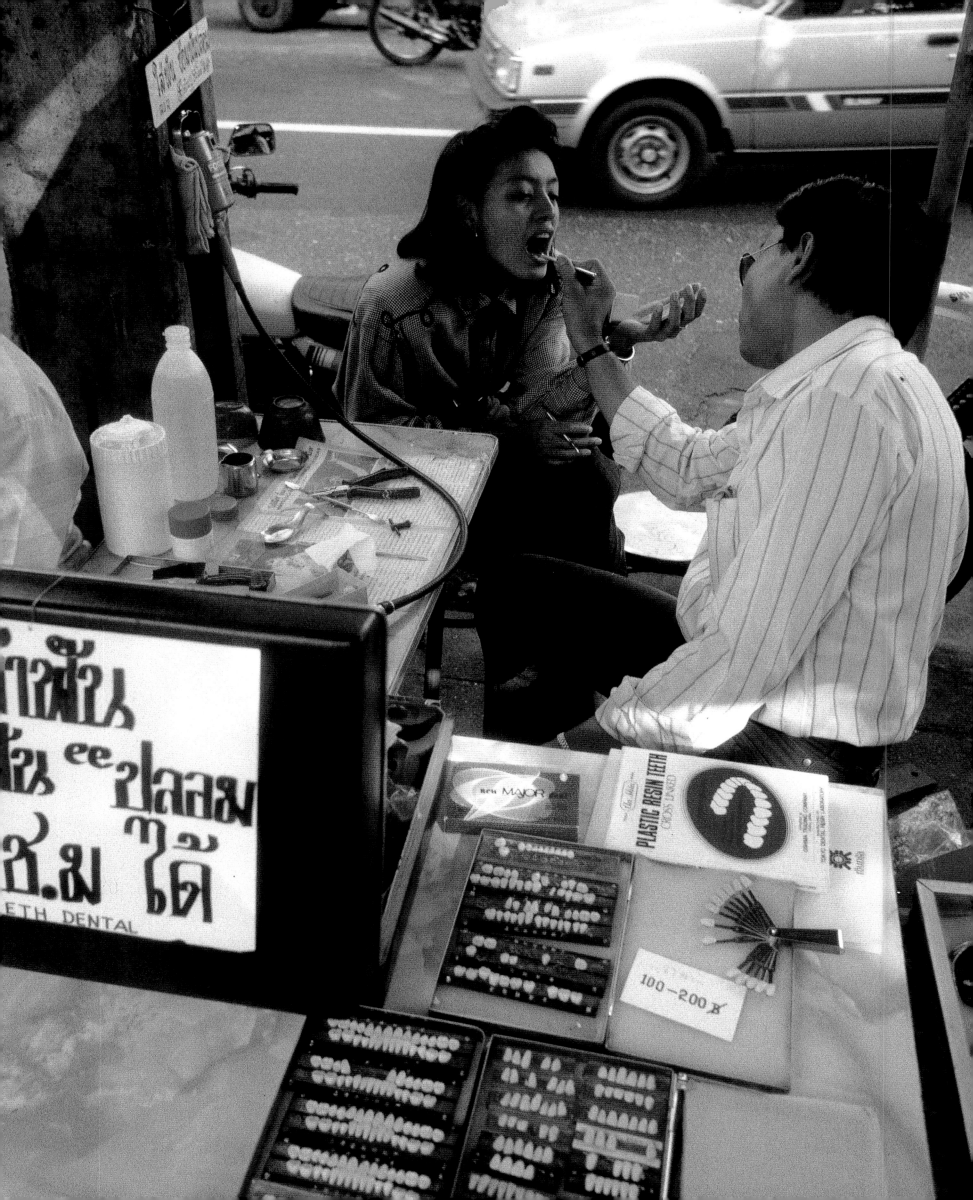

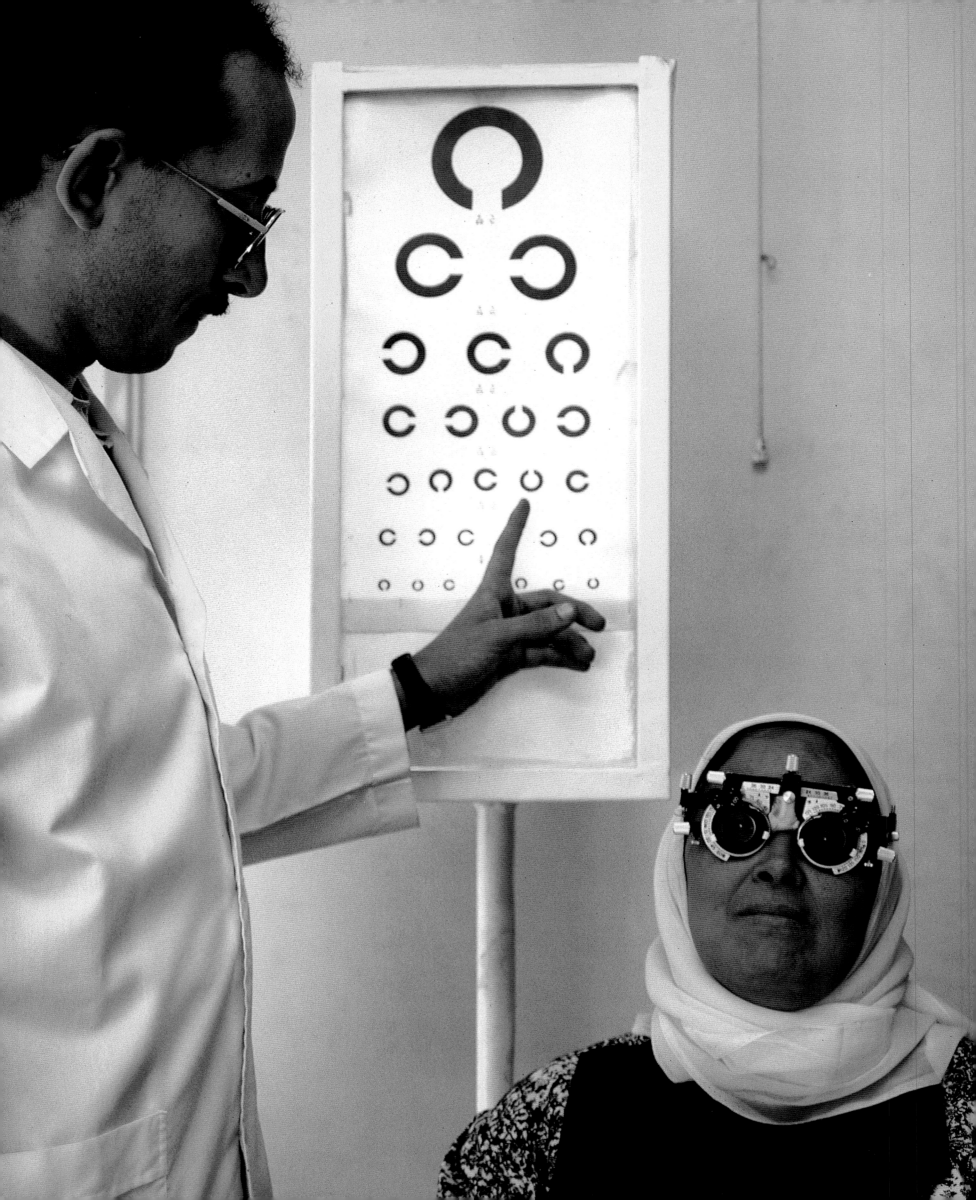

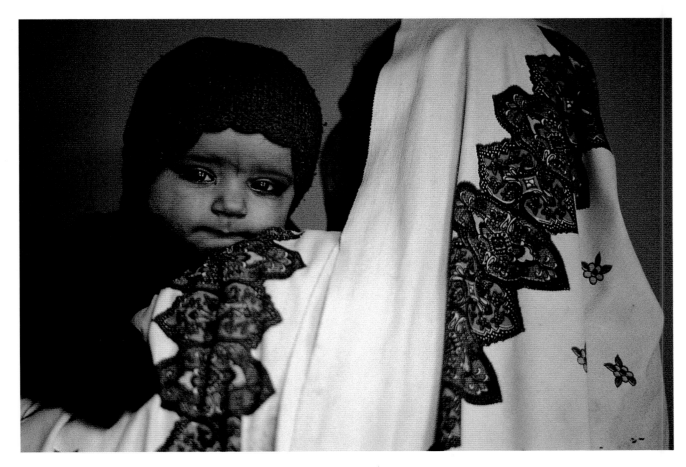

▲ **Wearing eye makeup as a health precaution,** a Pakistani girl takes part in a centuries-old tradition. A paste of hazelnut powder and several oils, known as *surma*, is spread in and around the eyes of children in rural Pakistan — in part to protect the eyes from the smoke from fires used to heat the homes, in part to cool and clean the eyes, and in part to ward off *nazar*, the evil eye. "Parents who use *surma* on their children to protect them from the evil eye don't like to talk about it, because they know people think it's backward," says Raymond Wallace, a resident of Lahore who runs a language program associated with the University of California. "But since infant mortality is so high here (107 per 1000 live births), they'll try anything."
Photo by Judy Griesedieck

◄ **Mixing Islam with modern medicine,** Dr. Ali Haffez gives a low-cost eye test at a state-of-the-art health clinic inside the Moustapha Mahmoud Mosque in Cairo. The health clinic's purpose, according to founder Moustapha Mahmoud, is "to embody and disclose the real Islam." More than a quarter of a million people use the clinic each year, usually paying about fifty cents a visit for the services. Donations from wealthy Moslems cover the majority of the clinic's costs.
Photo by Enrico Ferorelli

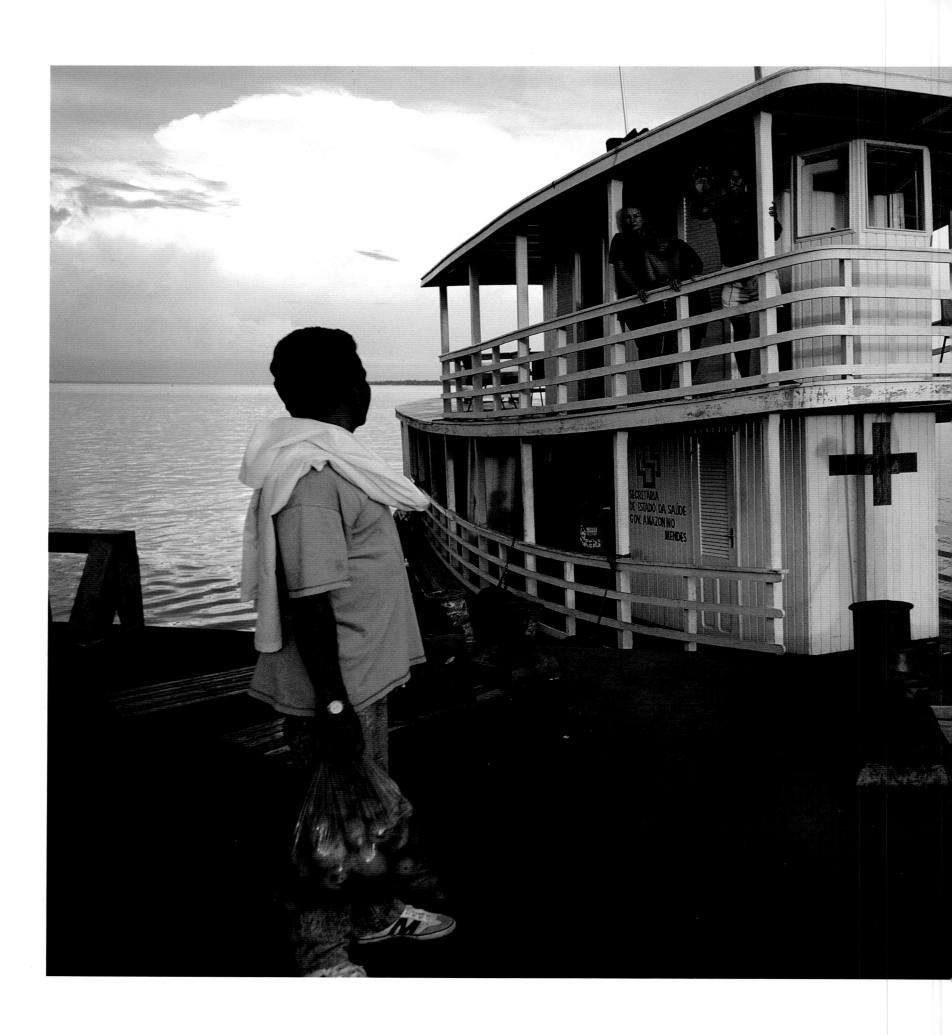

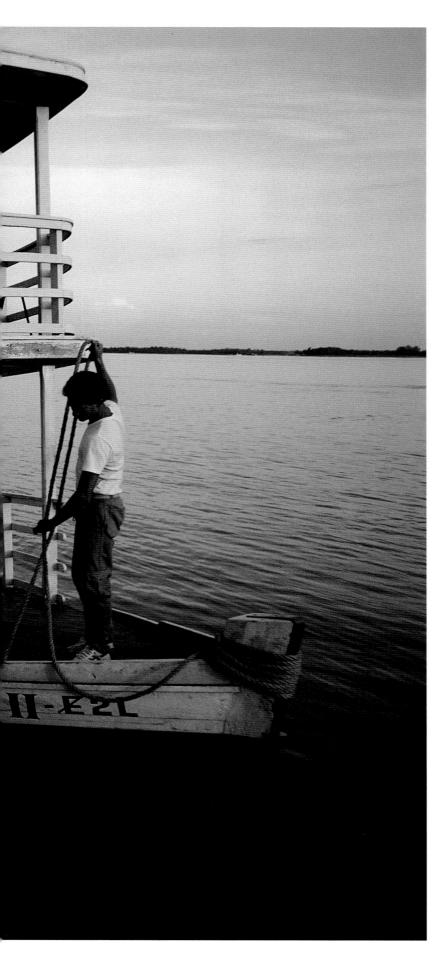

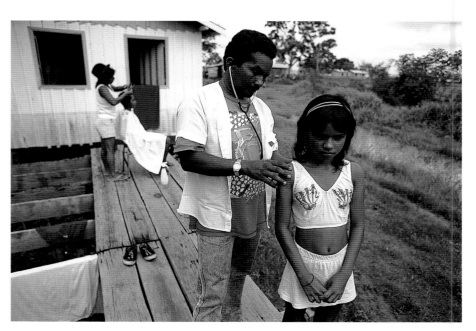

◄ **A floating ambulance on the world's second-longest river,** the Manaus Tropical Disease Hospital boat drops off Brazilian paramedic Miguel Passos at day's end. Passos visits poor and often otherwise-inaccessible communities along the Amazon each day, looking for cases of malaria, typhus, leprosy, hepatitis, tuberculosis, and various parasites. The ill are sent to the Brazilian city of Manaus on the boat; the relatively healthy get lectures from Passos on sanitation and AIDS. Passos gives a checkup (*above*) to eleven-year-old Rita Da Silva in the Amazon village of Careiro.
Photos by Doug Menuez

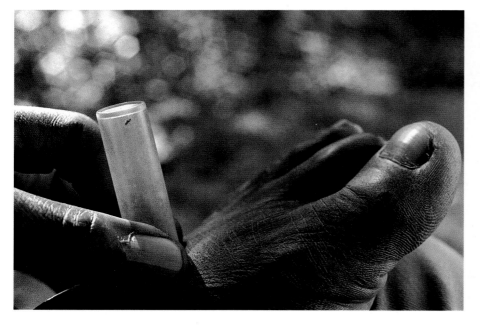

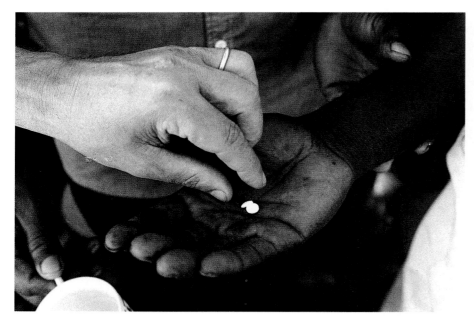

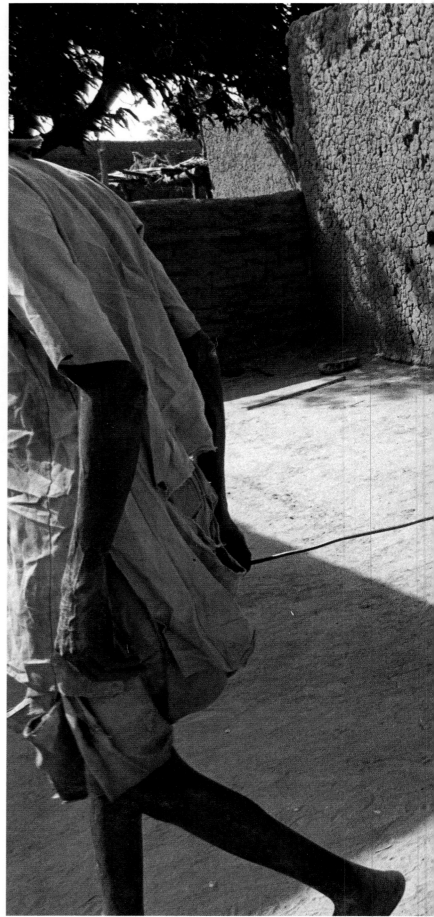

▶ **Young boys lead their blind elders in West Africa,** where river blindness, or onchocerciasis, affects millions of people. Now, for the first time, there is hope that the young can avoid the fate of their parents and grandparents: a U.S. drug company has given the World Health Organization, for free distribution, a drug that arrests the disease before blindness sets in. A volunteer uses a glass bottle to trap a black fly (*above top*), which breeds near water and spreads the parasitic worms that cause the disease. The drug ivermectin is distributed in several countries, including Guinea (*above*). One pill a year appears to be enough to halt the gradual progression towards the blindness that led one tribal leader in Mali to say, "Here it is normal to become blind before you have white hair." **Photos by Eugene Richards**

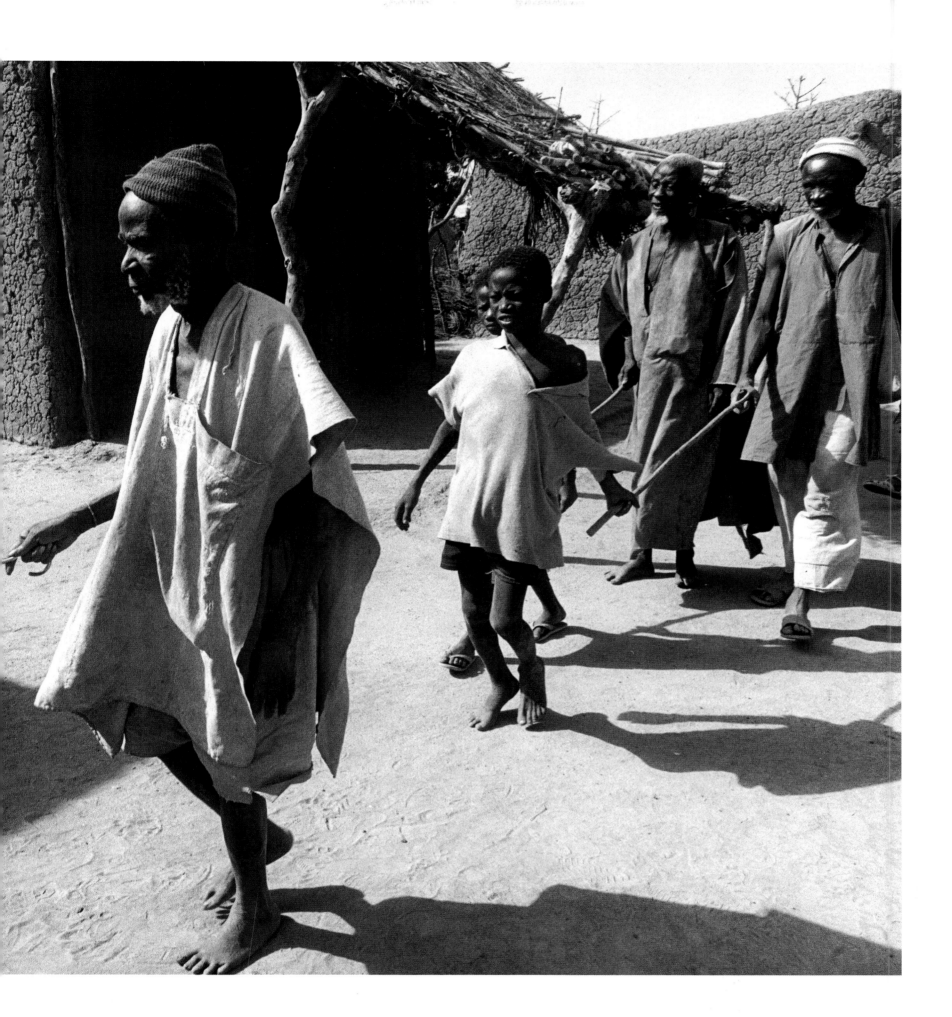

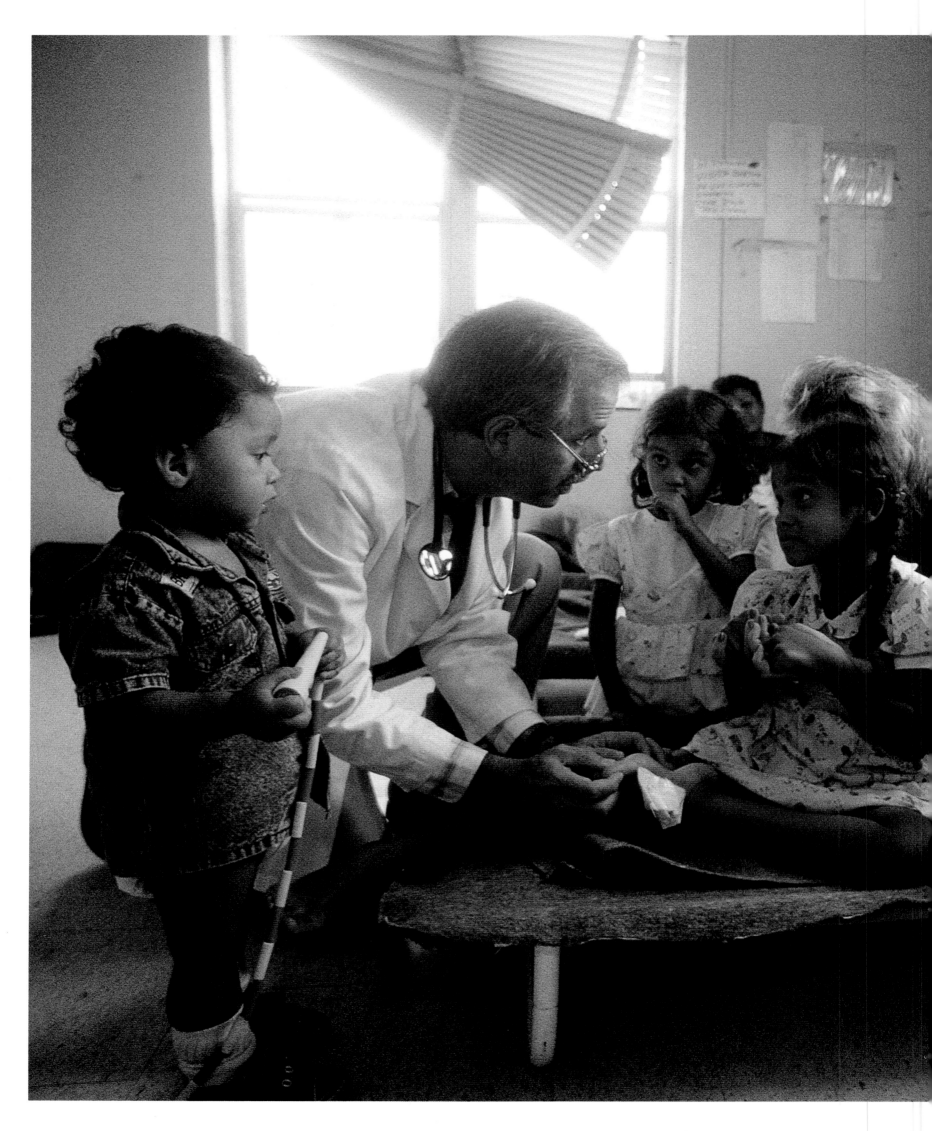

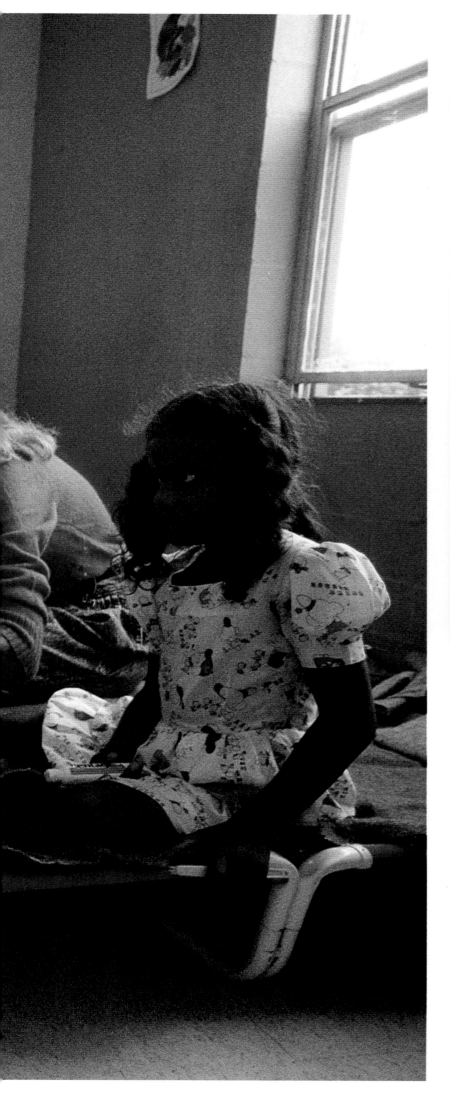

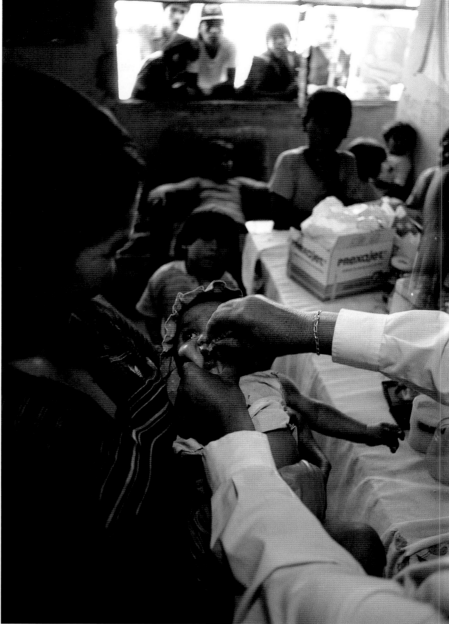

◄ **Doctor to the children without a country,** Cuban-born Lorenzo Pelly examines a girl at a Red Cross shelter for Central American refugees in Brownsville, Texas. At any one time, several thousand Central Americans live in shelters and detention camps in the lower Rio Grande Valley. As a physician for the Immigration and Naturalization Service detention center, the Red Cross shelter and the Casa Oscar Romero shelter, Pelly sees most of them. "My motto is to be nice to everyone," he says. "My role in life is that of a physician who sees people as human beings and will treat them no matter if they are good guys or bad guys."
Photo by Gerd Ludwig

▲ **A dramatic success story is built on millions of small steps,** like this dose of polio vaccine being offered to an Argentine child in Buenos Aires. The twentieth century has seen several epidemics of poliomyelitis, a viral infection of the motor nerve cells of the brain and spinal cord. Although an estimated 250,000 cases still occur annually worldwide, the World Health Organization says it hopes to announce the total eradication of the disease from the Americas by the end of 1990 — the most significant accomplishment in infectious disease prevention since smallpox was eradicated in 1980.
Photo by Diego Goldberg

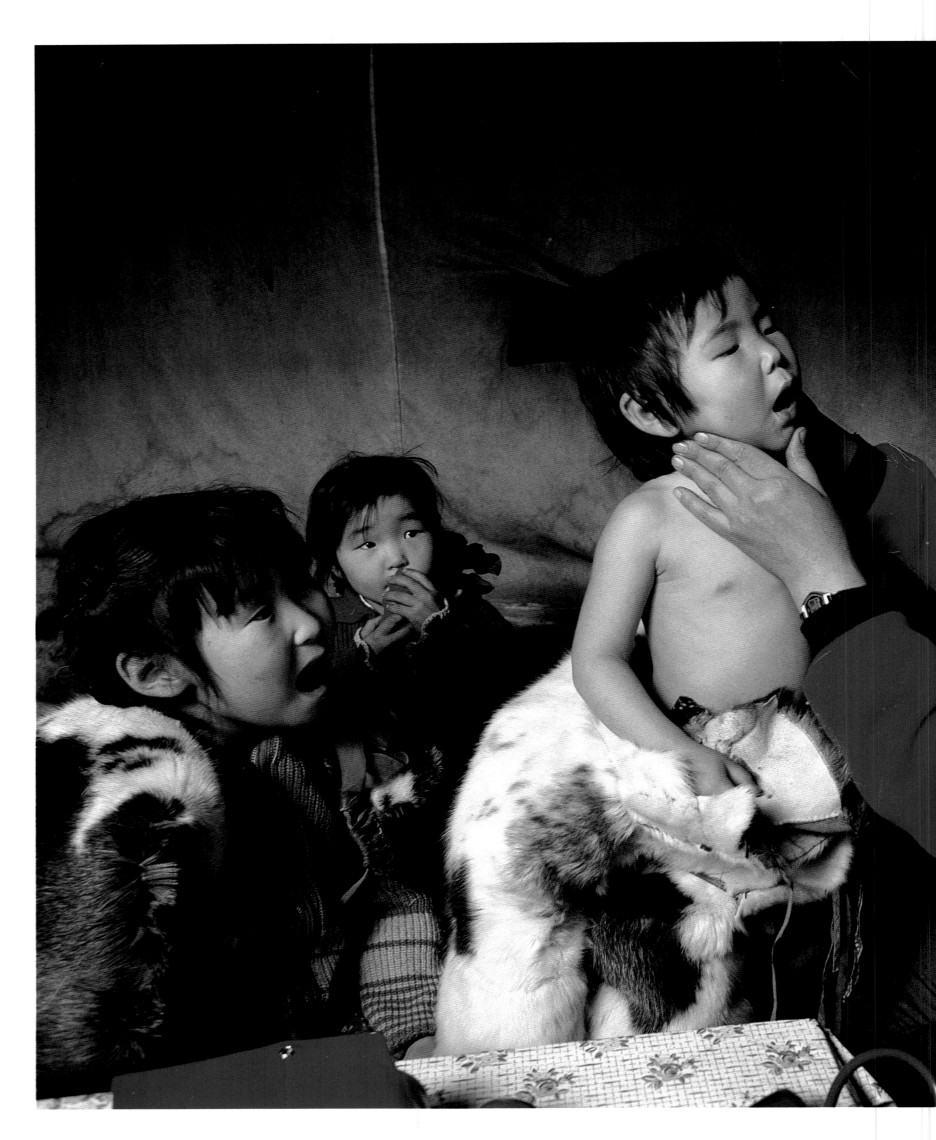

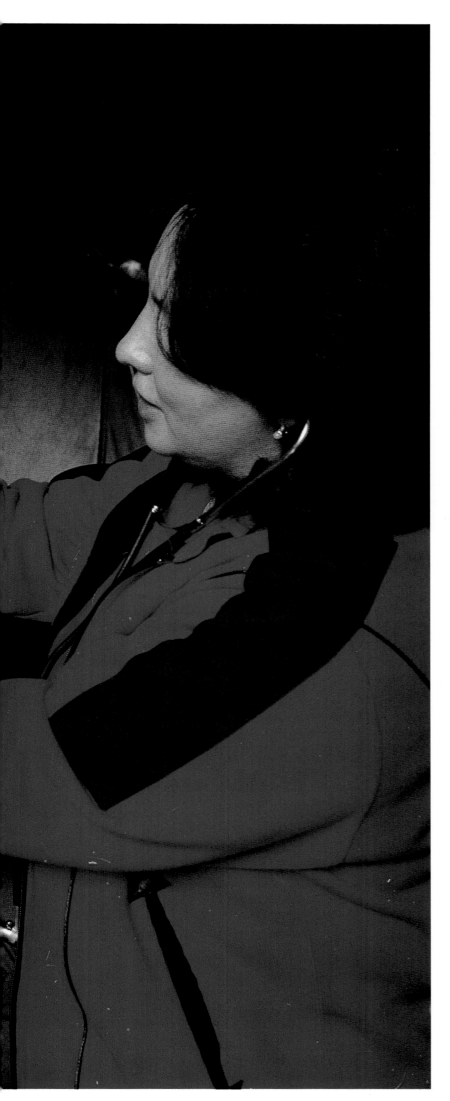

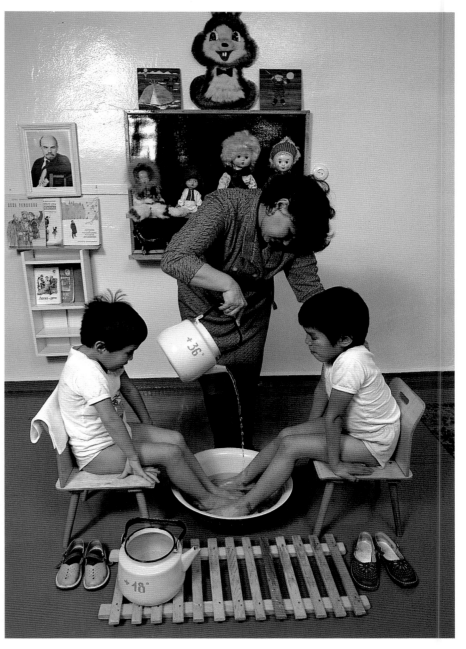

◄ **An Inuit child in the Soviet far north gets a checkup** from Dr. Larissa Abrutina, who travels by helicopter from reindeer camp to reindeer camp, carrying simple medical equipment and a small cache of drugs and medicines. In the summer months, she takes a mobile X-ray machine on her rounds.
Photo by Mark S. Wexler

▲ **In a land where the mercury can drop to sixty degrees below** zero, a schoolteacher alternately pours hot and cold water on the feet of Chukotka children in Ostrounoye, above the Arctic Circle in the Soviet Union. The water, at temperatures of thirty-six degrees centigrade (ninety-seven Fahrenheit) and eighteen degrees centigrade (sixty-four Fahrenheit), is meant to acclimatize the children to the extremes in temperature they're likely to find outdoors.
Photo by Mark S. Wexler

PHOTO ESSAY | *Portrait of a Healer*

For two weeks a month, flying doctor Anne Spoerry gives new meaning to the words "house call" by bringing medical care to the nomadic tribespeople of remote northern Kenya. Spoerry (right), a seventy-one-year-old native of France, has logged well over a million miles in her twenty-five years of flying with the Medicine by Air program of the Nairobi-based African Medical and Research Foundation, or AMREF. Equipped with a first-aid kit and a supply of basic drugs, Spoerry uses her Piper Cherokee to visit villagers and treat everything from spear wounds to malaria. She airlifts patients with serious ailments to regional hospitals.

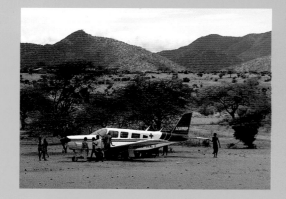

"Theirs is a very hard existence," says Spoerry of the 30,000 people who make up her caseload. "They live to care for their livestock. Their diet is usually milk, blood, and meat, and there is little medical help available to them.

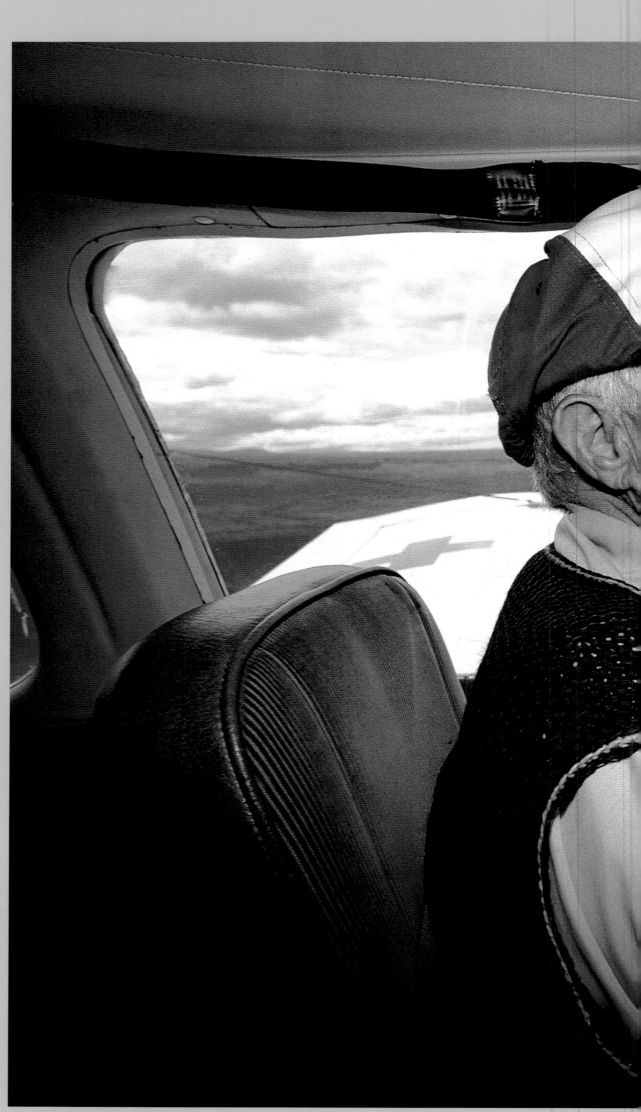

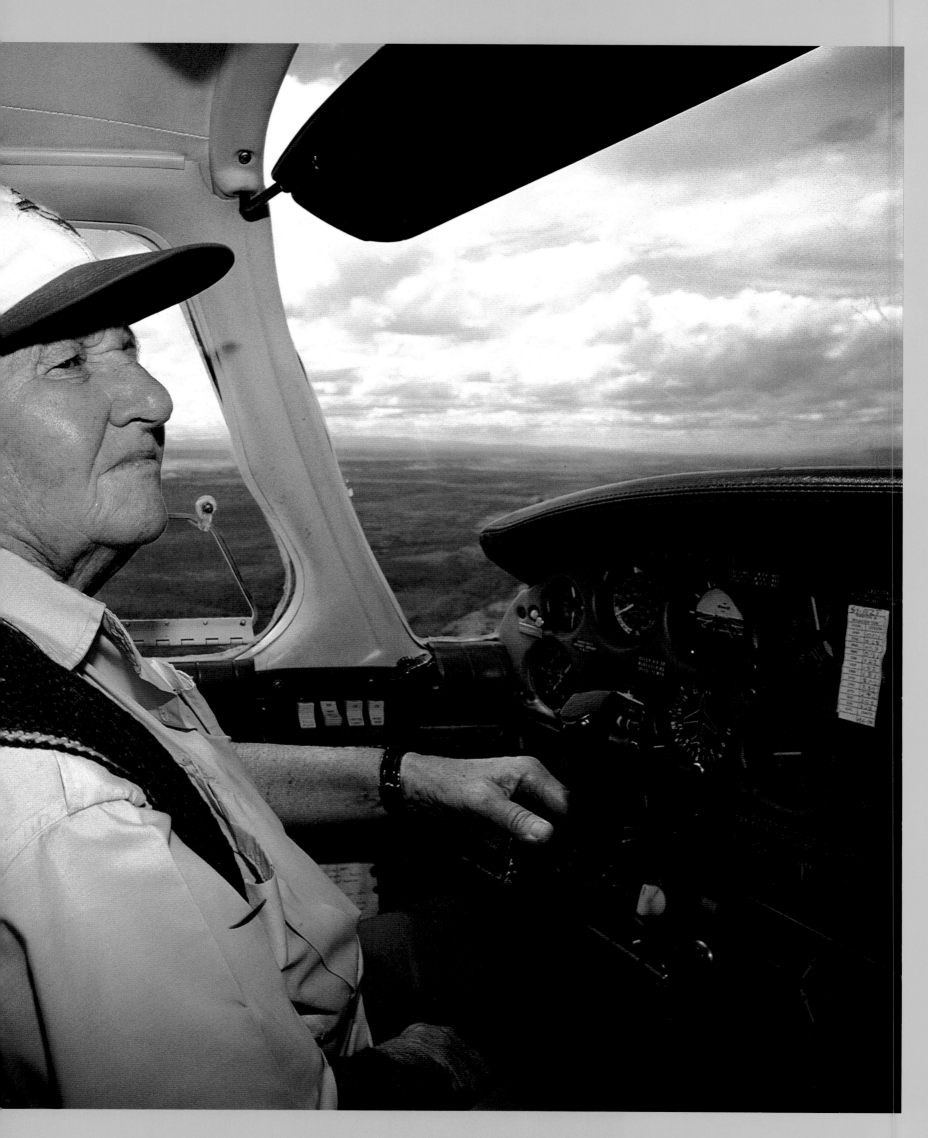

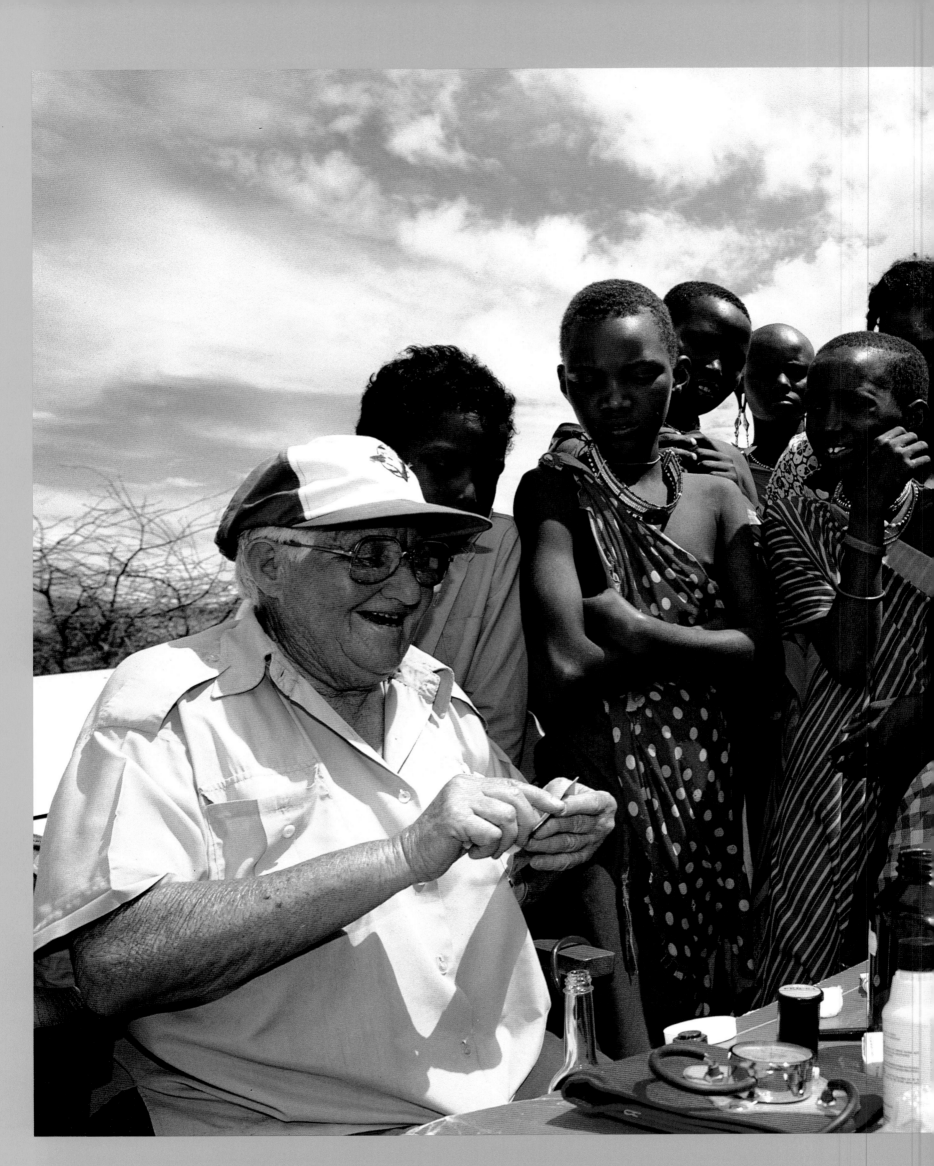

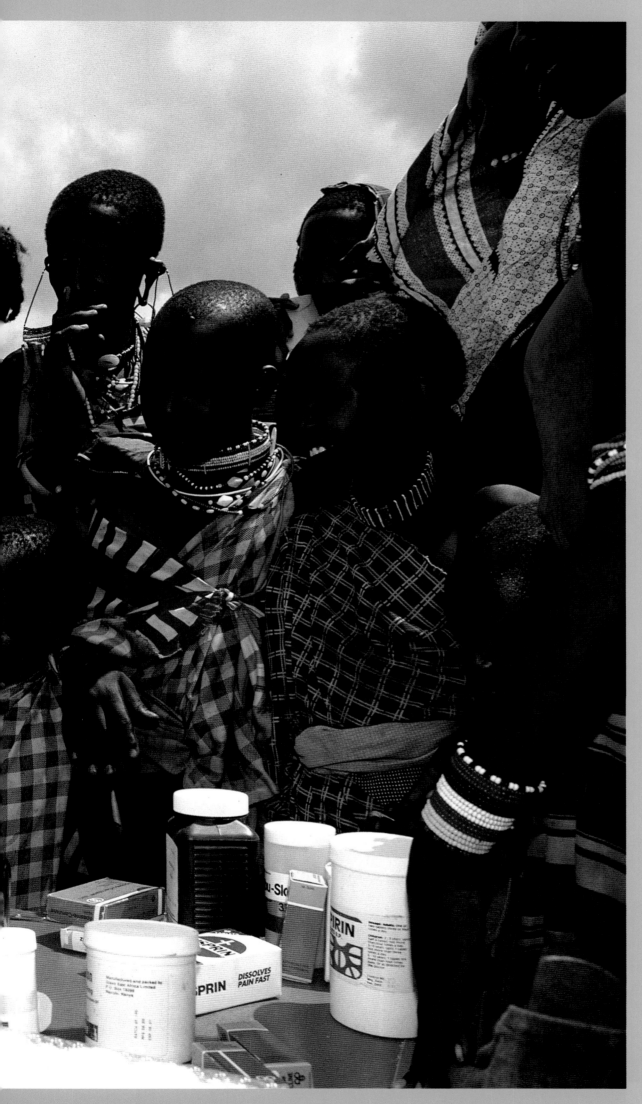

I found that it was here that I was most needed."

In addition to the flying doctor program, AMREF, which was founded in 1957, trains local residents as health care workers, sets up clinics, runs health education projects, and dispenses medical advice by radio with the Dr. AMREF program. Staff members travel to most of northeastern Africa, using laptop computers to collect data on malaria, sleeping sickness, and AIDS. The organization, whose motto is "It's people that matter," depends primarily on private funding for its operating expenses; says Spoerry, "The limitations and capabilities of my work are based entirely on how much money is available."

Children of the Masai tribe greet Spoerry (left) at a makeshift first-aid station in Oloika. Spoerry, who is fluent in Swahili, says that even as a child she dreamt of practicing medicine in Africa, and that she plans to continue as a flying doctor as long as she's physically able. Of her work, Spoerry says, "There are no sacrifices and the rewards are unlimited."

Photos by Rick Rickman

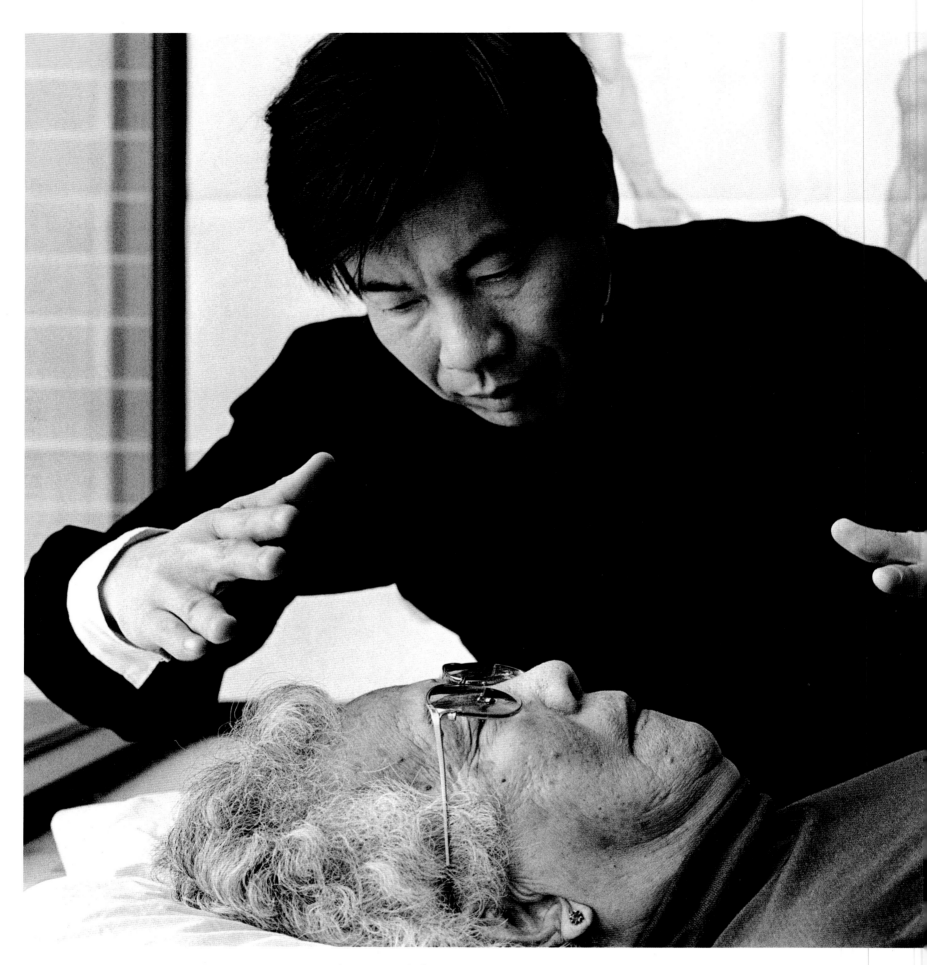

▲ **Old-style healing in the New World:** in the Canadian plains city of Calgary, Jin-Fa Zhang practices the ancient system of *qi-gong* on Shui Ying Wong. Sufferers of asthma, rheumatism, arthritis, and heart problems seek out Jin-Fa and his mentor, Philip Jiang, who study a patient's *qi*, or aura, before leading him or her into a meditative state. "Involuntarily," says Jiang, "the body then makes all sorts of movement, freeing up vital energy. After half an hour, the patient feels like an entirely different person."
Photo by Rodney Smith

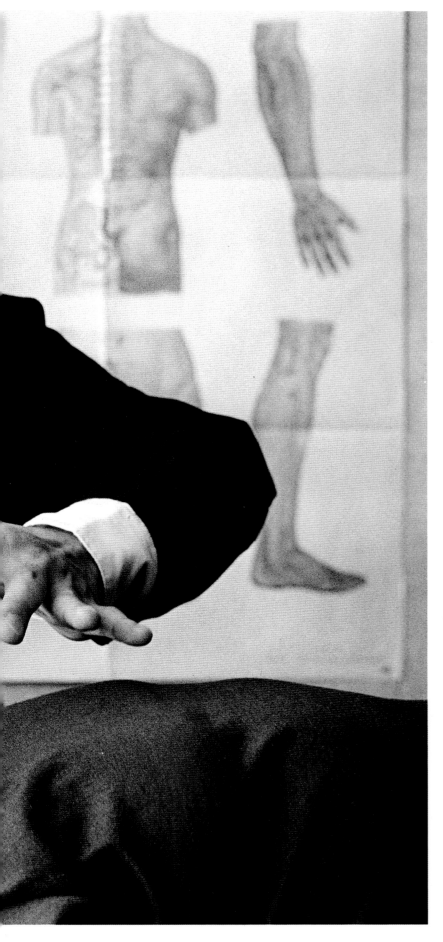

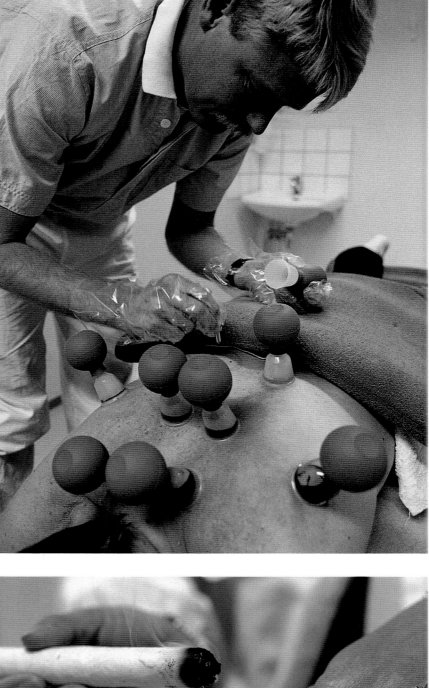

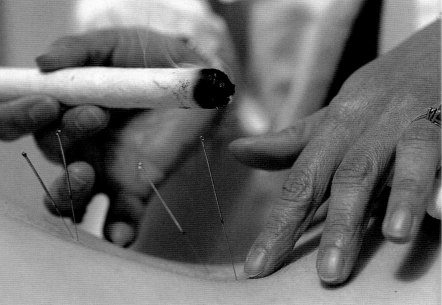

▲▲ **The centuries-old practice of cupping survives in modern Finland,** where physiotherapist Eero Kolehmainen works on patients who want to lower their blood pressure, improve their circulation, and relieve muscular pain. The cuppist pierces the skin and uses the suction cups to draw out blood, just as healers did in ancient China, India, Egypt, Greece, and Rome. *Photo by Stephanie Maze*

▲ **Combining two Eastern healing arts in a California setting,** Dr. Rong Zhou uses moxibustion and acupuncture at Emperor's College in Santa Monica. By using the acupuncture needle to conduct heat into the body, Zhou doesn't have to apply the burning moxa stick directly to the skin. The treatment is used for patients who are low in energy or suffer from noninflammatory pain. With 10,000 patients annually, Emperor's College is the leading treatment center among Eastern medicine schools in the West. *Photo by Alon Reininger*

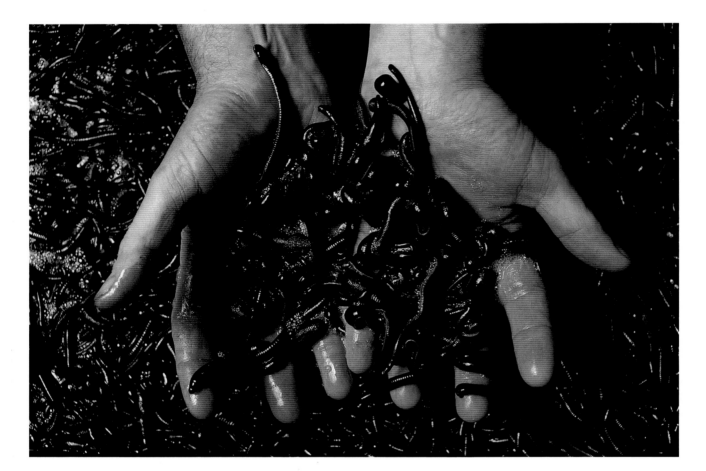

▲ Behold the lowly leech, once again the doctor's friend. Bloodsuckers like these, raised by Dr. Roy T. Sawyer and his Biopharm Ltd. in the Welsh village of Hendy, are back in vogue in many American hospitals, where they're used to drain excess blood after micro-surgical procedures such as the reattachment of severed fingers and ears. In the 1500s, the term "leech" was used to describe all healers; even into the 1800s, the tiny creatures played a major role in medical care, as doctors placed dozens at a time on an ill patient, believing that the hungry leeches would suck out only the patient's "bad blood."

With its rediscovery in the early 1980s by medical science, the medicinal leech, known more formally as *Hirudo medicinalis*, has also attracted the attention of bioengineers. The saliva contains an anti-coagulant, a local anesthetic, and an antibiotic, and bio-engineers hope to re-create the saliva for use in the treatment of various maladies, including arthritis, glaucoma, embolisms — even heart attacks and strokes.
Photo by Nick Kelsh

▶ East meets West at the Maharishi Ayur-Veda Health Center in Lancaster, Massachusetts, where warm, herbed sesame oil is poured on the forehead to reduce the body's stress and bring about a state of bliss. Dr. Deepak Chopra, the medical director of the Lancaster center and a former chief of staff at New England Memorial Hospital, hopes to foster the spread of the traditional Indian healing system in the United States. "The fundamental premise of ayurvedic medicine is that consciousness is primary, matter is secondary," says Chopra, whose ministrations are designed to trigger the body's "healing response."
Photo by Henry Hilliard

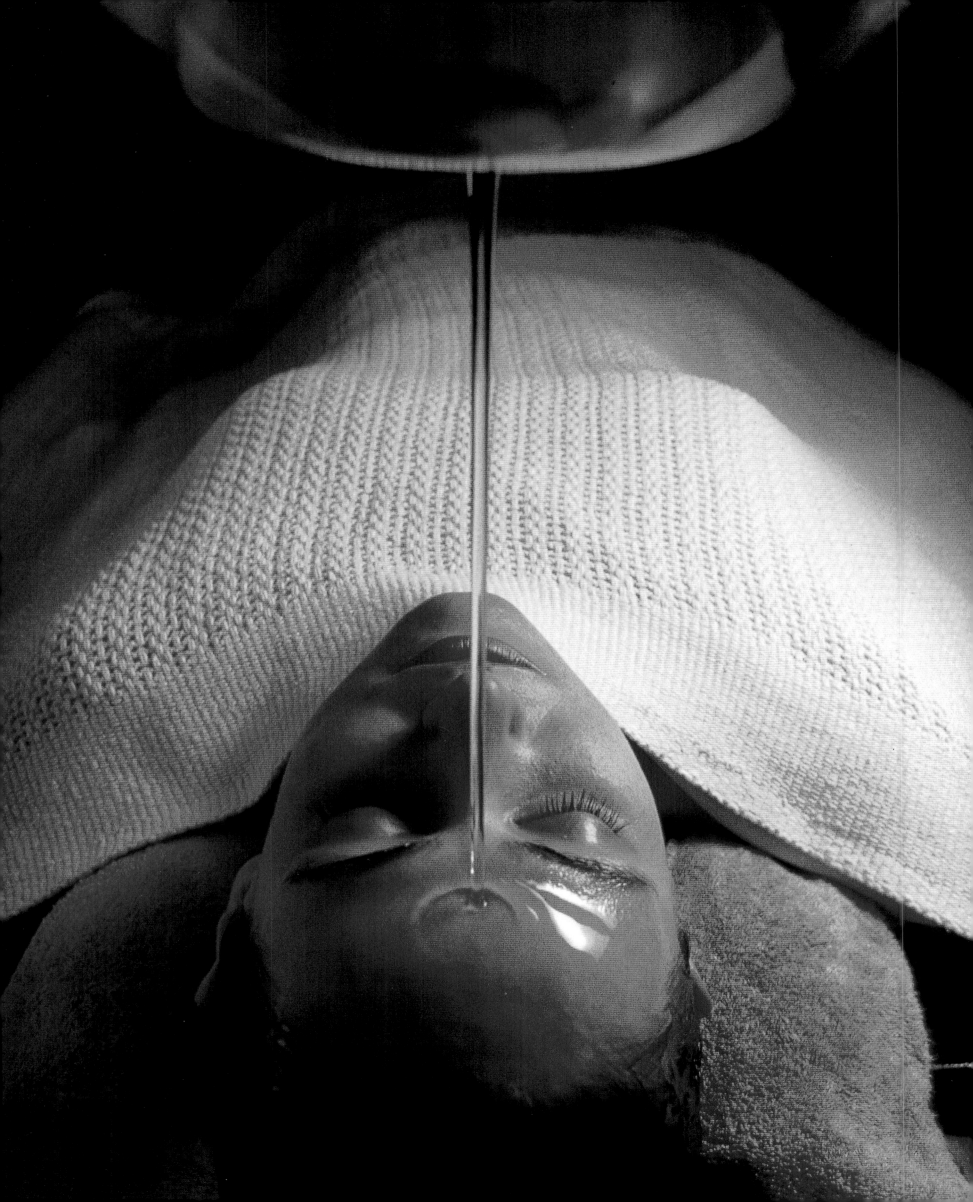

A surgical team at work at Tu Du Obstetrical and Gynecological Hospital, Ho Chi Minh City, Vietnam. *Photo by Monica Almeida*

THE HEALERS

These kinds of courage stand on another, deeper kind: the courage to make oneself responsible for an outcome. A healer is no passive observer. She or he sees people whose bodies are disintegrating, whose lives have lost their safety.... It is the impulse to commonplace courage and everyday heroism that the healer formalizes into a life's work.

—John Poppy

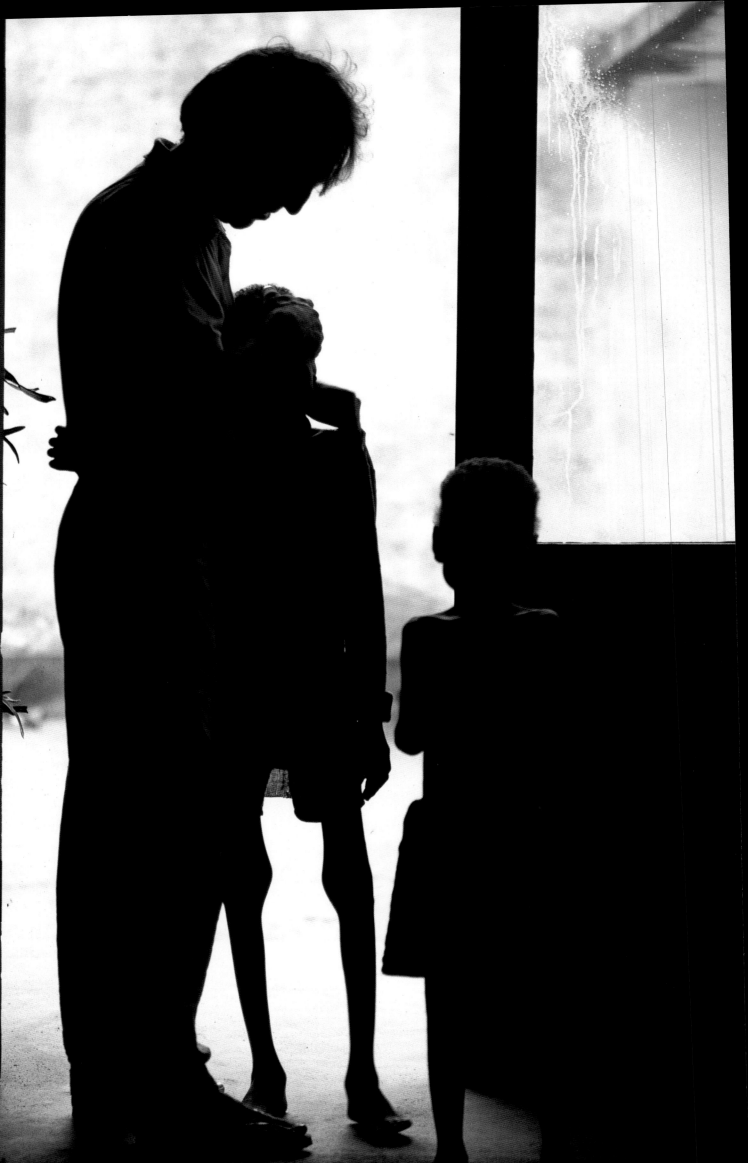

The Hero in the White Coat

JOHN POPPY

THE CHILD'S EYELIDS KEEP WANTING TO CLOSE. SHE IS SIX, AND MIGHT report some clues to what is making her so sick if she could speak, but consciousness is slipping away. Heat rises from her; her skin blazes dry and pink against the blue cooling blanket. Her arms lie at her sides as if she has forgotten them. The nurses and doctors crowded around the table, seven of them by now, see with relief that the stab of a needle into a vein makes her protest with a harsh little moan and try to pull away.

"I know, sweetheart, it hurts, it's okay," says the nurse who is taping a plastic tube to a hot forearm.

"You're going to be fine, Roxanne, we're taking good care of you." The chief of pediatrics bends to the child's ear to offer his assurance, and lays his hand on her cheek, hoping some comfort will penetrate her fever. Dr. Moses Grossman left his bed at 3:00 this morning when the hospital called, worried about the possible causes of this 106.5 degree temperature. He has studied medicine for almost fifty years so that he can help children. Infectious diseases are his specialty.

Standing beside Roxanne, he knows what he and the emergency-room team at San Francisco General Hospital can do for her. They measure vital signs and blood gases. They give her fluids for her parched tissues, oxygen to make her struggle a little easier, and an aspirin substitute to knock down the fever. They put mechanical coolers around her. They inject drugs that attack a wide spectrum of microbes, hoping to hit the one, or ones, that might have invaded her. And they send a sample of her blood to the lab. A superb team like this one does it all in five to eight minutes.

But, Grossman knows, these are just steps. What he doesn't know is the identity of the threat to Roxanne's life. A severe, possibly overwhelming, infection. But what kind? He needs to see the face of the monster.

The child's parents wait in the hospital's Family Room. Grossman goes to them. They had been enjoying a camping trip with their daughter; now they are terrified that she might lose the life they gave her. Their eyes beg this graying man in a green scrub suit to say he can save it. Grossman recalls times when he's had to force himself to go into rooms like this one and say, "Your child is going to die." He has seen health professionals on such occasions withdraw into a brisk formality or not show up at all. Feeling helpless to prevent a death that has not yet occurred but is coming, perhaps thinking of their own children's mortality, they cannot bring themselves to offer the comfort they are empowered to give. This morning, he does not speak of a possible death. He speaks of his hope that they've caught it in time, the nameless thing, and says he's waiting for the lab report.

Toward midday, a bacterium reveals itself in the blood culture: *Pasteurella pestis.* Plague. A demonic strand of memory from the Black Death of the fourteenth century survives in certain squirrels on the West Coast of the United States; a flea from one must have bitten Roxanne at the campground. A bubo—a swollen lymph node—appears on her neck. Now Grossman can sharpen his defense of her.

Among other things, he orders pus drained from the bubo. The surgeon, the anesthesiologist, and the nurses all admit they're concerned about plague contaminating the operating room. They take what precautions they can—extra gloves, masks, goggles—and perform the operation. Later, Roxanne is sitting up, able to drink some juice, starting to win.

Healers themselves, busy with the techniques and stresses of their art, often forget to wonder at what they can do. "I just wanted to get good training and be a good doctor," Moses Grossman says. The rest of us, except in moments of need or illumination, give little thought to the dimension in a healer's life that is, in a word, heroic.

We can count up plenty of reasons for disillusionment, with health care in Western nations now an industry as huge as others we've learned to be wary of: impersonality, expensive and exclusive insurance, malpractice disputes, and, as always, the doctor's high income and fabled Wednesday afternoon golf games. A career in medicine can produce material rewards, to be sure. But increasing standards of care, subtleties of research, and demands from patients make healing a more arduous calling now than it has ever been. A doctor likely spends that Wednesday afternoon not swinging a golf club but turning journal pages, studying to keep up. (The same is true for a nurse, who never got the money and prestige in the first place.) None of the rewards would exist without, first, the demands of a discipline that reveals the heroic side of the true healers.

Their heroism is not the antique kind made of superhuman strength and special favors from the gods. It is the plain human kind that you might also call courage, which Mark Twain defined as "resistance to fear, mastery of fear—not absence of fear." The hero knows fear and doesn't run away.

This courage encompasses more than physical bravery, though that has long been a part of it. It's nothing new for healers to expose themselves to the diseases of strangers. Hippocratic physicians in Greece 2,400 years ago, and

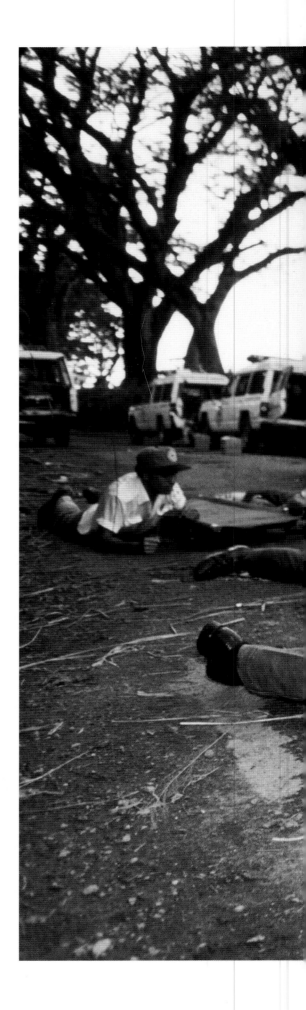

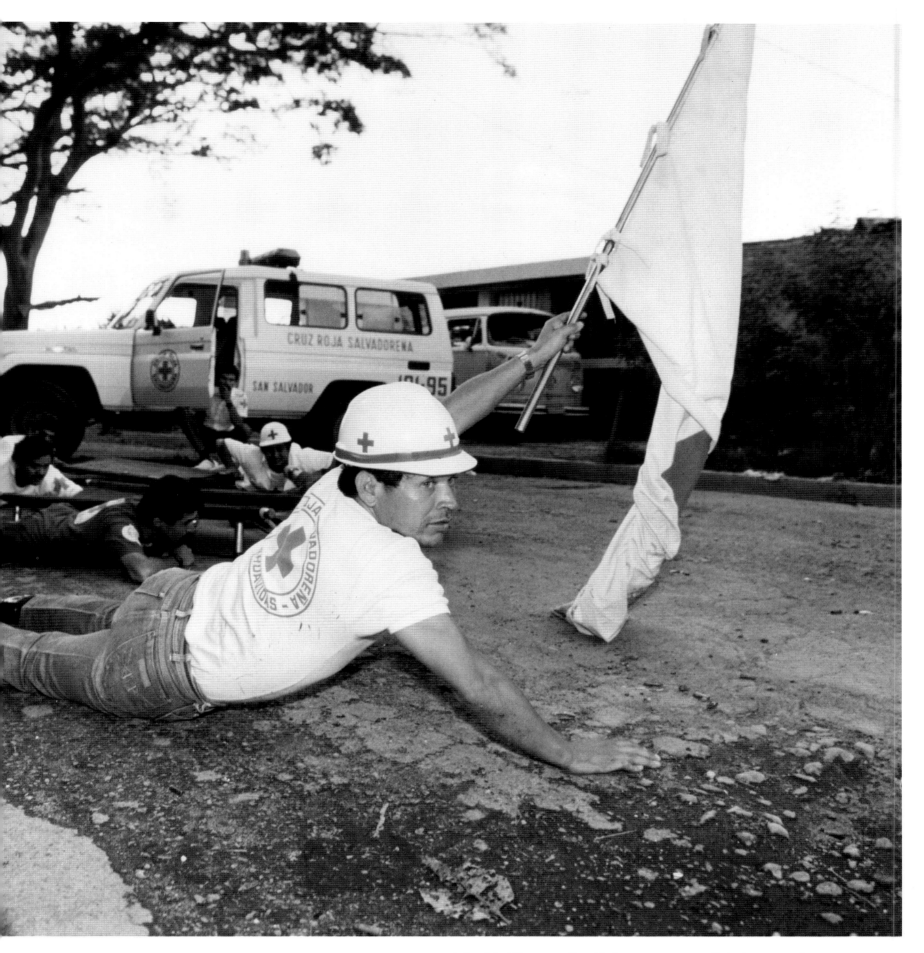

▲ **Ducking the cross fire, Red Cross workers attempt to reach the wounded** during fighting in El Salvador's decade-long civil war. The Geneva-based International Red Cross counts 149 member countries; besides being El Salvador's only ambulance service, La Cruz Roja also operates a clinic that treats thousands of people who might otherwise go untreated. "These Red Cross guys take incredible risks," says *Newsweek* photographer Bill Gentile. "The only defense they have is their white shirts and the red cross on the white flags."
Photo by William F. Gentile

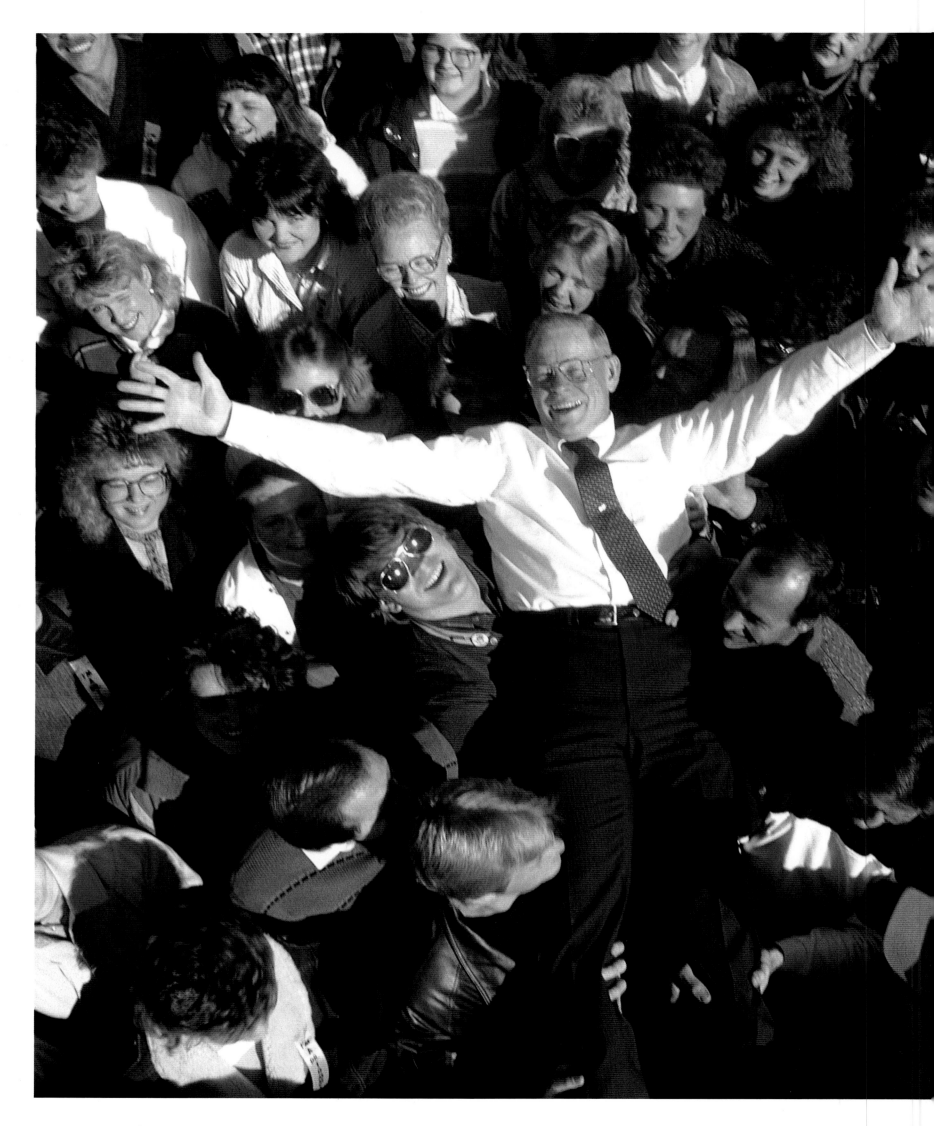

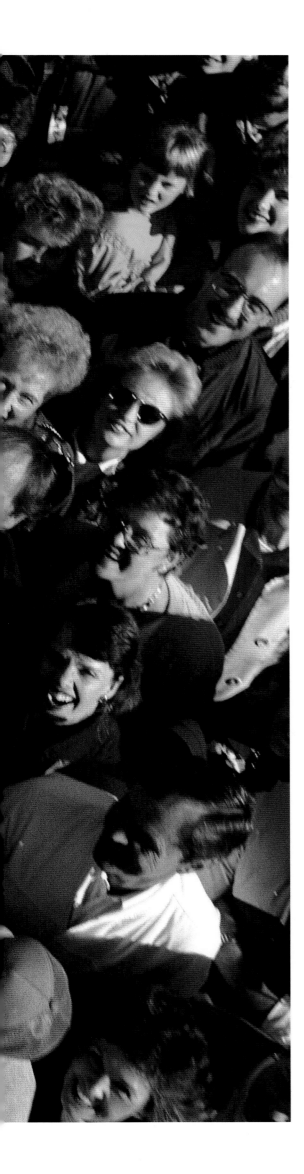

◄ **Held aloft by some of the 4,000 people he brought into the world,** Dr. Tommy Macdonnell celebrates a reunion with several hundred of his "babies" in Marshfield, Missouri. During his more than thirty-five years as a general practitioner, Macdonnell delivered some 2,500 babies in Webster County alone, creating a built-in constituency for his second career as a Missouri state representative. Ever the doctor, Macdonnell — whose campaign slogan was "We need a doctor in the House" — is pushing a bill that would require half of each Missouri workplace to be set aside as nonsmoking. *Photo by Jay Dickman*

their counterparts in Asia had their own version of today's lab tests. They tasted the blood and urine of their patients, the nasal mucus, ear wax, tears, sputum, and pus. Closer to our own time, cholera stampeded whole populations with its messy deadliness and mysterious origins; until the *Vibrio comma* bacterium was discovered in 1883, theories of cholera's causes ranged from atmospheric "miasma" to moral defects among slum dwellers. Most citizens of New York who could afford to flee did so in the epidemic of 1832. Most doctors, however, stayed. In fact, at the news weeks earlier that cholera had broken out in Montreal, American physicians had ridden north to study it. Granted, few at the time thought the disease was contagious, but still they rode into the heart of the miasma. Today, AIDS provokes caution if not fear in any doctor or nurse who gets near a patient's bodily fluids, yet all but a tiny minority lay hands on the ill with the attitude that some risk comes with the license.

Those kinds of courage stand on another, deeper kind: the courage to make oneself responsible for an outcome. A healer is no passive observer. She or he sees people whose bodies are disintegrating, whose lives have lost their safety. One may think the ordinary impulse would be to turn away, to act as if the disposition of another person's pain were God's business, not one's own. Yet anyone who has seen a toddler fall off a boat knows that the ordinary impulse is something else: to want to help, at the risk of one's comfort and even one's life. It is the impulse to commonplace courage and everyday heroism that the healer formalizes into a life's work.

Of course, physicians know it is not they who do the healing. When the immune system eats up viruses and bacteria, when collagen bridges a wound with new tissue, the living body and mind are performing miracles that science may assist but cannot yet copy. So here is the final element, the most poignant, in the healer's courage: humility.

"I cannot endure this," an afflicted person may say, or "I cannot recover from this." The physician may hesitate, then dares to say, "Yes, you can," and, blending carefully learned skills with that faith, attempts to become a companion in suffering and a companion in healing.

Volunteering to make a difference opens the healer to both triumph and failure—to "rejoice with them that do rejoice," as the Apostle Paul advised the Romans, "and weep with them that weep." Moses Grossman can rejoice with Roxanne. But first, he had the courage to make himself an accomplice to a miracle.

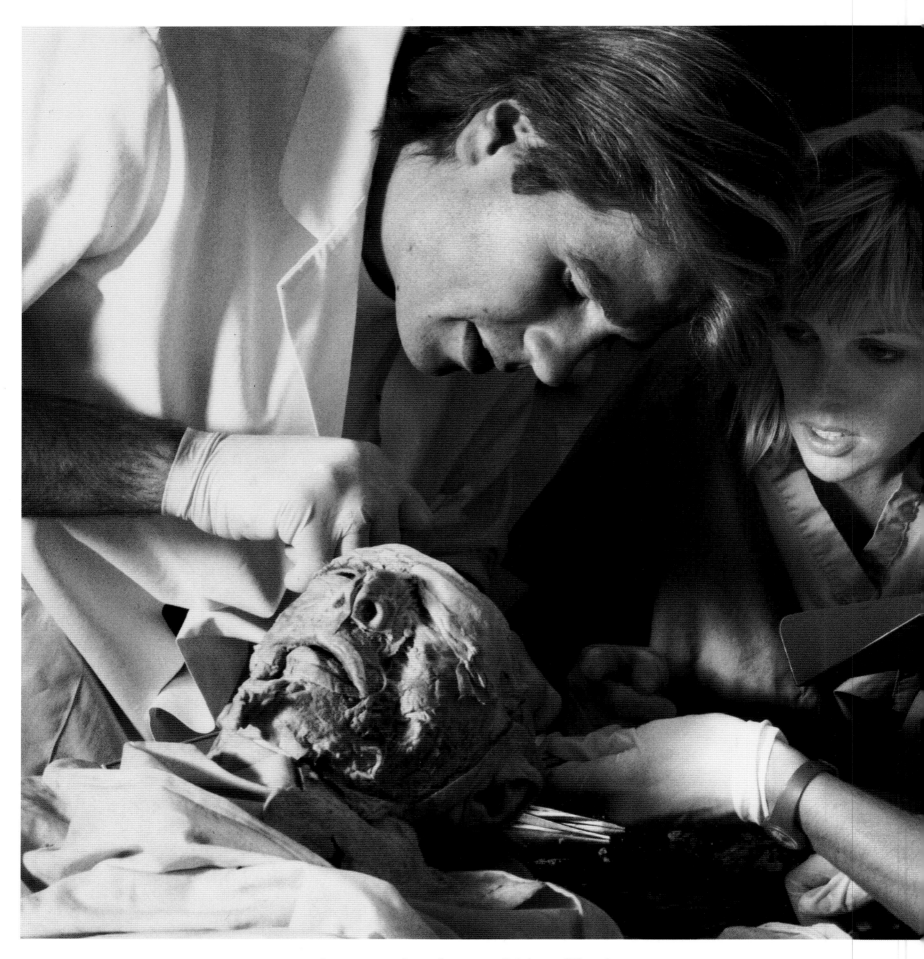

▲ **"It's an eerie feeling the first time you work with cadavers,"** says Erik Barton, removing the skin from the head with fellow second-year medical students Diane Hutchinson and Wendy Patton, to study the blood vessels, nerves, muscles, and bones in the head and neck. Over the past twenty-three years, more than 9,000 people have arranged to have their bodies donated to the University of California at San Diego School of Medicine. When the semester is over, the bodies are cremated and buried at sea. According to Dr. Roger Marchand, Barton's professor at UCSD, "we couldn't teach medicine without cadavers." *Photo by Doug Lewis, M.D.*

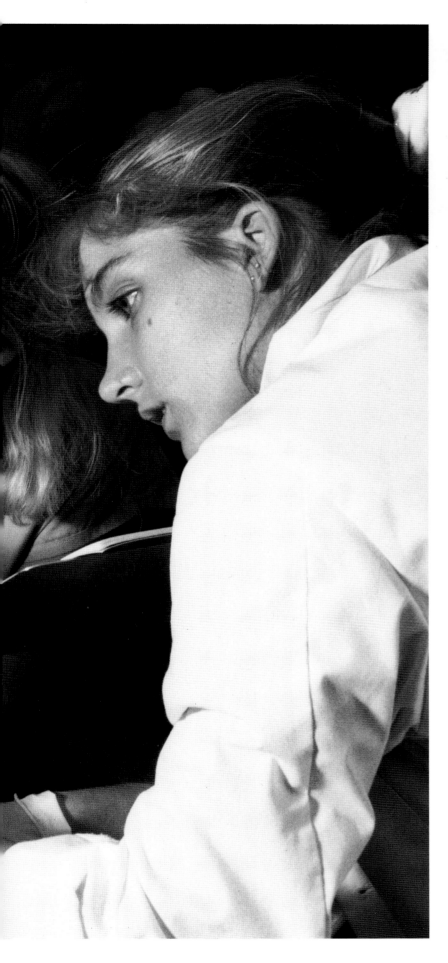

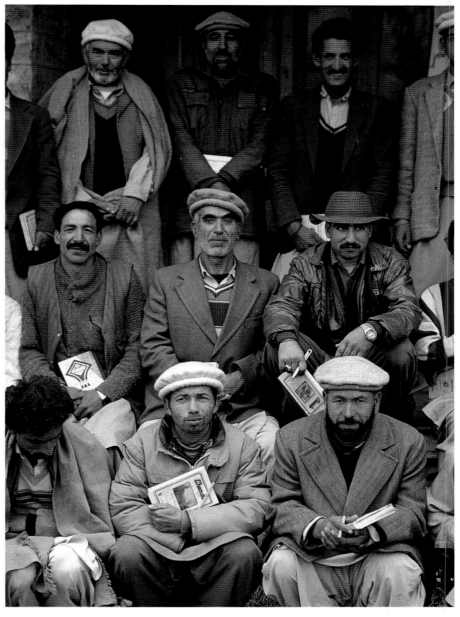

▲ **The first graduating class of primary health care workers** at the Aga Khan Health Services clinic, high in the mountains of Pakistan, poses for a class picture before taking their health kits back to their villages. The kits contain aspirin and other simple medicines, thermometers, and what is perhaps the key element: oral rehydration solution. In Pakistan, more than half a million children under the age of five die each year from dehydration brought on by diarrhea.
Photo by Judy Griesedieck

▶ **Soviet nurses in training steal a moment to gossip** at the Magadan Nursing Institute in Siberia. Some 450 students are enrolled in the school's two-year program, which features lectures and hands-on work in physics, chemistry, anatomy, hygiene, internal medicine, pediatrics, and surgery. After graduation, the nurses will join the huge hospital work force in the Soviet Union, whose 1.5 million doctors account for about one-third of the world's total.
Photo by Mark S. Wexler

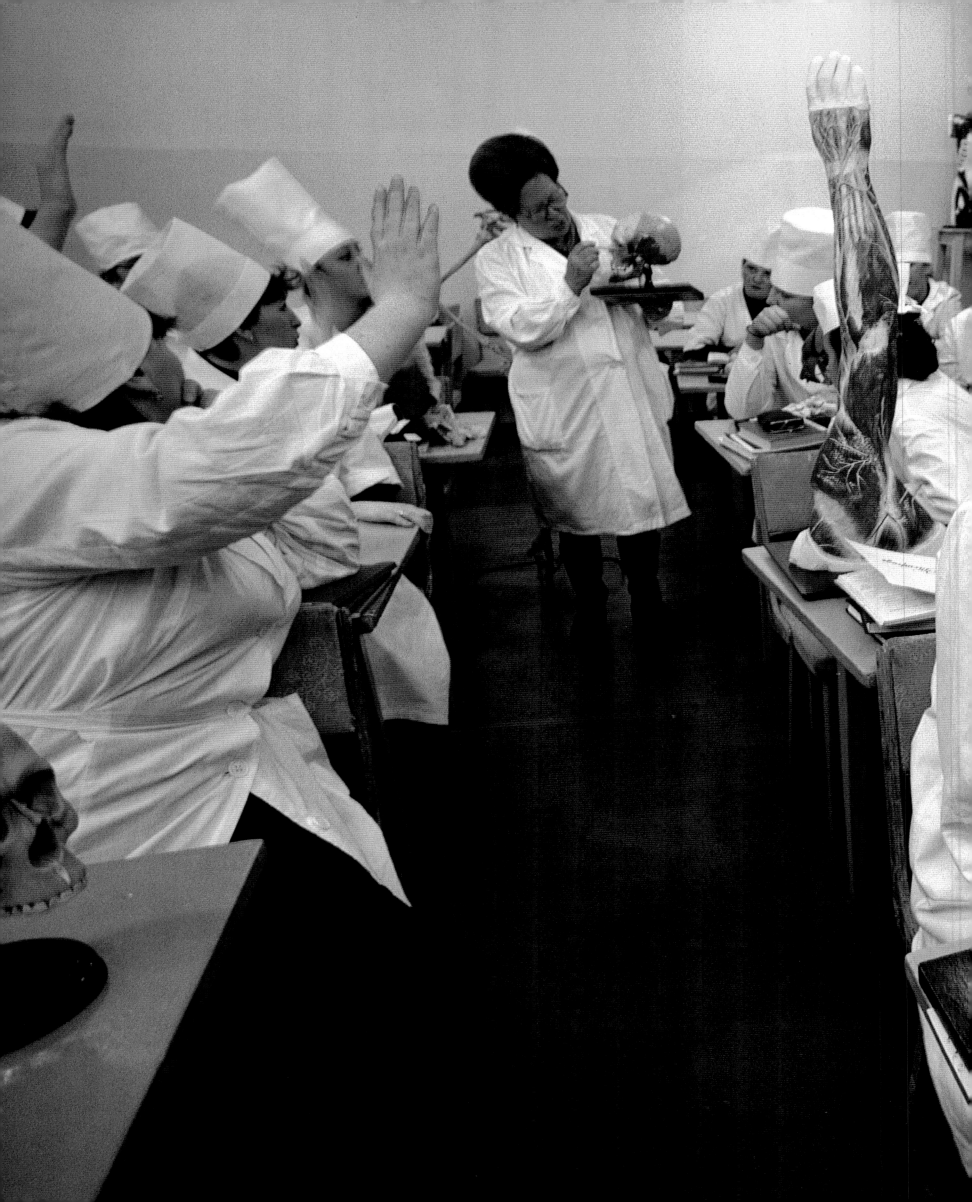

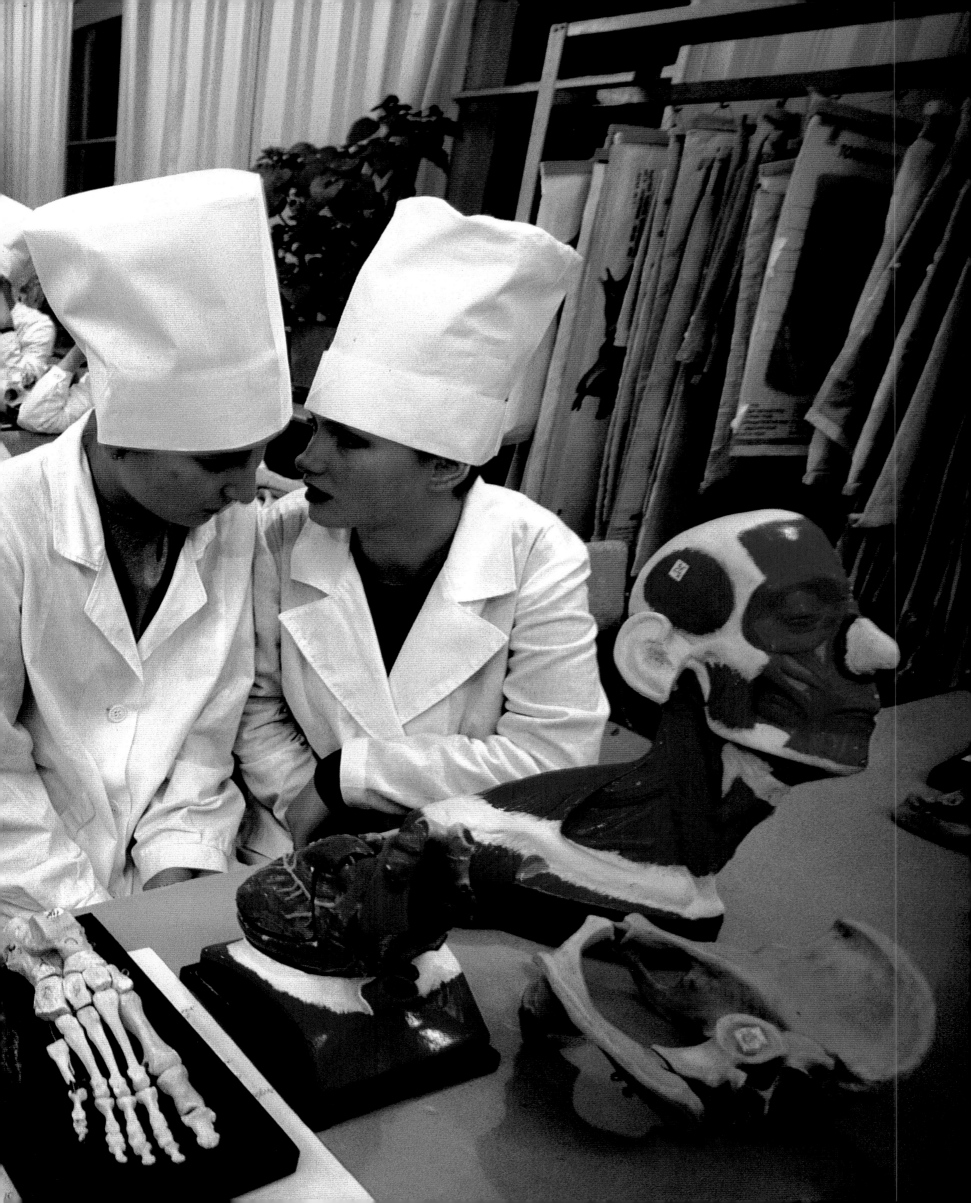

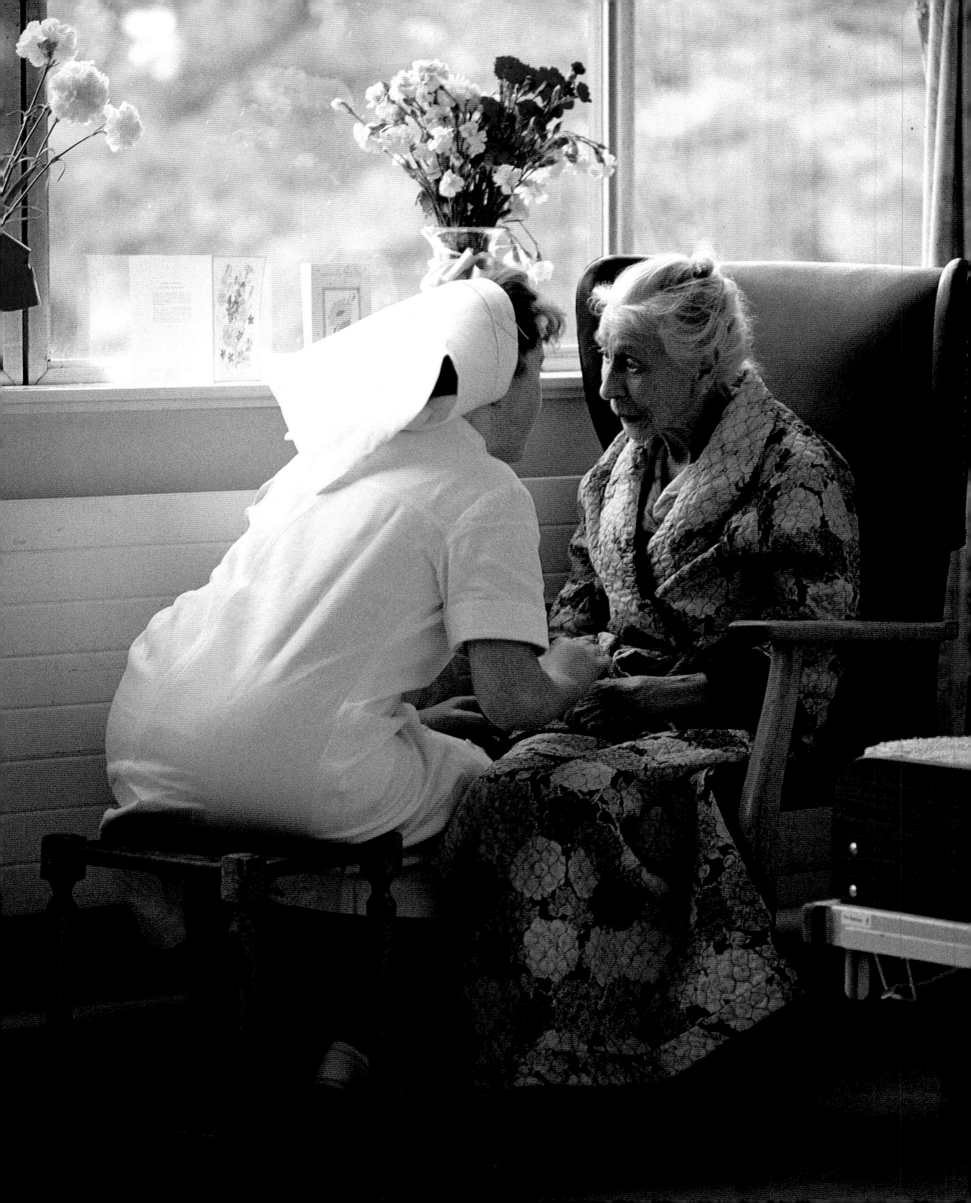

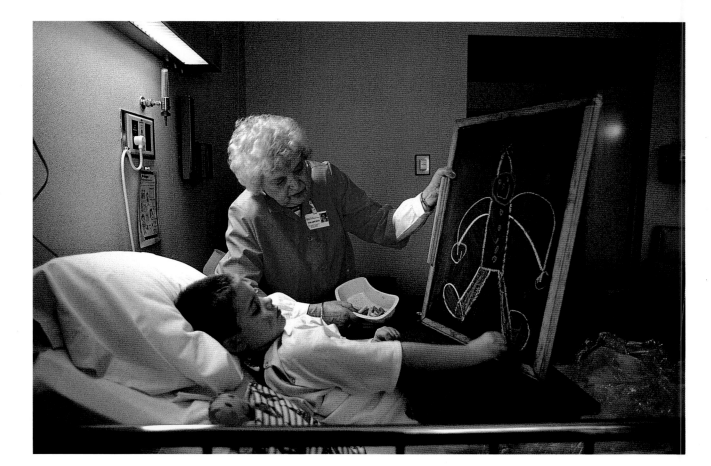

▲ **One in ten adult Americans is a volunteer in the health care field.** Here, energetic grandmother Charlotte Miller plays with six-year-old asthma patient Jonathon Dolieslager during one of her two weekly visits to West Suburban Hospital Medical Center outside Chicago. Jonathon went home a few days later, but Miller keeps coming back. "There's just so much out there for me to do that I can't sit at home," she says. "I want to make a difference."
Photo by Gary S. Chapman

◄ **Administering to the sick, as nurses have done for centuries,** Siobhán Magner talks with ninety-four-year-old Neta Shortall at St. Vincent's Hospital in Dublin, Ireland. Although nursing wasn't established as a profession until the nineteenth century, the medical philosopher Charaka, who lived several hundred years before Christ, had already identified four key characteristics of a nurse: "knowledge of the manner in which drugs should be prepared or compounded for administration, cleverness, devotion to the patient waited upon, and purity." Magner, one of 300 nurses in training at St. Vincent's, will become a practicing nurse in May of 1991.
Photo by Nick Kelsh

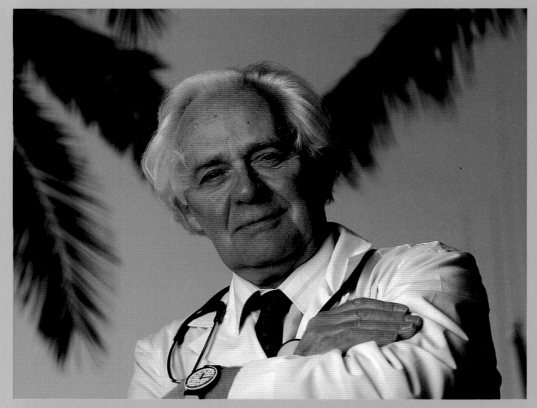

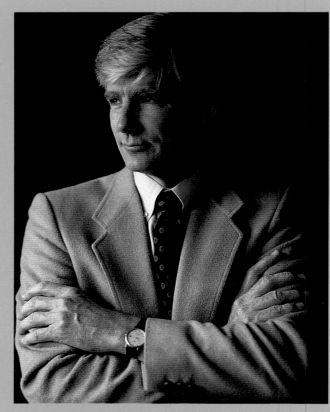

"It's important to get involved with patients, because you can't always solve their problems just by looking at X rays and being scientifically correct." Dr. Frank Catchpool, family practitioner, Sausalito, CA. *Photo by Doug Menuez*

"The emotion and appreciation of the patients is the greatest reward." Dr. William DeVries, heart surgeon, Louisville, KY. *Photo by Bradley E. Clift*

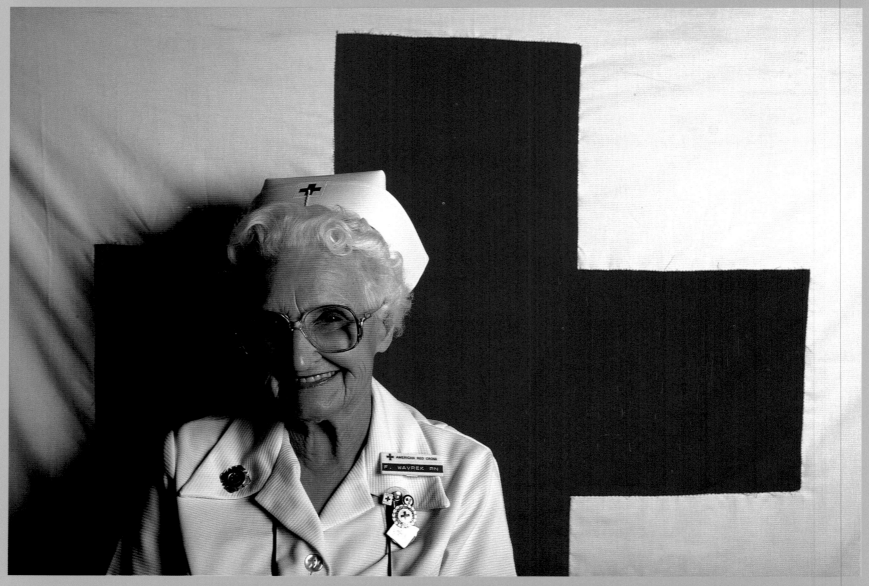

"The cap is your dignity. Today nurses don't wear it like they used to. I tell them to put it on; otherwise patients don't know whether it's a nurse or a cleaning woman who's coming to take care of them." Frances Wavrek, American Red Cross volunteer and retired nurse, Quincy, IL. *Photo by Gary S. Chapman*

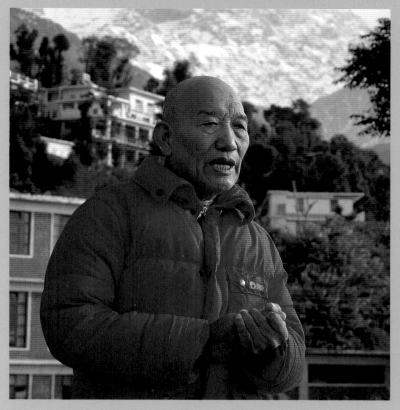

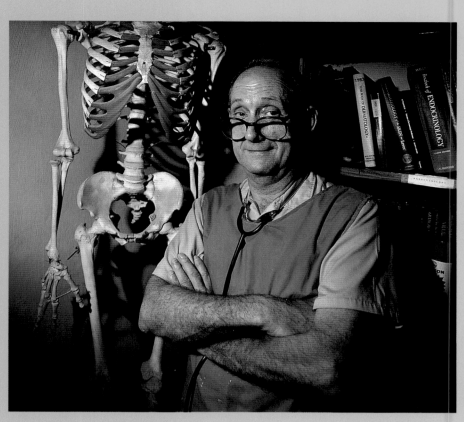

"The cause of illness is all one. It is the ignorance arising through not recognizing the meaning of selflessness." Dr. Tenzin Choedak, senior physician to the Dalai Lama, Dharamsala, India. *Photo by Galen Rowell*

"A lot of the people here don't really understand what I do for them. They just know that it helps." Dr. William Hodges, family practitioner, Limbé, Haiti. *Photo by P.F. Bentley*

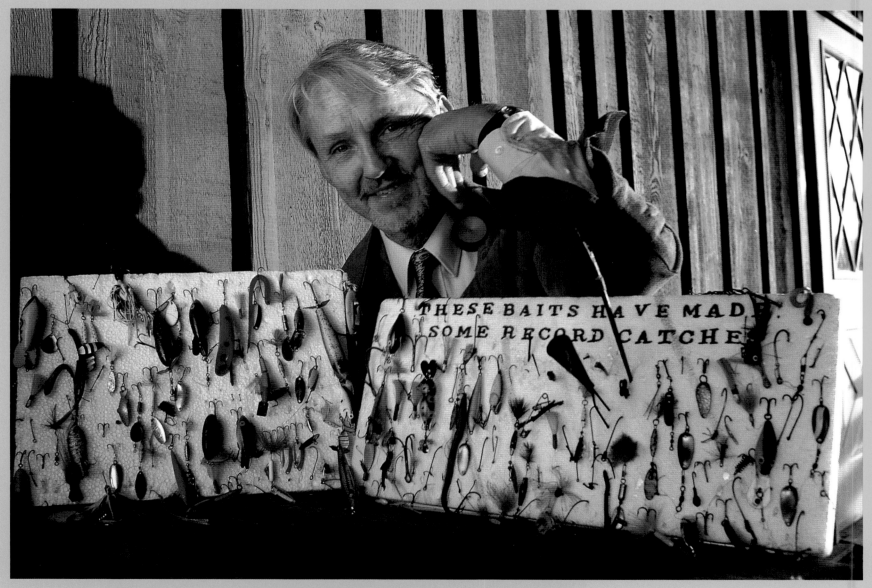

"I've removed about 500 fishhooks from people. I used to give them back, but now I keep them. I have about 300. I worked in an emergency room for twenty-two years, and I took a lot of things out of people." Dr. Carroll Traylor, family practitioner, Calvert City, KY. *Photo by Jay Dickman*

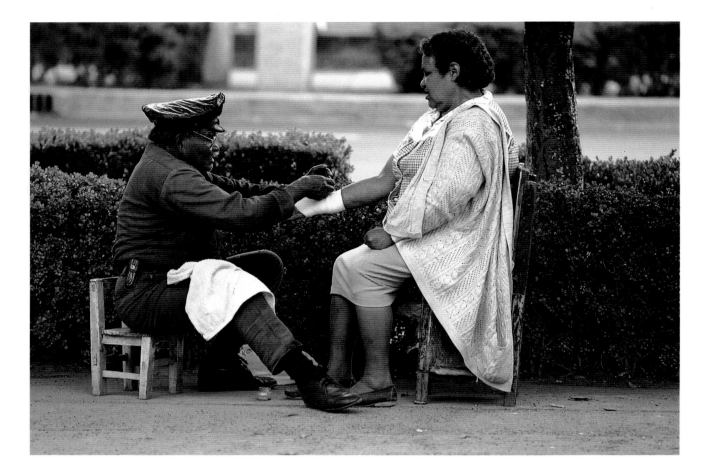

▲ **Massaging muscles and wrapping bones as he has for more than twenty years,** "The Boneman" of Mexico City tends to a customer at his post across the street from Los Venados Hospital. Mexicans come from throughout the sprawling metropolis to search out former shoeshine man Florencio Martínez Morales and his trademark wintergreen balm.
Photo by Eric Lars Bakke

▶ **A nurse at a Siberian maternity hospital holds one of the more than 14,000 babies** born in the Soviet Union each day. The nurse and her Soviet medical colleagues will provide the newborn citizens with free, state-sponsored health care from these cradles to their graves. But, says Dr. Mark Field of the Russian Research Center at Harvard University, "the Soviet medical system is in bad shape. The number of doctors and hospitals is impressive, but the Soviets spend less than four percent of their gross national product on health care." The U.S. figure is about twelve percent.
Photo by Feliks Soloyov

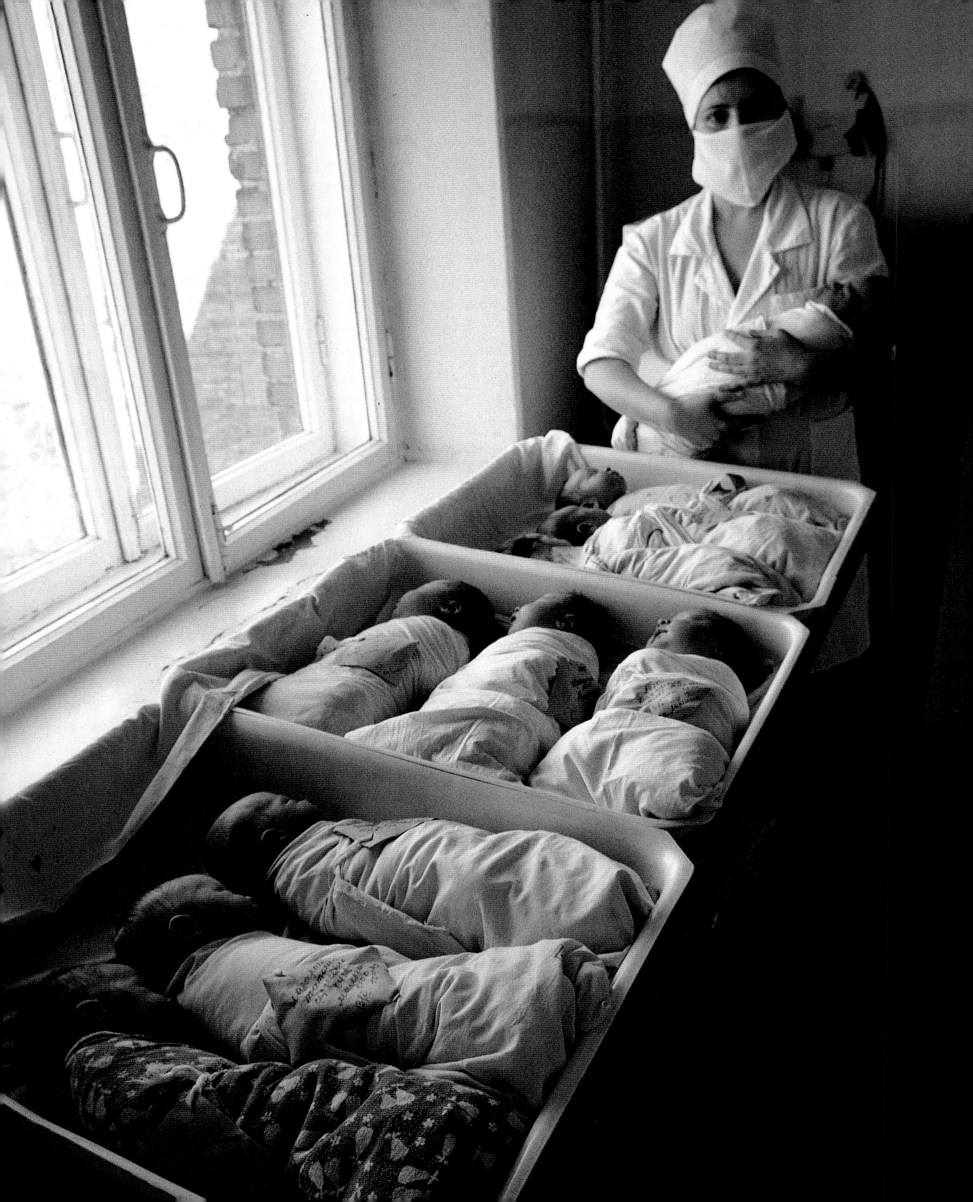

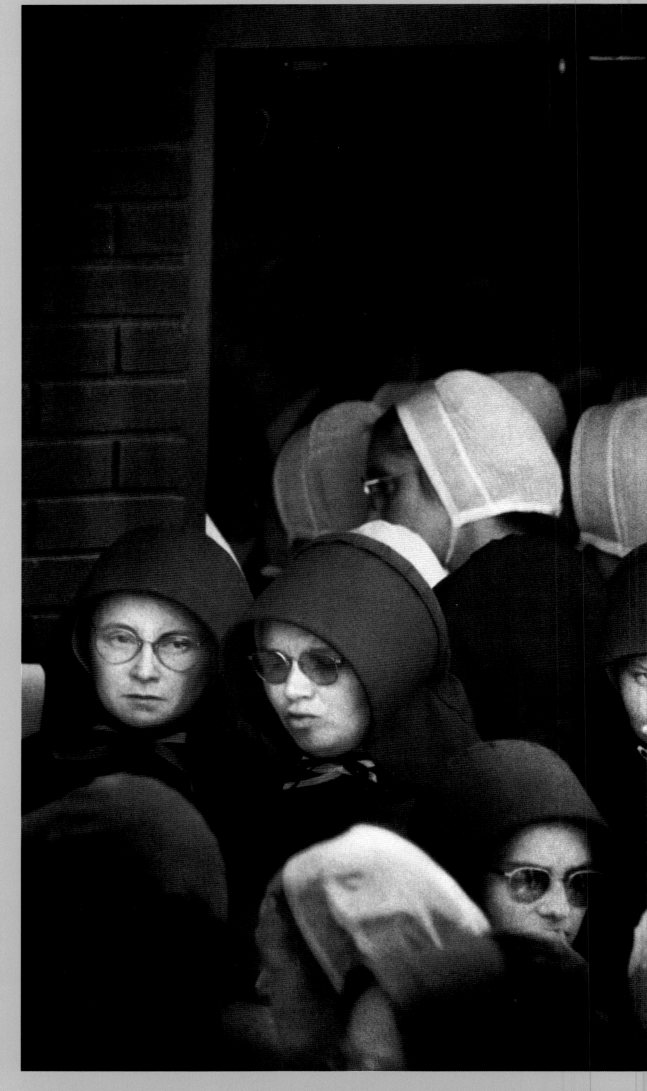

Nearly 700 babies have come squalling into the world in the hands of midwife Lucille Sykes over the past fourteen years—most of them born to Amish parents in Ohio and Pennsylvania. So when Pennsylvania's Mercer County brought charges against Sykes for practicing without a license, hundreds of normally publicity-shy Amish crowded into the county magistrate's office for the hearing (right), at which the charges against the forty-nine-year-old Sykes were dropped because of ambiguous language in the state's Medical Act. Sykes, a member of the Midwives Association of North America, apprenticed as a midwife for a year and a half before setting out on her own, and plays down criticism of her lack of formal medical training. "Pregnancy is not an illness," she says. "There are women with high-risk pregnancies that have no business using a midwife, but for a healthy mother with a good diet, there should be no problem."

Most Amish women prefer to give birth at home or in a home-like

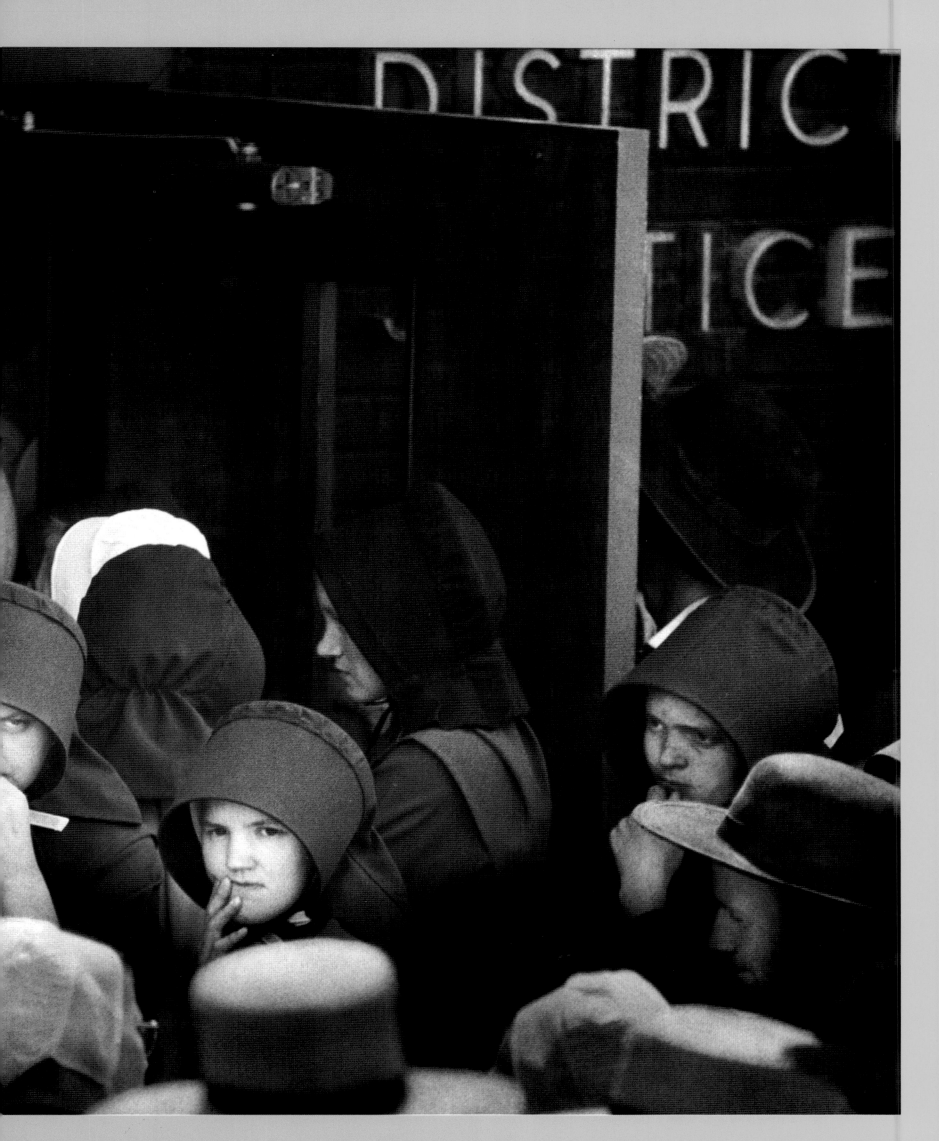

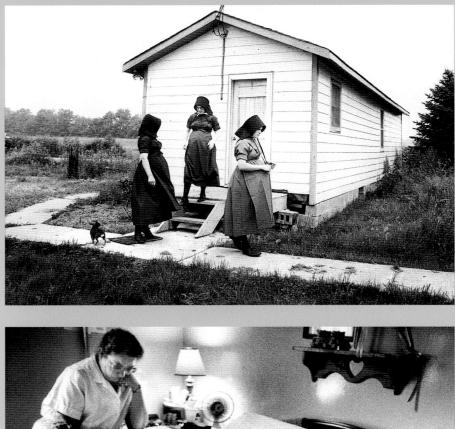

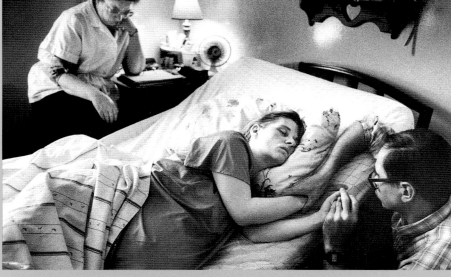

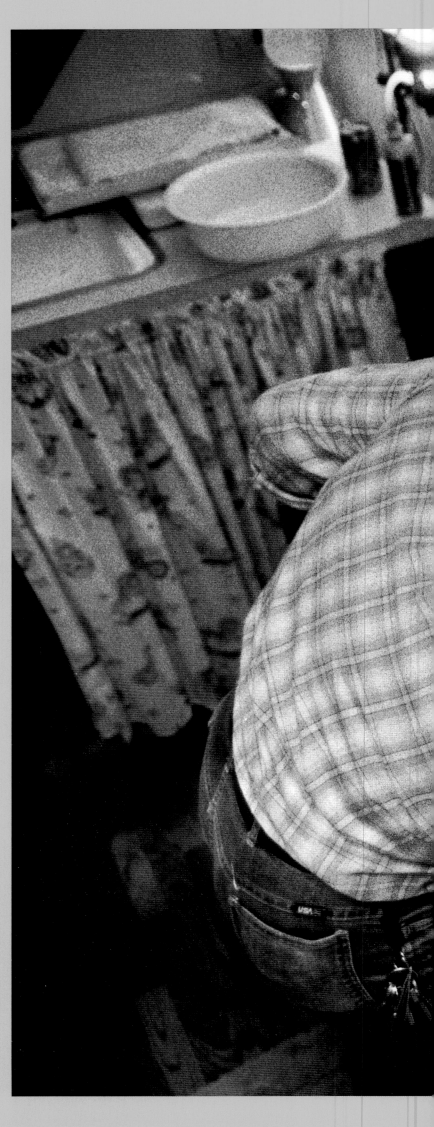

atmosphere, making Sykes's Cradle Time Birthing Center (above top) a popular spot. Sykes, whose standard fee is $600, insists that the mothers-to-be see a doctor for prenatal checkups and does not hesitate to call paramedics if any trouble arises. "I'm not afraid to have a doctor help out," she says. "I don't know everything. But doctors don't either."

Sykes watches as the Reverend James Brewer, the pastor of Sykes's own Cooperstown Evangelistic Tabernacle Church, comforts his laboring wife, Lolly (above). With the help of her daughter Cyndee (right), Sykes delivers Valerie Michelle Brewer—the fourth child and first girl for James and Lolly. "I'd recommend using a midwife to anyone," says Lolly. "I had hospital births and because of the

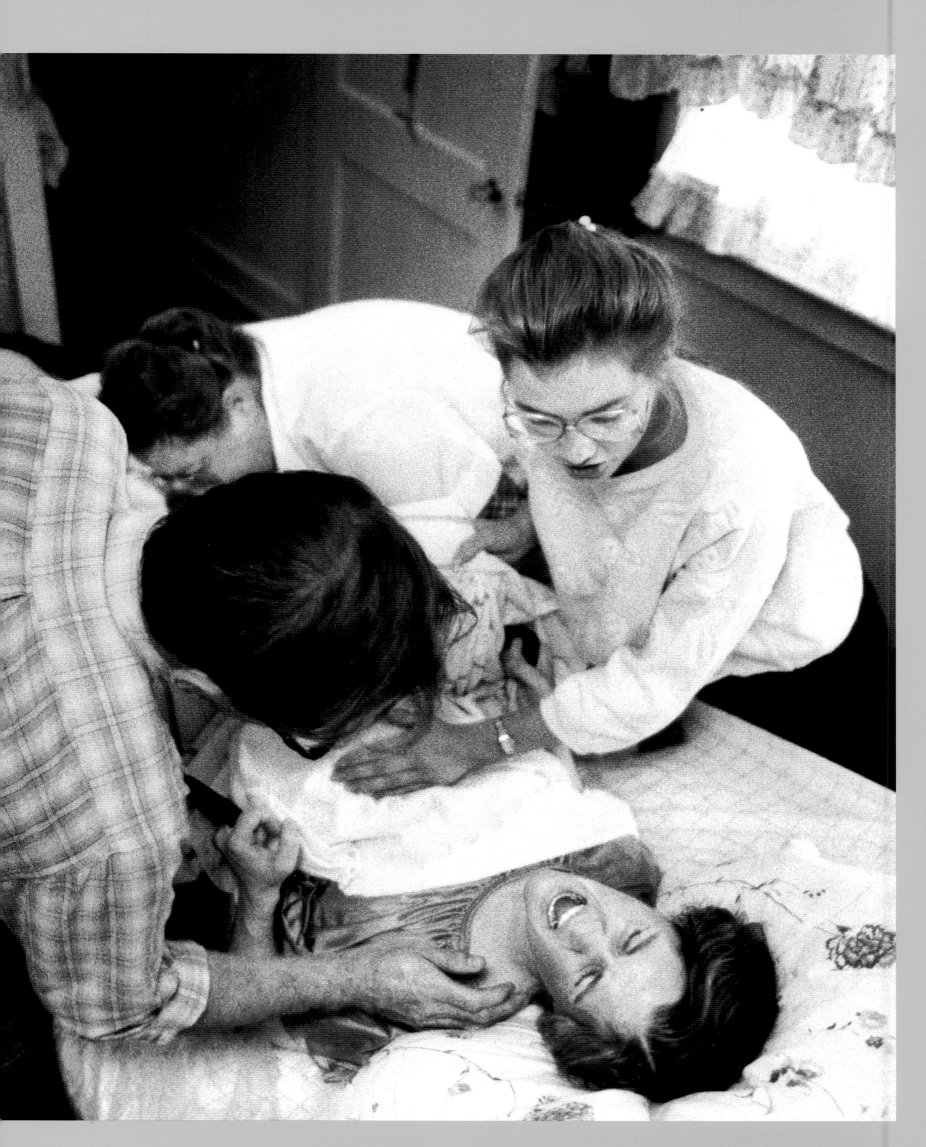

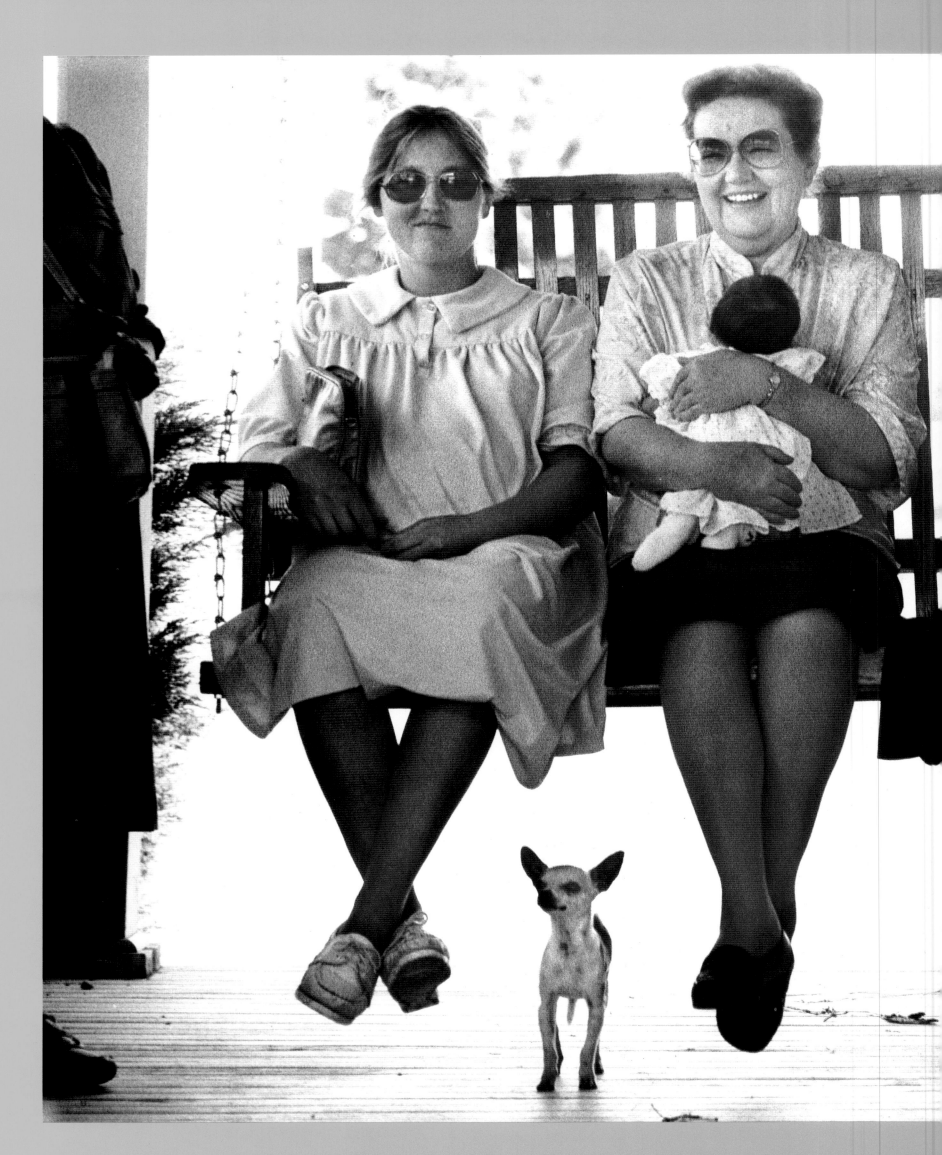

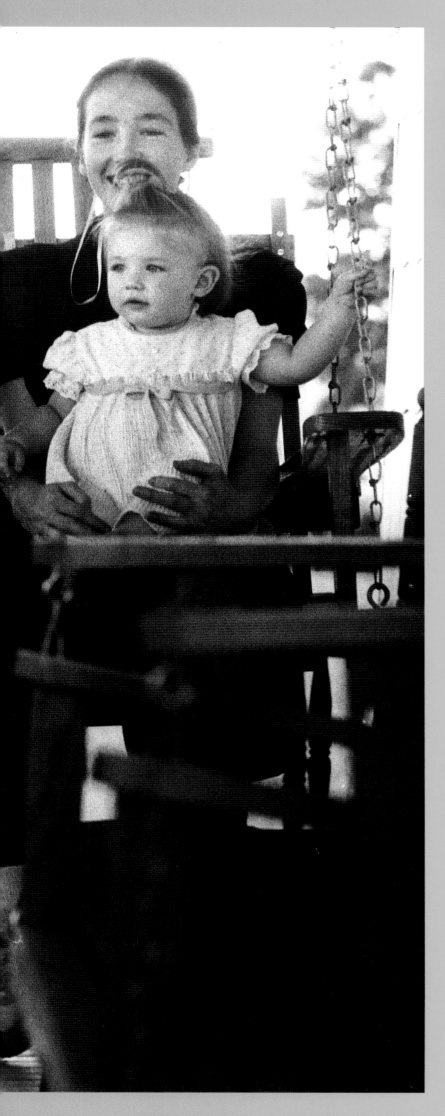

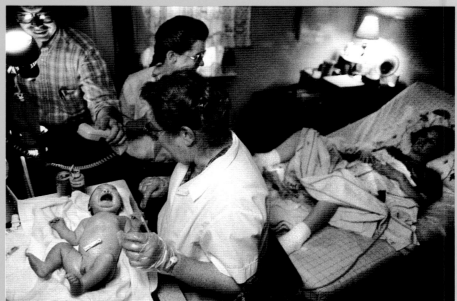

drugs I couldn't understand the doctors and nurses. This time I was very aware of everything that was going on."

After the birth, Sykes weighs the newborn as James Brewer holds the phone so that Lolly's mother, in Apache Junction, Arizona, can hear her new granddaughter cry (above). Sykes, who is one of about 3,000 lay midwives practicing in North America, often stays in close touch with the families she serves, and relaxes (left) by holding a baby she recently delivered. During the two months between her initial arrest and the charges against her being dropped, Sykes says, "My arms ached to hold a baby again."

Photos by Randy Olson

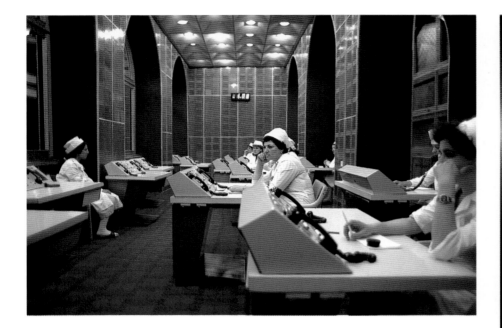

▲ It's a slow night for these Soviet ambulance dispatchers in Baku, the capital of the southwestern republic of Azerbaijan. Dispatchers are on duty aroundthe-clock in this oil-rich port city of 1.7 million people and, as in the United States, they can be reached by dialing a simple emergency number.
Photo by George Steinmetz

▶ Medics rush a patient across the rooftop heliport of the Maryland Institute for Emergency Medical Services System's Shock Trauma Center in Baltimore. Nearly sixty percent of the 3,500 patients received here annually arrive by medical evacuation helicopters, which are capable of carrying two critically injured patients at a time and are equipped with monitors, a ventilator, a hoist mechanism, and intravenous pumps. The copters can travel up to 520 miles, and a special on-board infrared system for detecting body heat helps medics locate injured accident victims in water or in hard-to-see wooded areas. Remarkably, more than ninety percent of the patients brought here survive; twenty-five years ago, only about one in ten lived.
Photo by Michael J. Bryant

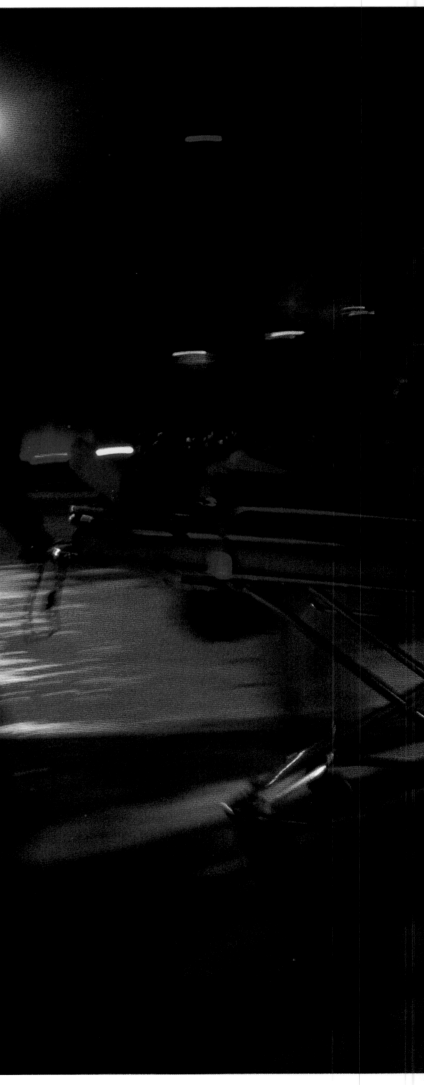

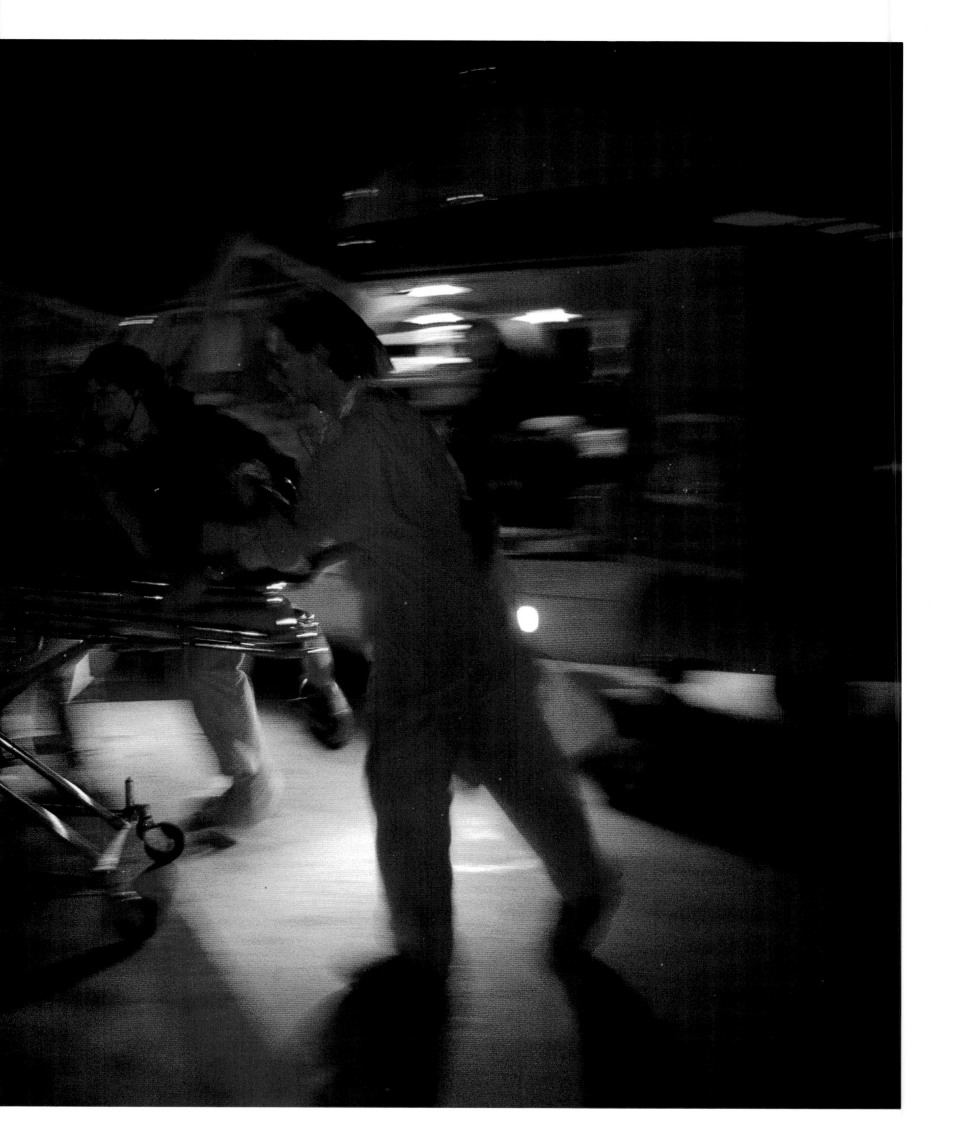

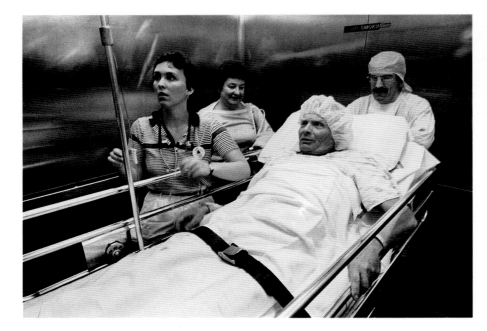

▲ After seven months of agonizing waiting, it's time to hurry for heart patient Bob Shaw. The fifty-two-year-old man's doctors at Stanford University Hospital in California have just learned that a heart suitable for transplantation has become available, and "timing is key," says transplant surgeon William Frist. Most adult hearts will last about four hours after being taken from the donor and before they begin pumping in the recipient's chest. Shaw was one of the more than eighty percent of heart transplant patients at Stanford to live at least a year with a new heart.
Photo by Sam Forencich

▶ As precious minutes tick away in the world's largest shock trauma center, Dr. David Gens, center, reviews a computerized axial tomograph, or CAT scan, of a patient's head. Gens, one of the team of doctors who worked on then-President Reagan after he was shot in 1981, says his job at the Maryland Institute for Emergency Medical Service System's Shock Trauma Center "gives me a kind of instant gratification." The forty-five-year-old Gens plans to keep up his current pace of sixty-five-hour weeks for another ten years, but he says a policy change by the automotive industry would change his life. "About seventy percent of the cases we see here involve cars or motorcycles," he points out. "If there were air bags in every car, I'd be out of work."
Photo by Michael J. Bryant

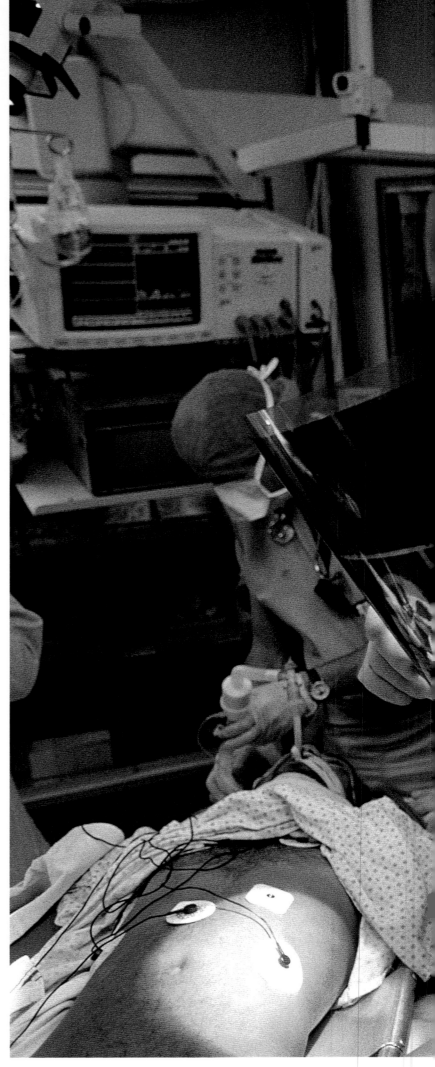

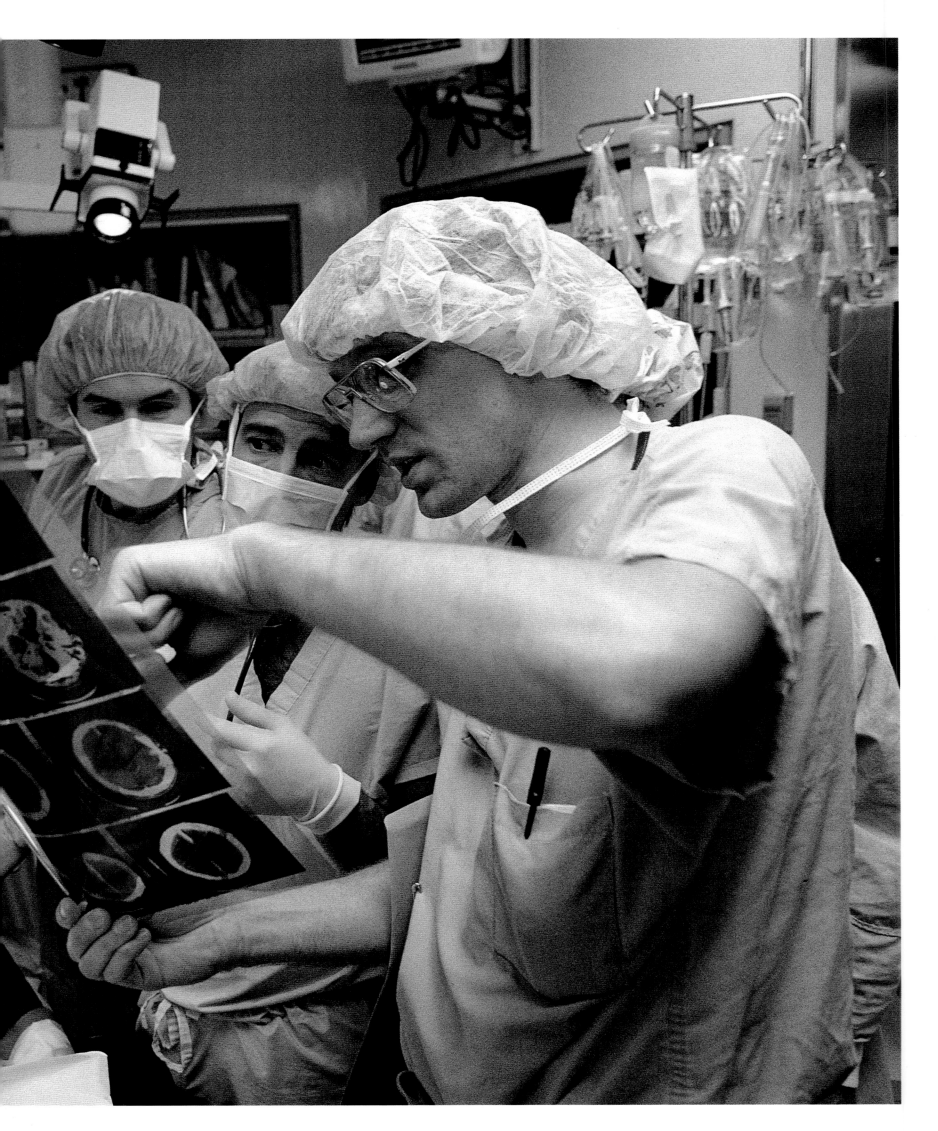

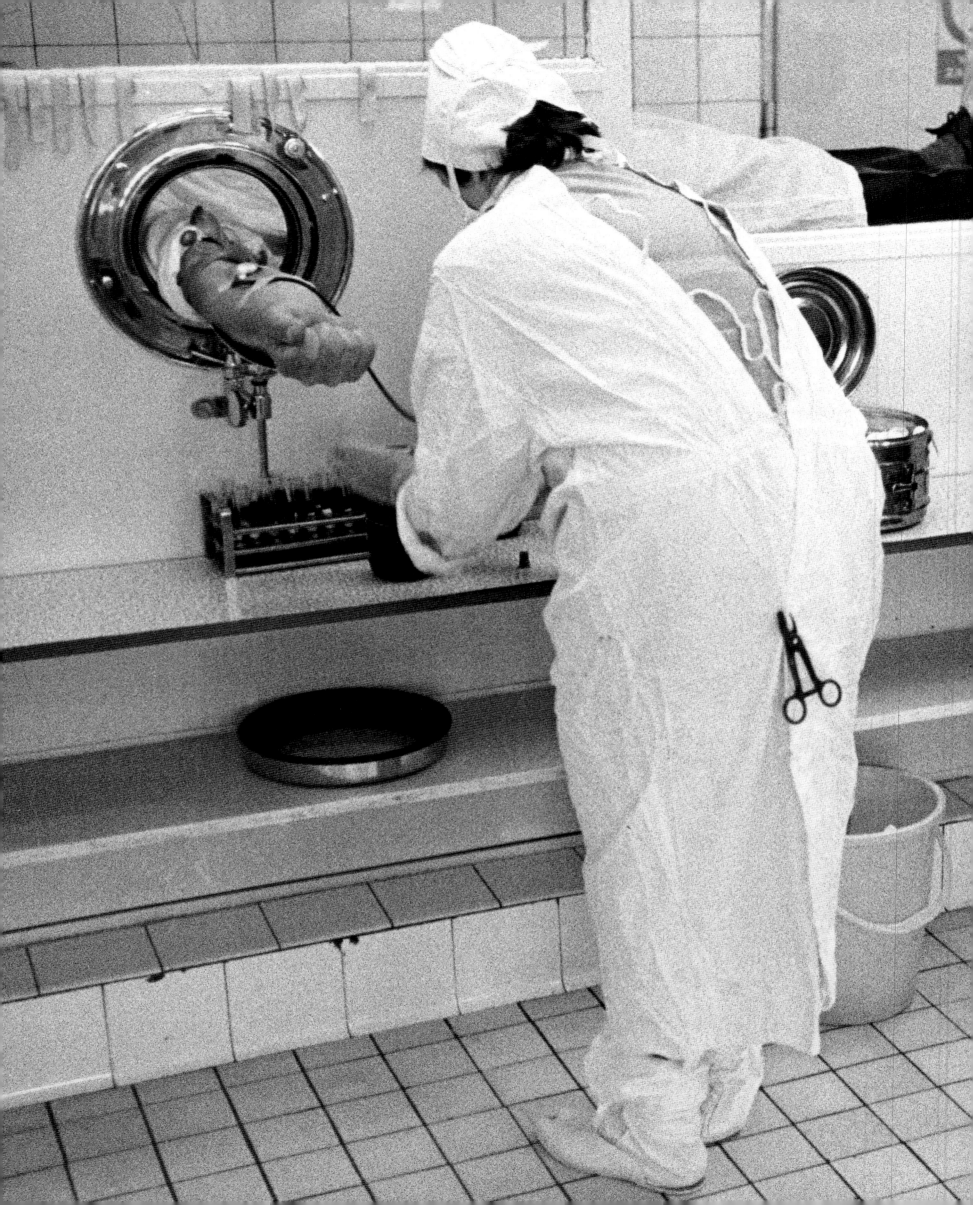

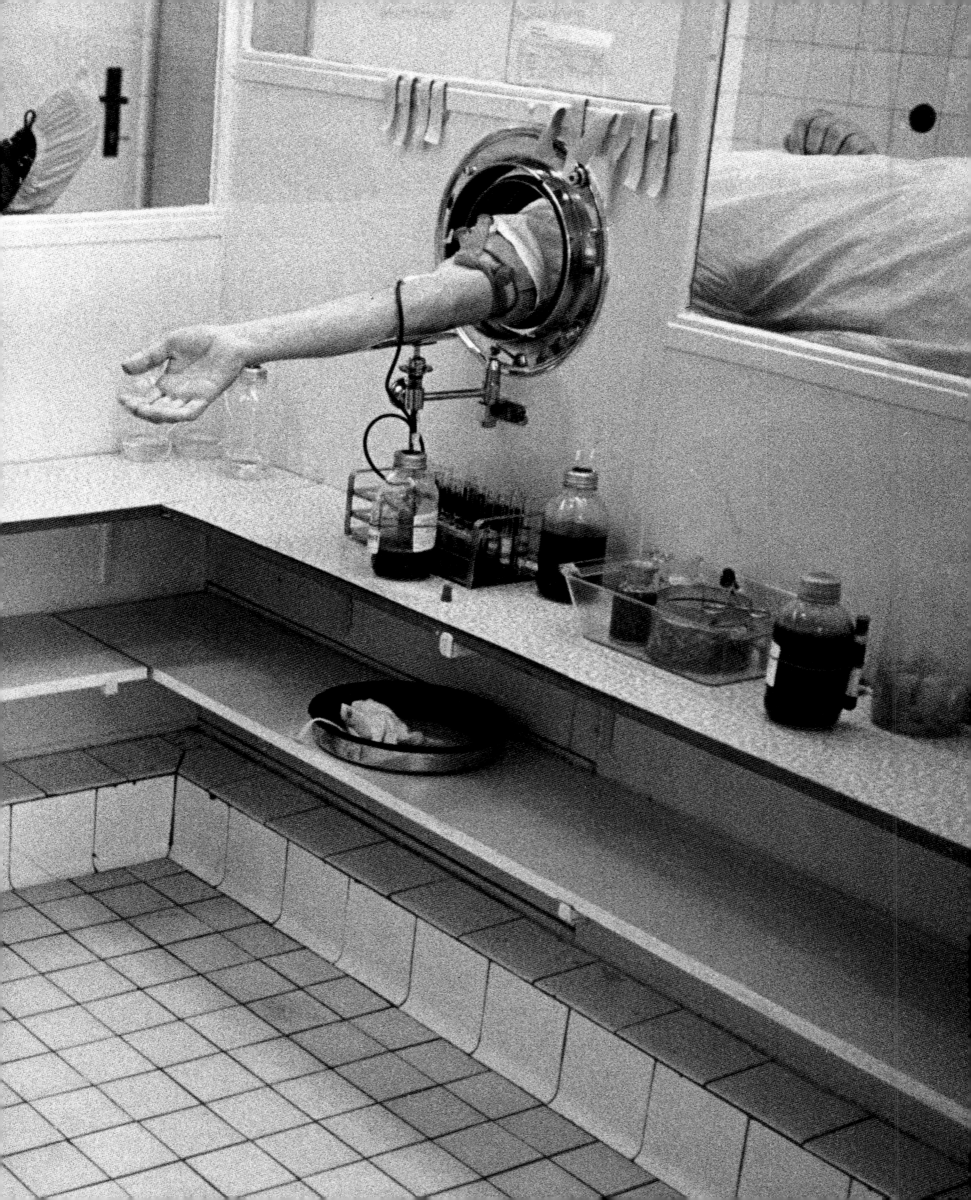

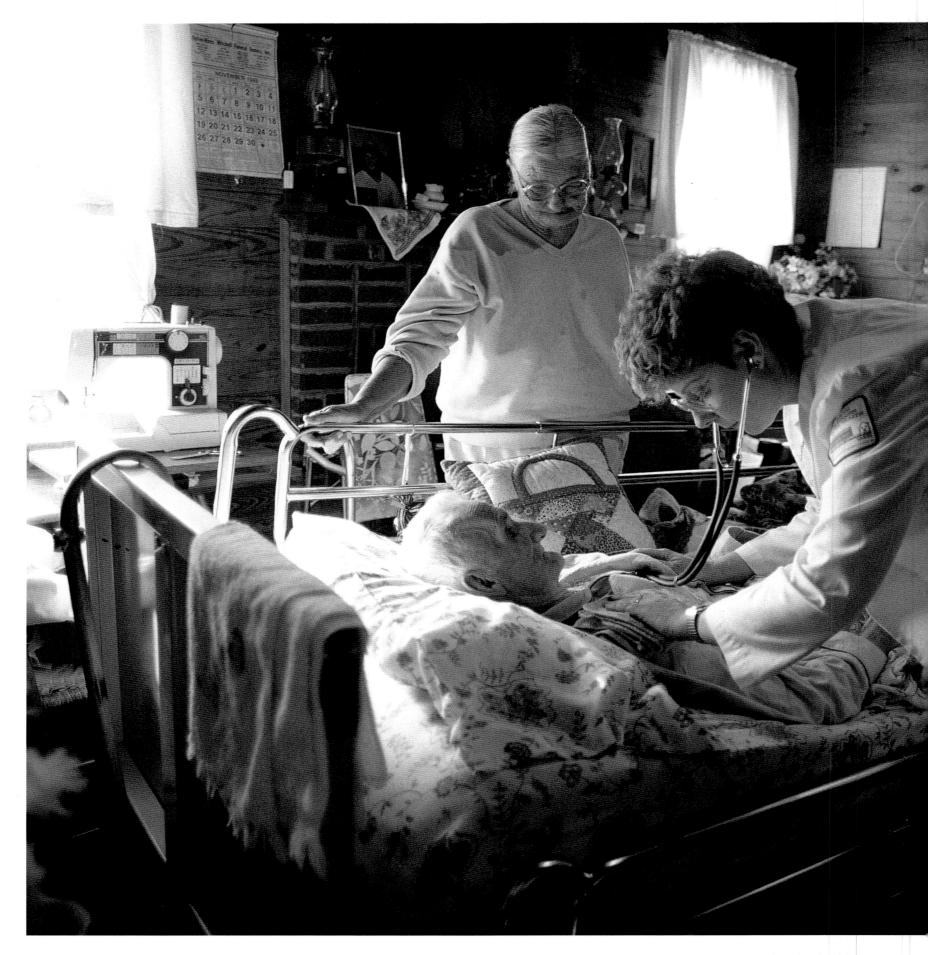

◄ **A nurse monitors two blood donors at a hospital in Czechoslovakia.** Unlike in nearby Romania, where transfusions with infected blood have resulted in a large number of AIDS babies, hospitals here screen blood donors for the AIDS-causing HIV virus.
Photo by Karel Sláma

▲ **Home is where the heart is** for Mississippi nurse Maureen Raubert, who puts about 100 miles a day on her compact car visiting patients. "I love it," says Raubert, here with Boyd McCallum and his wife, Gladys. "I treat patients in their own environment, and they get very attached to me." Raubert is one of nearly 200 nurses who work for South Mississippi Home Health, a private agency credited with pioneering organized home-health services in the late 1960s. The days of house calls may seem like the stuff of nostalgia, but health care providers now say that home visits by trained health professionals could play an important role in cutting health care costs in the years to come.
Photo by Andy Levin

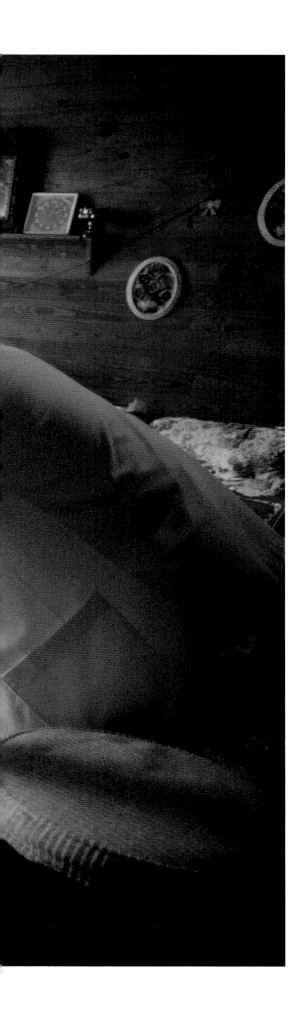

The Women
Who Heal

BARBARA EHRENREICH, PH.D.

WOMEN HAVE ALWAYS BEEN HEALERS, AND IN TRADITIONAL CULTURES, women are often the principal healers—the first resort against illness or disease. The Latin American *curanderas*, the "wise women" of the old French countryside, and the midwives who delivered many American babies until well into the twentieth century all represent the ancient tradition of female lay healing. Even in modern societies, mothers are expected to be alert for signs of illness, to nurse the sick, and to monitor the health needs of their families.

Traditional female healing was markedly different, in spirit and approach, from the professional medicine that has by and large replaced it. Female lay healers were not formally trained; they learned their skills from other women, often their mothers or grandmothers. Nor did they undertake healing as a "career" in the modern sense; more commonly, they saw it as a community responsibility, even a divine calling. The African-American lay midwives who until recent times served the rural South, for example, report that they took up their vocation in response to a call from God. The responsibilities of the midwife in colonial and nineteenth-century America went far beyond delivering babies. She often remained with the family for a week or two after the birth, helping to run the household until the mother regained her strength. Payment might be in kind—a couple of chickens or whatever the family could afford.

Through their role as healers, women have often gained respect and authority in their communities. Balm healers in Jamaica are also spiritual leaders, and demand high standards of moral behavior from their clients. Women in modern Benin can win status as members of spiritualist healing cults, the sambani cults. In American history, healing skills often went hand in hand with other forms of leadership and achievement. Anne Hutchinson, the dissident religious leader who was banished from the Massachusetts Bay Colony as a heretic in 1637, first gained a following through her successful practice as a midwife. Harriet Tubman, the African-American leader who led hundreds of slaves to freedom on the Underground Railroad, was known for her healing skills as "Dr. Tubman."

Women have also been feared and repressed for their power as healers. Female healers were prime targets of the witch-hunts that swept northern Europe in the fifteenth and sixteenth centuries and may have resulted in the deaths of more than a million people, most of them women. The *Malleus*

Maleficarum, which served as the Church's official guide to witch-hunting until late in the eighteenth century, singled out female healers, especially midwives, for persecution.

Throughout most of the world, the tradition of female lay healing has been eclipsed more peaceably with the rise of modern, scientific medicine. The transition to modern medicine did not, however, always bring an immediate improvement in care. In the United States, for example, midwifery was outlawed in the early twentieth century—a time when midwives in some cases were achieving lower rates of maternal mortality than the physicians who replaced them.

In the United States, women suffered a double setback with the rise of the emergent, scientifically based medical profession: not only was midwifery outlawed, but the medical profession itself was conceived by its members as a distinctly masculine vocation. Nineteenth-century American doctors campaigned against the admission of women to medical schools, and theorized that women's intellects were too small—and their bodies too delicate—for the rigors of medicine. Women who did gain admission to medical school often faced harassment from students and hostility from professors, who would refuse, for example, to teach anatomy to female students. Most women were steered toward less autonomous—and less lucrative—roles as nurses. As recently as 1970, fewer than ten percent of American doctors were female.

In the last two decades, however, American women have been reclaiming their traditional role as healers. Young women, inspired in part by the feminist movement, have been entering school in force, so that today almost forty percent of American medical students are female. The nursing profession has been demanding expanded roles and greater autonomy. And midwifery, that traditional stronghold of female lay healing, has undergone a striking revival.

The women who are entering health professions today may have a larger healing role to play. For all its advantages over any pre-technological approach to healing, modern medicine has lost much of the traditional healer's sense of spiritual commitment and community responsibility. In the tradition of "Dr. Tubman," who helped awaken the soul of an entire nation, today's women healers may help revive the soul of modern medicine.

▶ **"Once I had someone's life in my hands,"** says Dr. Ellen Mahony, left, who started her career in health as a physical therapist, "I knew surgery was for me. It's a dance. You move quickly, constantly. When you put your hand out and the instrument hits it, there's a distinct smack. When you put your glove on, there's a snap. When you're with someone you work well with, everything flows.

"I hate to hear someone refer to a 'routine' operation," she adds. "Nothing is routine. No two problems are ever the same."
Photo by Stephen Shames

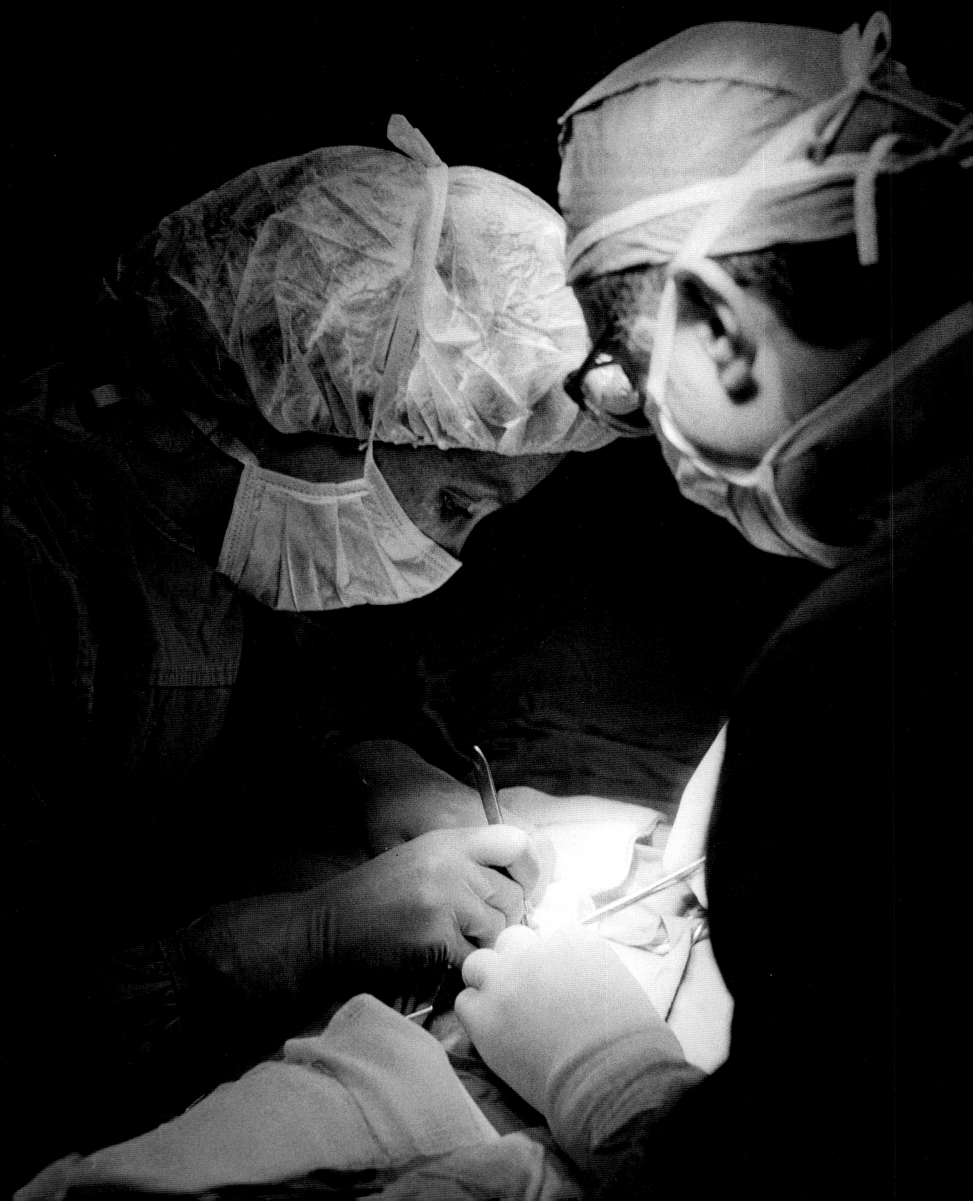

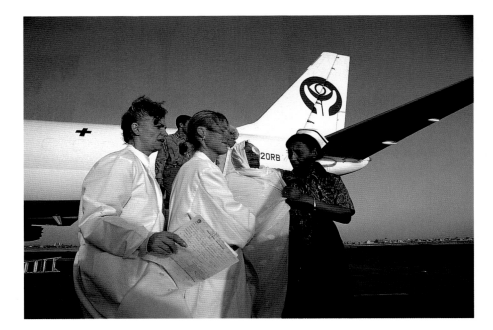

▲ **The world's only flying teaching hospital** unloads its cargo of doctors and nurses in Khartoum, the capital of Sudan. The converted DC-8 jet of New York-based Project Orbis includes an examination and laser treatment area, an operating room, a recovery room, an audiovisual television studio, a classroom, and a library. The plane spends about ninety percent of its time in developing nations, where ophthalmologists teach their local colleagues the latest surgical procedures, and donate medical supplies and educational materials.
Photo by Peter S. Greenberg

▶ **Working in their jet, members of an Orbis mission restore the gift of sight** as part of a three-day stop in Varna, Bulgaria. Orbis doctors and nurses have carried out more than ninety missions in fifty-five countries since the first flight in 1982, with the administrative staff raising the multi-million-dollar operating budget from various international agencies and private sponsors. According to Project Orbis statistics, about two-thirds of the forty-six million cases of blindness worldwide could be surgically treated or prevented.
Photo by Peter Freed

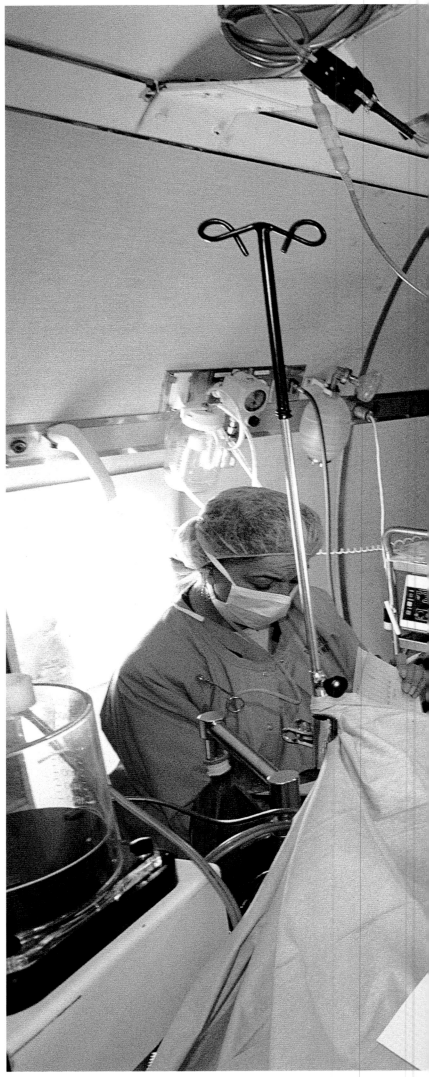

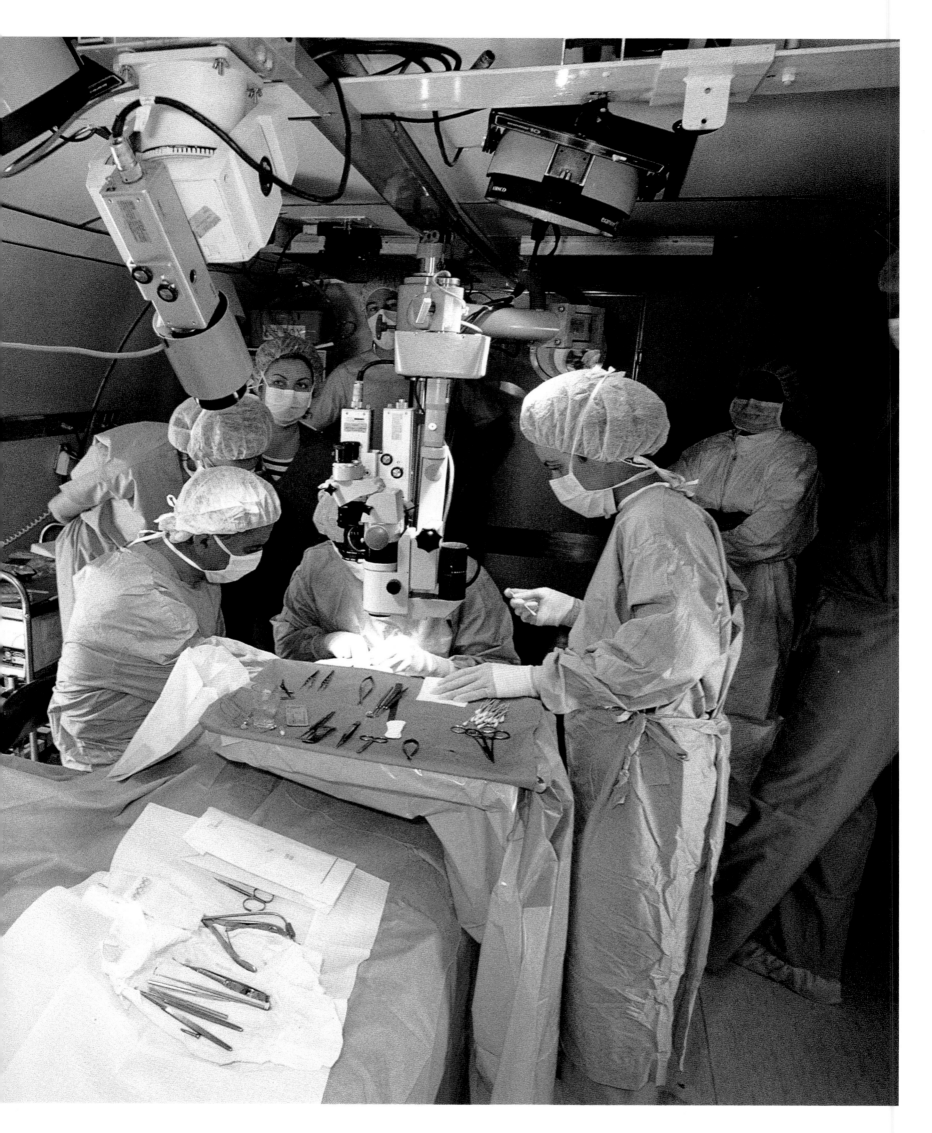

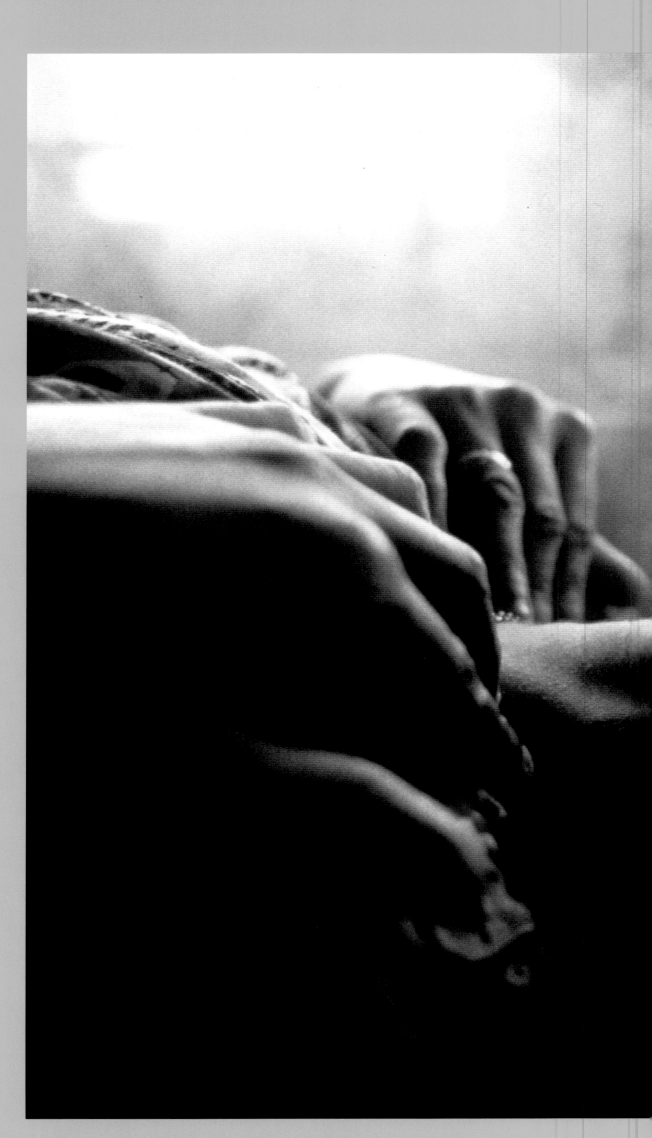

Touch starts as a reflex, an instinct, a healing language that we all understand. We learn this language as early as any other, and it is the source of many of our earliest sensations.

Study after study tells us that babies crave human touch, and common sense tells us that the need continues throughout our lives. In the world of healing, perhaps the highest praise we can give our doctor is to say that he or she has "a human touch."

The power of touch is one of the oldest of the healing arts, although what we now call massage was known for centuries as medical rubbing. For patients at the Ayurvedic Institute in New Delhi (right), the power of touch means hands working everywhere on the body, finding the aura, moving it, and freeing it. The 6,000-year-old tradition of ayurvedic (literally, "the science of life") medicine is practiced by more than 350,000 physicians in India, and includes a regimen of meditation, massage, yoga, and herb preparations, combined with diet and sleep modification.

Specialists aren't the only ones to heal through touch, of course; the beauty of the power of touch is

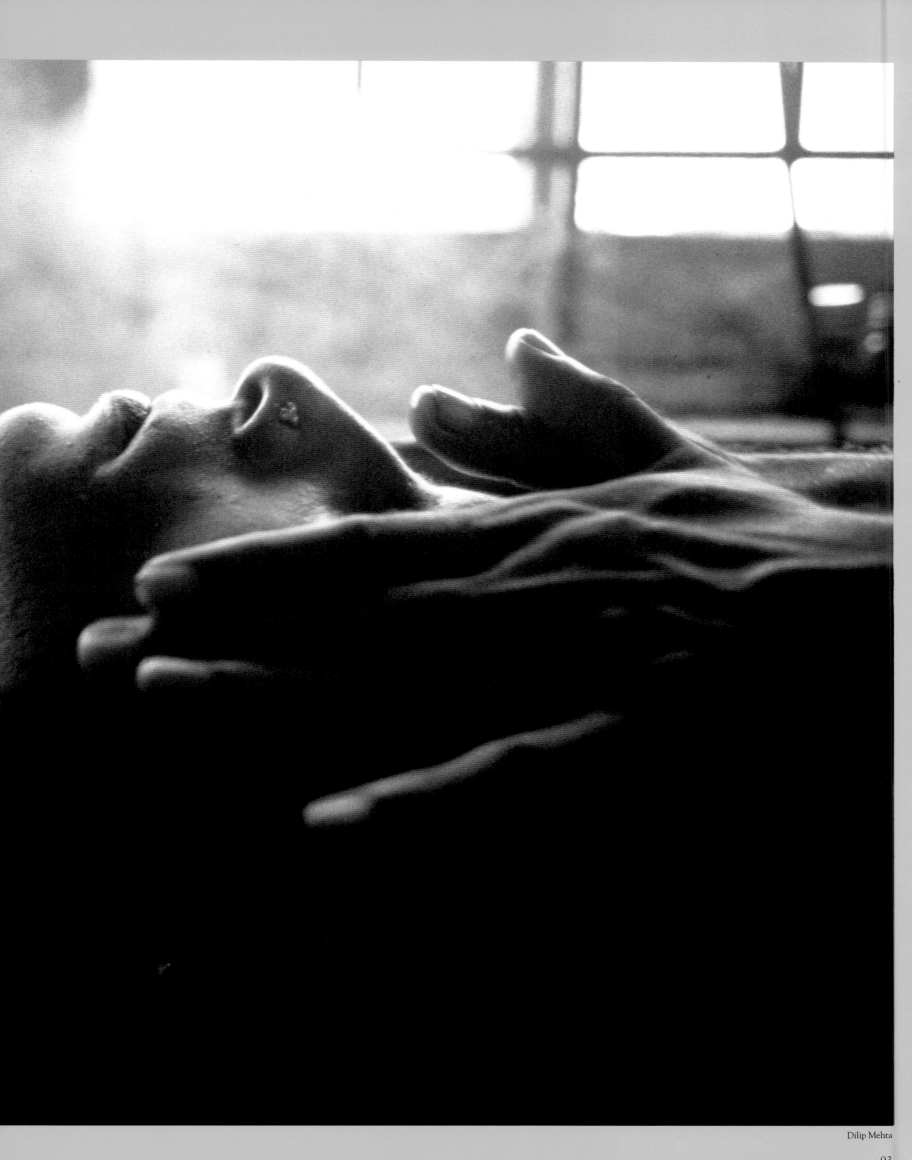

Dilip Mehta

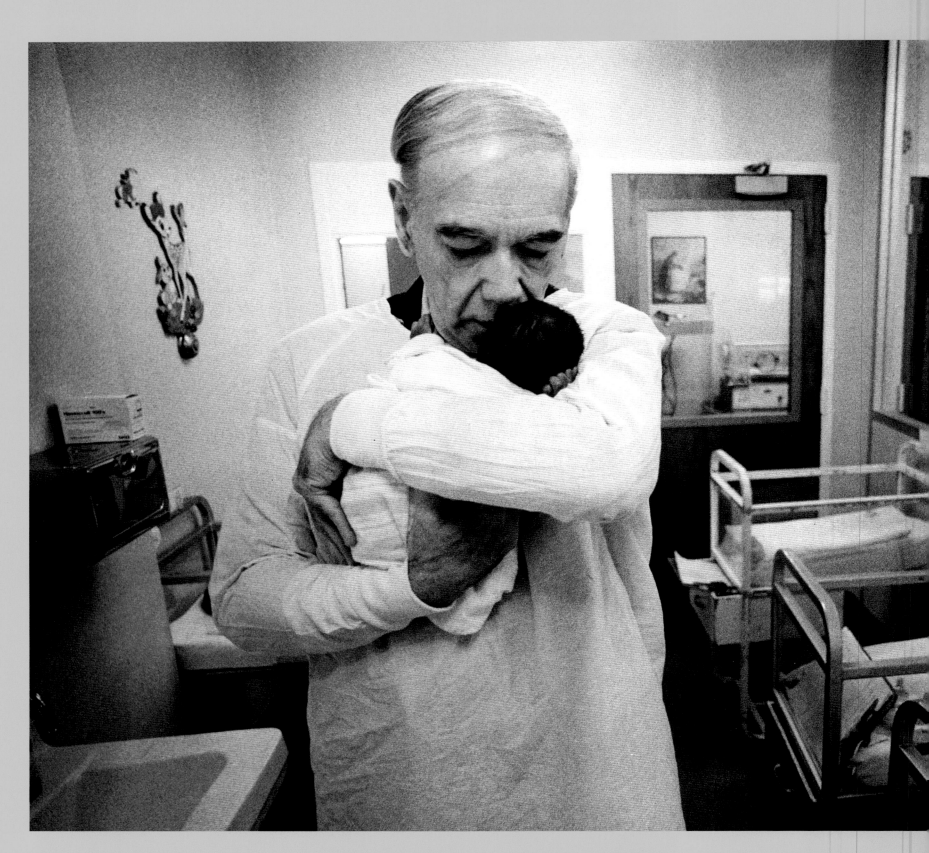

that it requires no special training. "I get a feeling of giving something to the most vulnerable people in the world," says writer Bill Gale (above), who visits St. Luke's Hospital in New York City eight hours a week to care for newborns. Gale is one of a growing number of volunteer "baby holders" in American hospitals; most of the babies he cuddles are "crack babies," born to mothers addicted to crack cocaine. Stark evidence of an infant's need to be held was supplied at American foundling institutions earlier in this century, when orphans sometimes died of a condition called "failure to thrive" syndrome. The number of such deaths dropped when attendants began holding the infants more regularly.

Animal touch, too, can be part of human healing. At Oakland Children's Hospital in California, seven-year-old Andy Davis (above right), who suffered a severe spinal cord injury in a 1988 car accident, is visited by animals who come to the hospital once a month as part of the regular rounds of the Friendship Foundation, which takes animals to hospitals, nursing homes, mental institutions, and day care facilities. "Whenever I have a choice between physical therapy and the animals," says Andy, "I choose the animals."

Contact with animals is even more important for autistic teenager Jackie Stephens (right). Jackie comes regularly to Dolphins Plus in Key Largo, Florida, where dolphin handler Bobby Easom works with him to break down his aversion to touch and increase his spontaneous behavior. Says anthropologist Betsy Smith, who

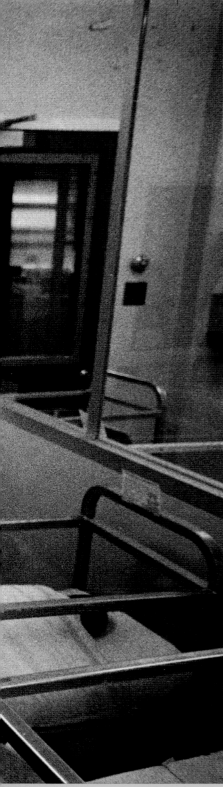

James McGoon

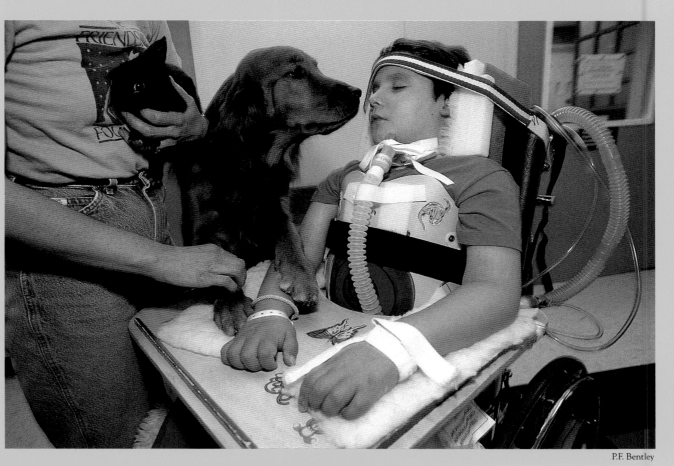

P.F. Bentley

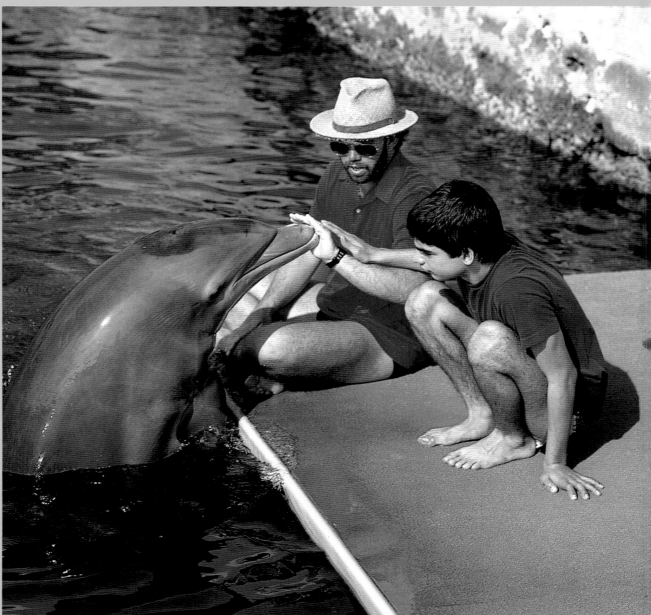

Randy Olson

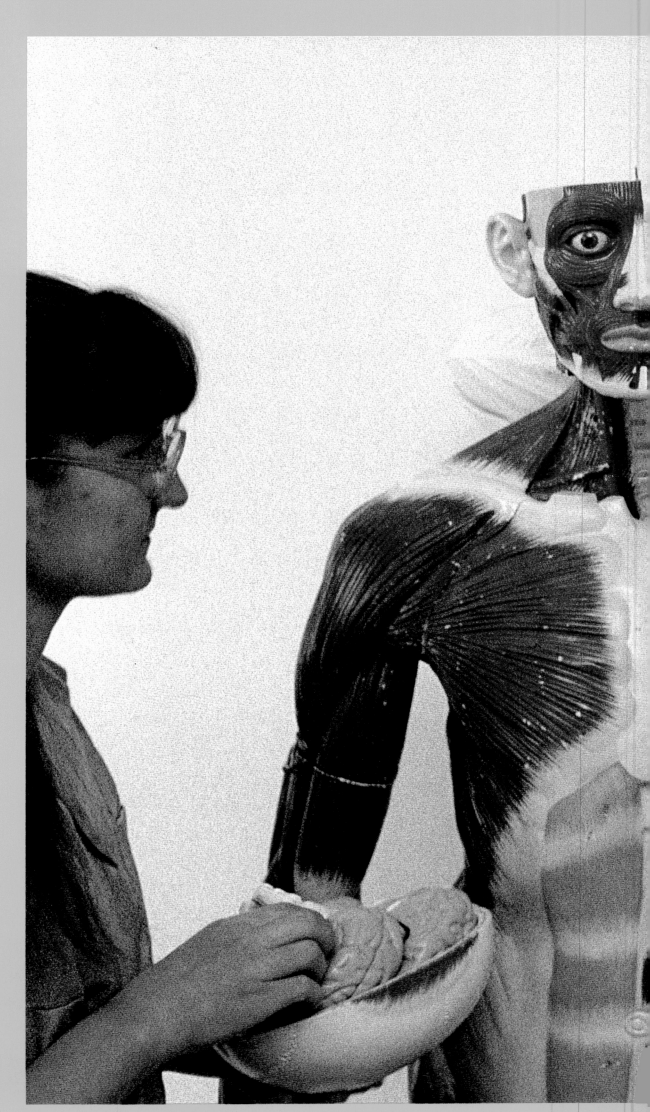

started the dolphin-assisted therapy program here in 1979, "Jackie wouldn't even touch people when he came here three months ago, so we started him stroking and touching the dolphin. Through this initial touch, we try to open his universe, to bring out the inner spontaneity that makes him an individual and that's locked up in there." Now, she says, Jackie will touch people, although he remains absorbed, for the most part, in the mysterious inner world of autism. The dolphins sense his pain, says Smith: "They don't test him right away like they would you or me. They want to bond but they're very patient."

Touch can become more acute when one of the other senses is missing. Throughout history, and in every corner of the globe, many masters of medical rubbing have been blind, their sense of touch enhanced by their lack of sight. Here, two young Poles study the art of massage by learning human muscle structure and pressure points at the Institute for the Blind outside Warsaw.

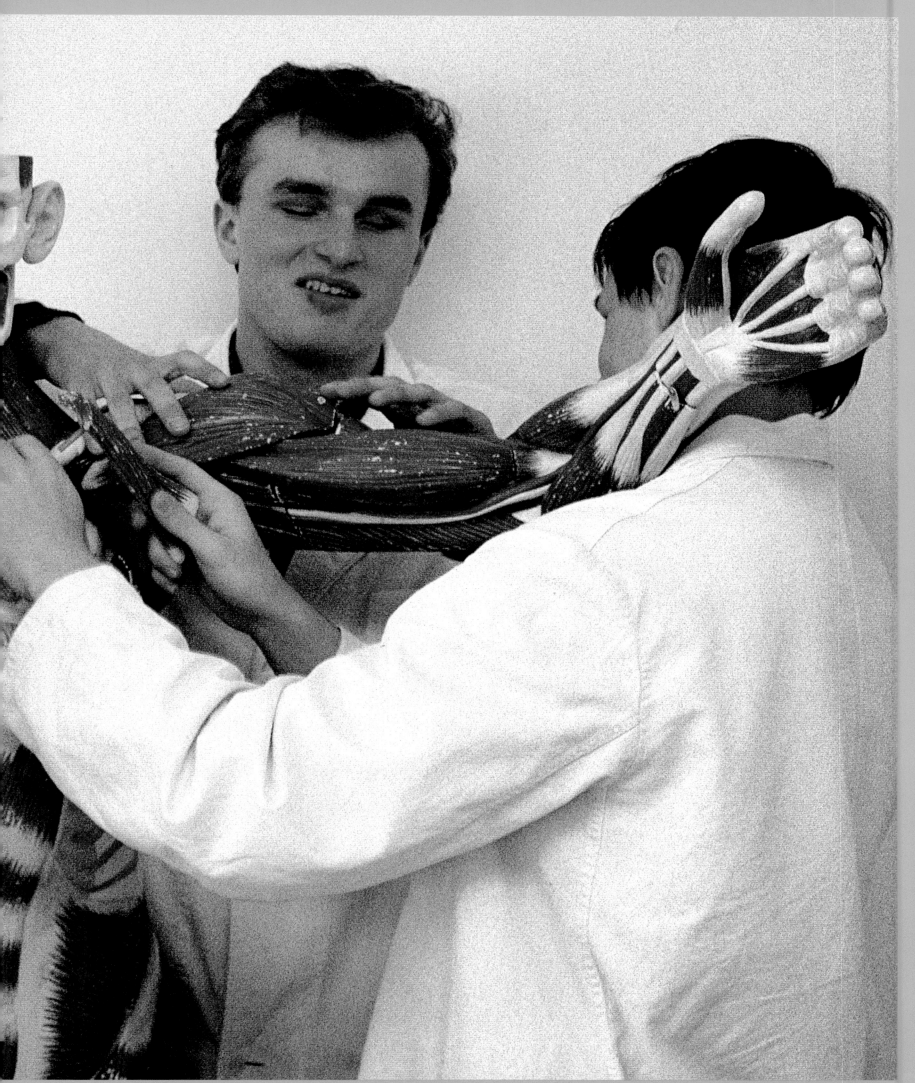

Pregnant women exercise in the pool at the University of North Carolina in Chapel Hill. *Photo by Annie Griffiths Belt*

THE PULSE OF LIFE

Despite all the hard scientific knowledge we have accumulated, the heart still retains its mythic, metaphoric role as the bodily center of courage and love.... A living heart "is...the pulsing energy that is the essence of all life, whether atoms and electrons or two people making love or the whole universe expanding and contracting. It's the vital force. It's life itself."
—George Leonard

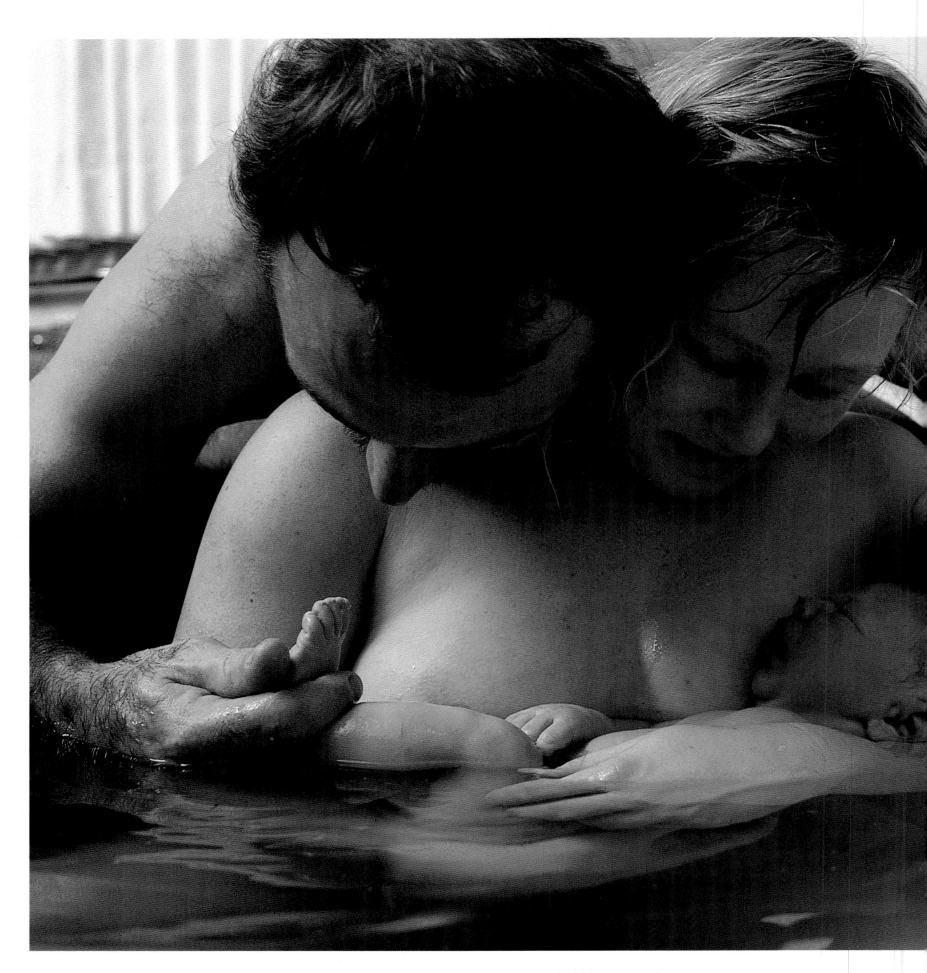

▲ **Minutes after being born underwater** at a southern California birthing center, Jeremy David Cox greets his parents, Terrie and Dave. Terrie gave birth to Jeremy squatting in a huge tub of warm water, with Dave's arms around her. Although many of the nearly 600 babies born underwater at the Family Birthing Center of Upland stay submerged for up to two minutes after birth, according to attending physician Michael Rosenthal, the umbilical cord remains attached so "there's no cause for concern about the baby drowning." Many doctors are critical of the practice of underwater births, but none of the major medical associations have taken a position against it. Says Terrie, "This was so much more comfortable than giving birth in the hospital."
Photo by Dana Fineman

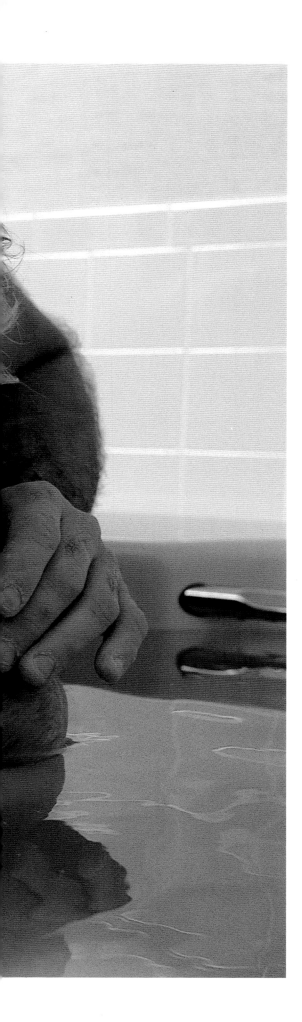

The Heart That
Never Rests

GEORGE LEONARD

It is the toughest inhabitant of the body, and the most tremulous, the furnace of animal passion and the seat of the most exquisite sensibilities. It is a dauntless pump that sustains life on a moment by moment basis, and a delicately poised seismograph that responds to every fleeting change of mood, every unexpected sound, sight, smell, or touch; quick to take offense or alarm yet capable of profound composure. What we have shaped in our innocence as a valentine candy, a jewel, a piece of soap, is actually a slimy, throbbing mass of muscle entwined in its own veins and arteries, a tender, fearsome instrument of love and power—the heart!

In traditional and esoteric thought, this organ is most often associated with heat, fire, courage, passion, empathy. The Chinese system of the five elements—wood, fire, earth, metal, and water—gives fire to the heart and holds that it rather than the brain is the center of feeling and thought. In the kundalini yoga of India, the heart center, or fourth chakra, expresses love, devotion, and compassion for others. Astrology links the heart with the sun sign Leo: the flaming golden lion of courage, generosity, and love. The sixteenth-century Swiss alchemist and physician, Paracelsus, saw the heart as the "sun in the Microcosm"—the fiery center of the body, the seat of the imagination, the dwelling place of the soul.

For the Indians of North and South America, the vital powers of a warrior resided in the chest and heart. To embody the will, strength, and courage of a particular animal or human, the warriors of some tribes would eat the heart of a bear, sometimes of a valiant enemy. But the heart in primitive culture also expressed good will and caring love, and shamans throughout the world knew that to gain the power of vision and healing they would have to "see with the heart" as well as the mind.

More than 2,000 years ago, the Chinese figured out that the heart is a pump sending blood on a round-trip through the maze of vessels in the body. Physicians and anatomists of the West, through the time of the Renaissance, clung to an ancient Greek misconception. Aristotle taught that blood was elaborated from the food in the liver, sent from there to the heart, then dispersed through the veins over the body. The Greeks believed that the arteries (the word means "air pipe") functioned mainly to carry a subtle kind of air or spirit. Though that theory was revised somewhat over the centuries, it was not until 1628, when Charles I's court physician, William Harvey, published

and contracting. It's the vital force. It's life itself."

And also death. Heart disease, with nearly 800,000 casualties a year, is far and away the leading cause of death in America. Most of the deaths come as a result of atherosclerosis, a narrowing or obstruction of the coronary arteries that provide the heart itself with blood, caused by deposits of fatty plaque inside the arteries. This carnage is strictly a twentieth-century phenomenon; surprisingly, there was very little heart disease in America before 1900. The greatest rise occurred between 1940 and 1967.

What has caused this modern plague? Some factors are easy to specify: the increased consumption of cigarettes and rich, fatty food; the reduction of everyday physical exercise due to automation and the automobile; the resulting increase in obesity. Other factors are harder to measure but hold perhaps a deeper significance: we have weakened or entirely broken our connection with family and community, separated ourselves from nature, become a nation of consumers. Our gains in prosperity and convenience have been paid for by a dangerous rise in alienation, stress, and cynicism, which have been shown to release just the kinds of hormones into the blood that damage the coronary arteries.

The good news is that since 1967, a watershed year for lifestyle changes, the rate of heart disease in America has declined significantly. Exercise enthusiasts attribute this to the fitness boom. Dieticians point to a growing awareness of good nutrition. Cigarette smoking, no question, is down. And medical experts proudly cite advances in emergency heart care and new corrective procedures such as bypass surgery.

Still, the noble organ now beating tirelessly in the chests of all who read these pages has the last word. The heart holds within it the power of life and death, and can be neither deceived nor cajoled. Drugs and technology, no matter how effective in repairing damaged hearts, can't stop the plague that caused the damage in the first place. Ultimately, the remedy lies not in our machines, but in our behavior and our values. It might not be easy, but it's simple. To heal the heart, we must change the way we live.

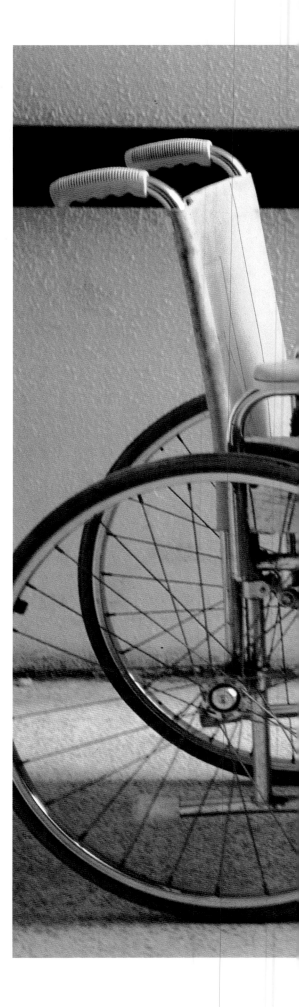

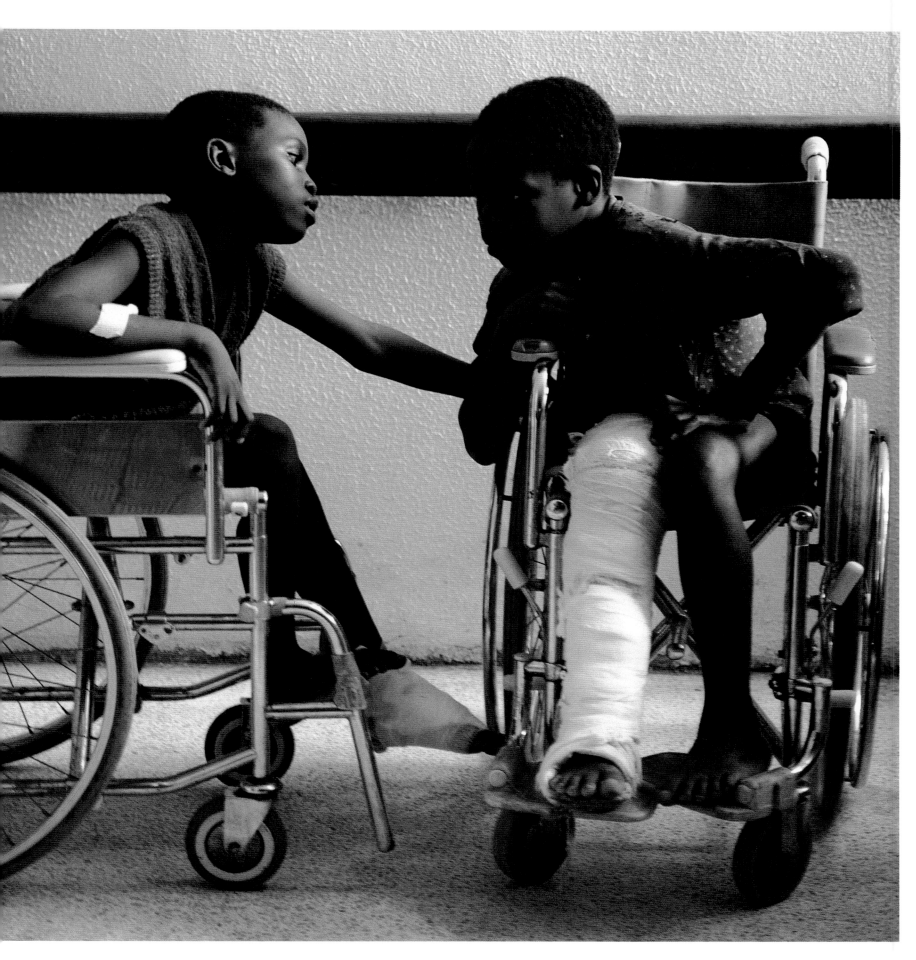

▲ **A word of solace is passed**
between broken-bone sufferers
in Mozambique's largest hospital,
the Hospital Central in Maputo.
Photo by Larry C. Price

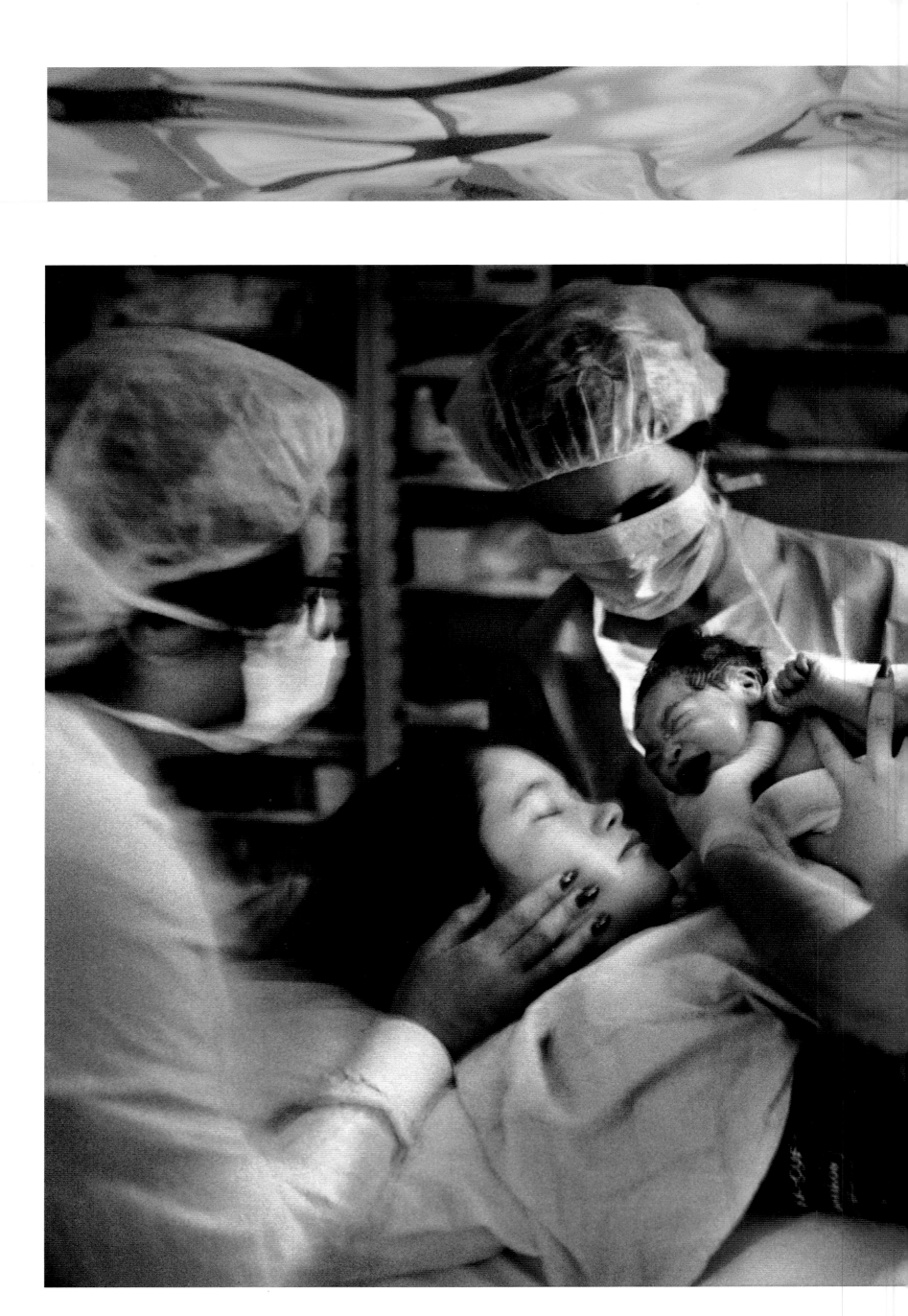

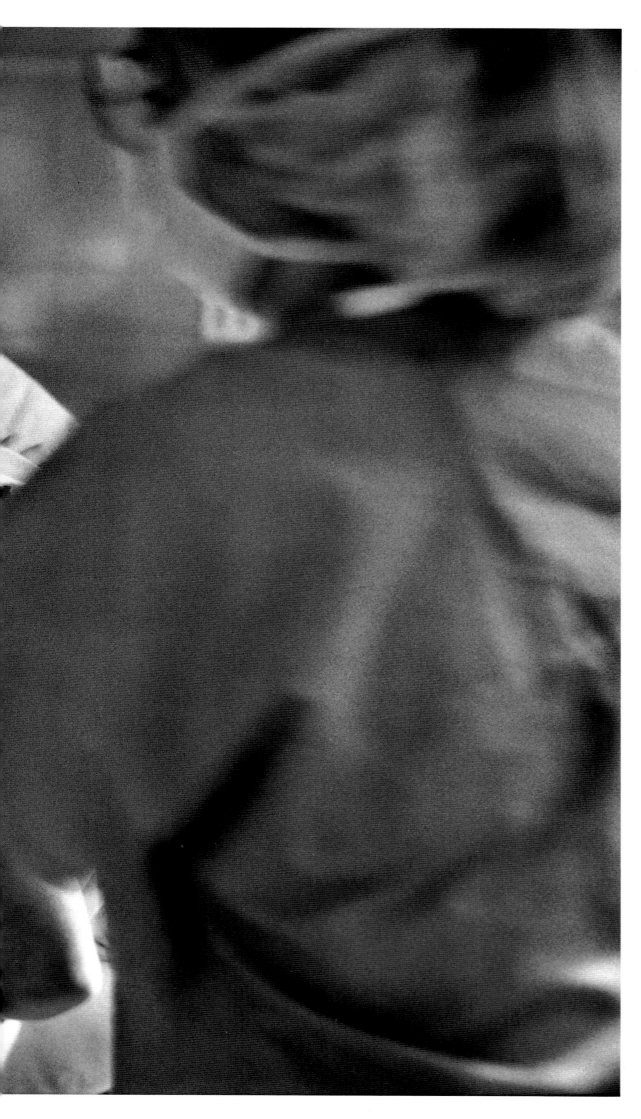

◀ **A mother at fifteen, Jessica LePak holds her baby for the first time** in the delivery room at Kaiser Hospital in San Francisco. Jessica's mother, Fran, rests her hand on the face of her exhausted daughter, who was in labor for twenty-five hours. About 3,000 adolescent girls become pregnant each day in the United States, where the teen pregnancy rate is the highest in the industrialized world. About half of the pregnant teenagers in the United States give birth; the other half have abortions. Jessica gave up her daughter, Allison Nicole, to a couple she met through an adoption agency during her pregnancy.
Photo by Steve Ringman

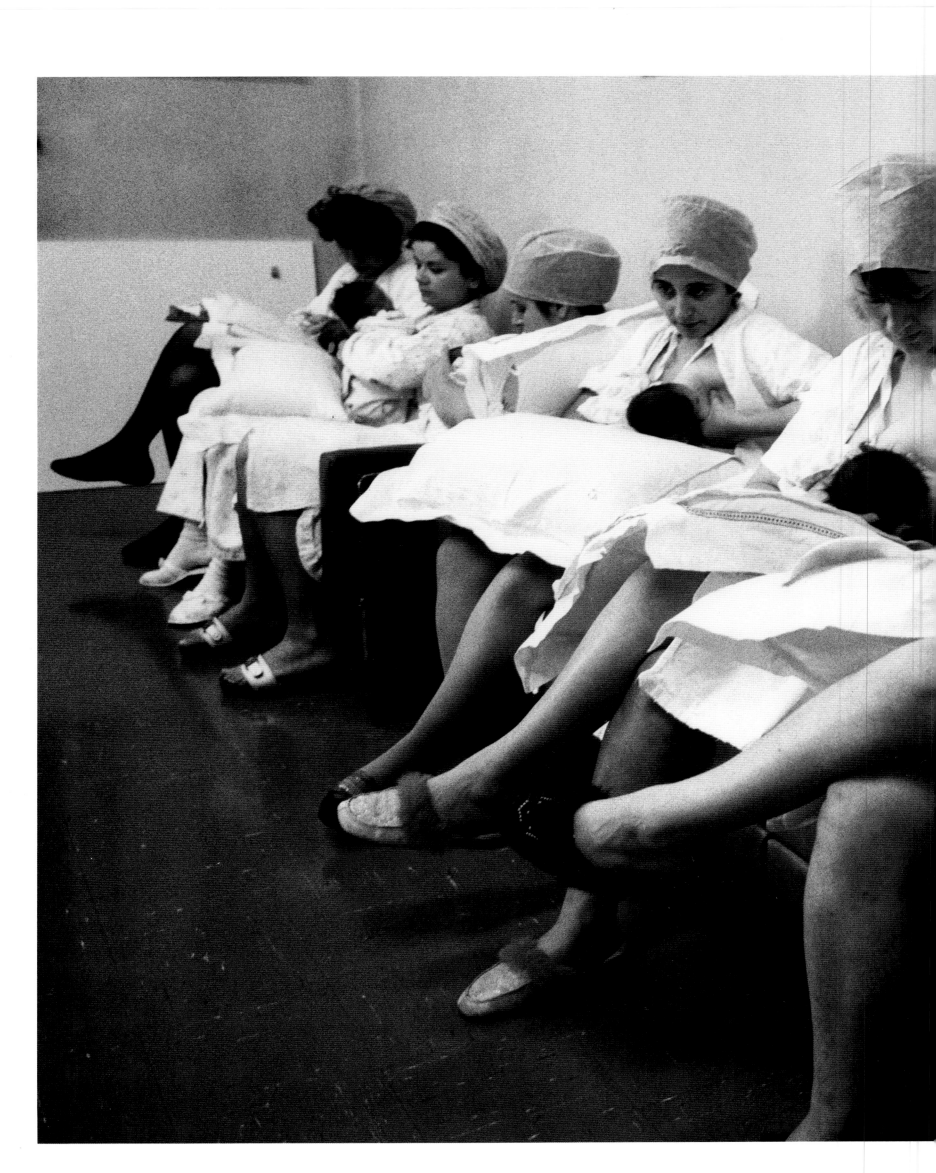

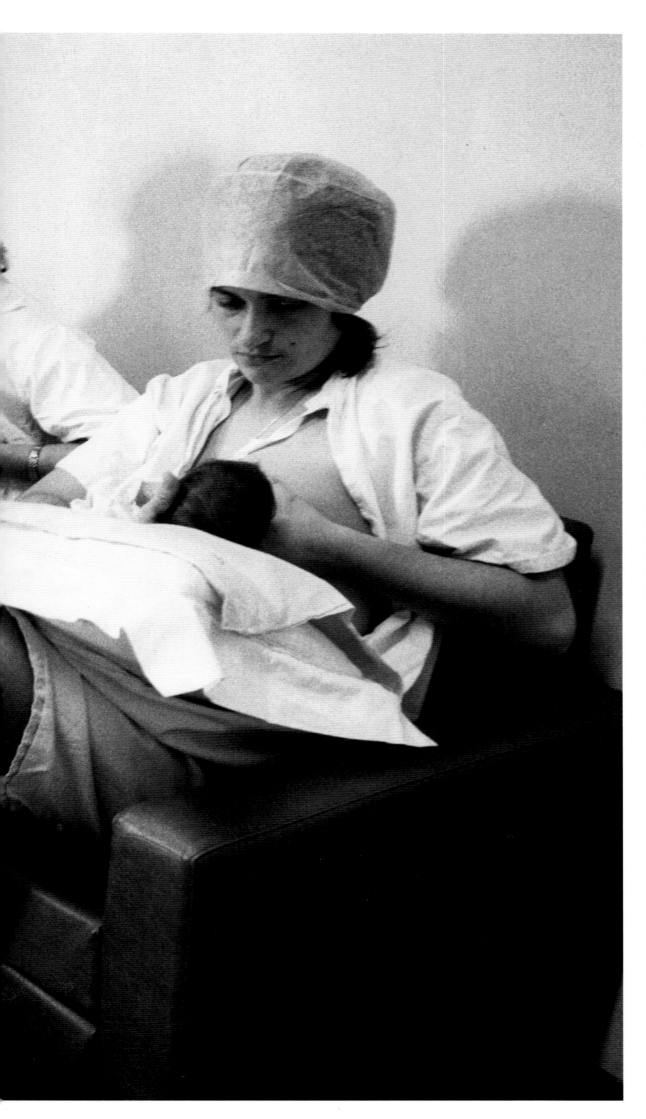

◄ **It's feeding time at the Elena Maternity Hospital milk bank in Athens,** where Greek mothers give their newborns one of a dozen daily helpings of mother's milk. Once their babies are full, many of these mothers will express, or pump, their breast milk into a container for later feedings. Mother's milk is the healthiest food a baby can eat, and in the United States, breast-feeding has soared in popularity: more than fifty-five percent of American mothers now breast-feed their babies, as opposed to about twenty percent in the early 1970s. *Photo by Misha Erwitt*

PHOTO ESSAY | *The Power of Persistence*

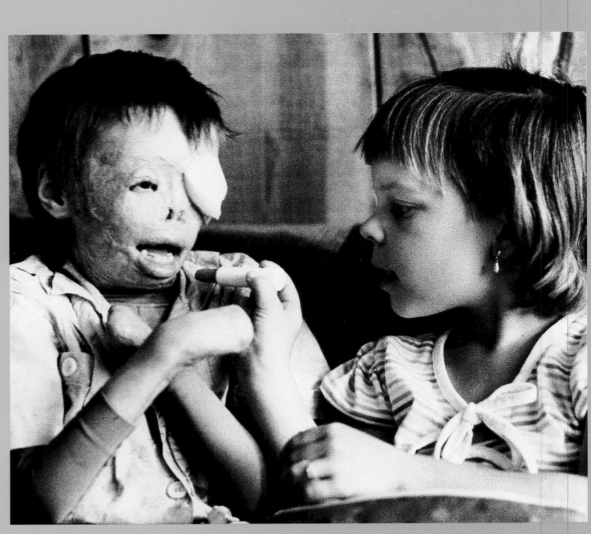

Sage Volkman was a happy kindergarten student in Bernalillo, New Mexico, when she posed for a school portrait (below). She had just scored her first soccer goal and was beginning to learn acrobatics.

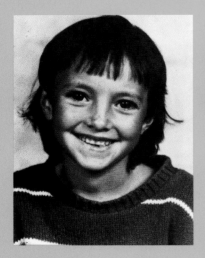

She loved to draw and color, play with Barbie dolls, and tease her older brother.

Then, on October 24, 1986, fire swept through the family camper where she was sleeping. Michael Volkman, who had just left camp to go fishing, rushed back and pulled his daughter from the flames. Sage's sleeping bag was partially melted; her body was lifeless. The desperate father pumped Sage's chest so hard he broke one of her ribs, but he saved her life. Six weeks later, when Sage emerged from a coma, she could remember nothing about the fire.

Forty-five percent of Sage's body was charred or burned to the bone. She had lost her nose, her left ear,

both eyelids, and all her fingers. The fire had melted the skin on her face, chest, arms, and legs. "When I first saw her, I wouldn't have known that was my child if they hadn't told me," says Denise Volkman (far right), who was not with Michael and Sage on the fateful camping trip.

"When I first saw her, she was different," says Kate Scott (above). "But it's okay, because we're best friends."

Sage's rehabilitation includes wearing a Jobst garment (right), a nylon and rubber suit that applies constant pressure to her skin to minimize scarring. When Sage began physical therapy, she was in a wheelchair. Scars made movement difficult and painful. She had suffered nerve damage in her legs and feet, leaving them too weak to support her weight. But within six weeks, she was walking. Now she skis, bikes, and jumps rope, and wants to return to the soccer field.

"I'm happy I can walk," says Sage. "I can walk because I

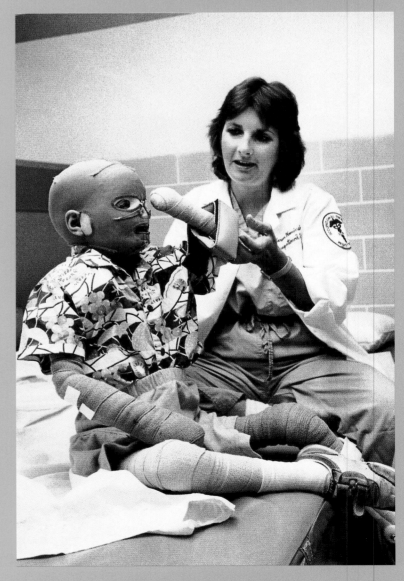

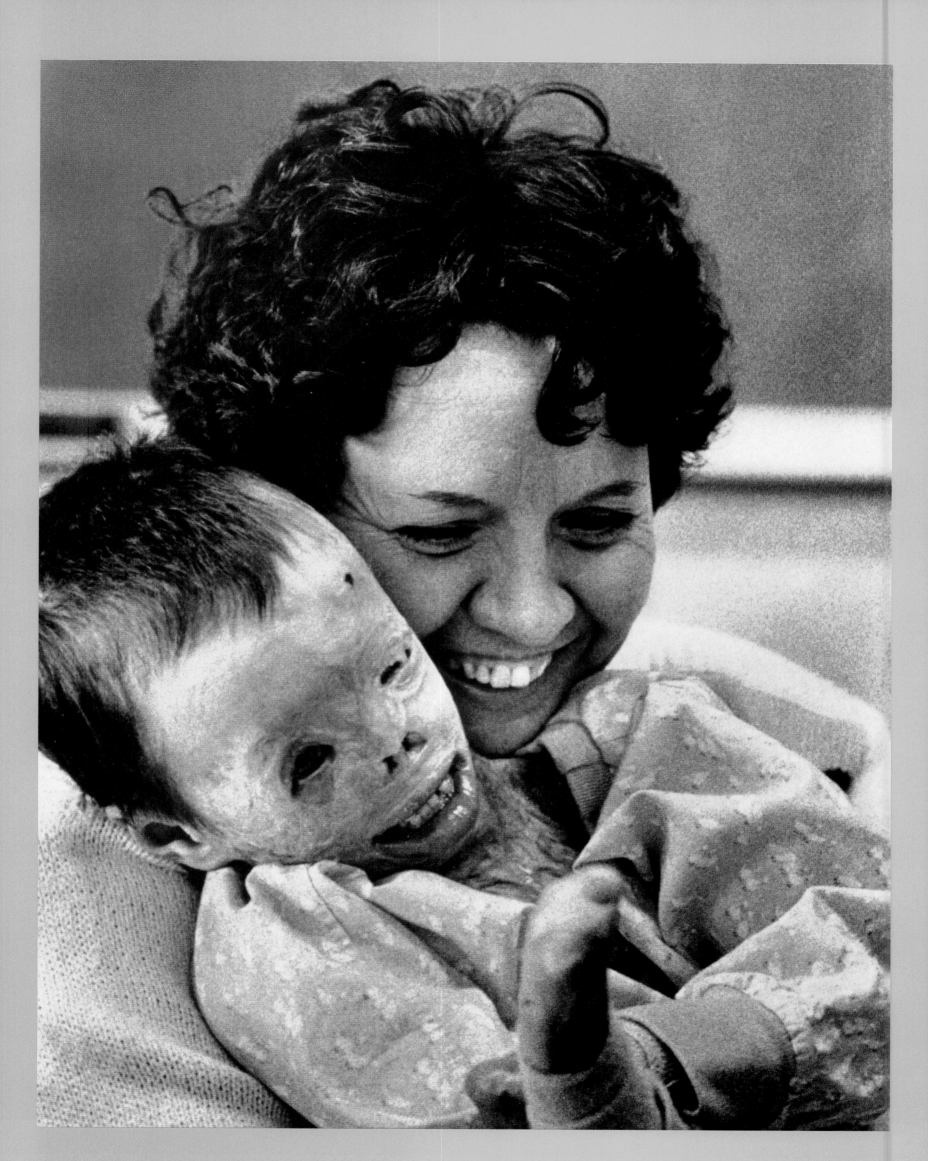

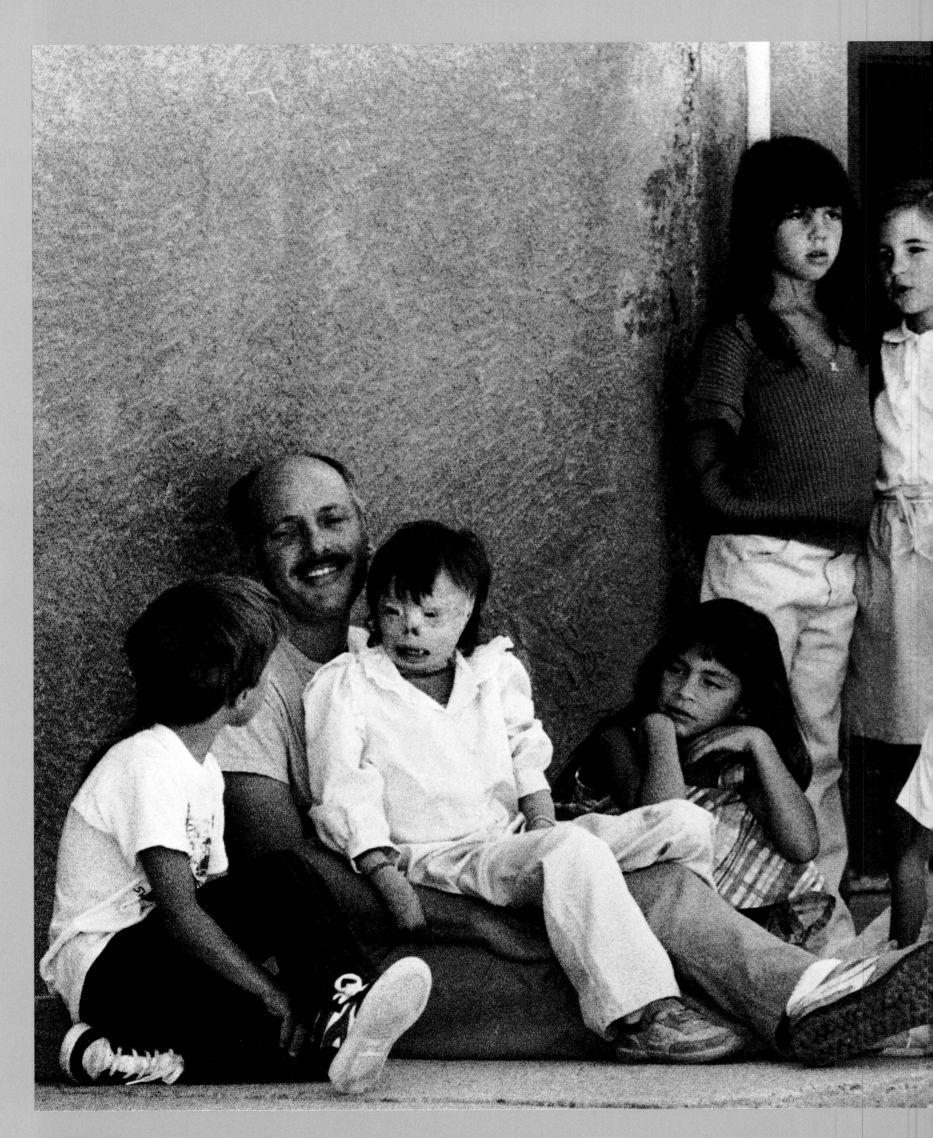

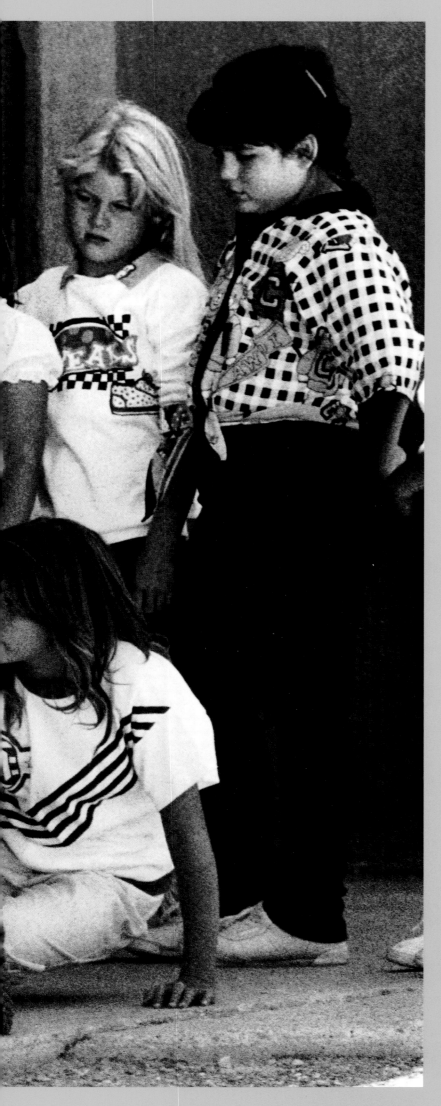

practiced and practiced and then one day, I thought I could do it and it happened."

In the years since the fire, says Michael, "she's never once complained or felt sorry for herself. Not once. I think it's normal to feel sorry for yourself once in a while, but she says, 'It's easy for me to be a burned girl.'"

Not so easy were Sage's twenty-six spinal operations. Recently, surgeons at New York University took skin from Sage's back and reattached it to her neck so she could flex and swivel normally. In yet another operation, excess skin was taken from her forehead and shaped into a nose. Michael says Sage has a "Karl Malden look" now because the doctors gave her an adult nose that will require further surgery to shape, and they must still add bone and cartilage. In addition, Sage faces surgery to attach fingers to her hands.

To help Sage and her classmates adjust, Michael accompanies Sage to her first day at Placitas Elementary School (left). Michael spoke to a school assembly about Sage's burns, and answered questions from the students. "Denise and I try to protect her," says Michael, "but we made a determination to go out and do everything we did before as a family."

As Sage grows older and prepares to enter adolescence,

the Volkmans hope the openness they've fought hard to maintain will bolster their daughter through hard times. Michael believes his daughter can face any obstacle and overcome it. "Sage handles people's

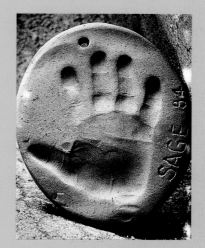

reactions better than we do," he says. "It's no big thing for her.

"Once we were at a pizza parlor and a group of kids were staring at her," he recalls. "One of the kids said, 'Look at that ugly boy over there.' The 'ugly' part didn't bother her. She was upset that they'd called her a boy."

Photos by Vickie Lewis

121

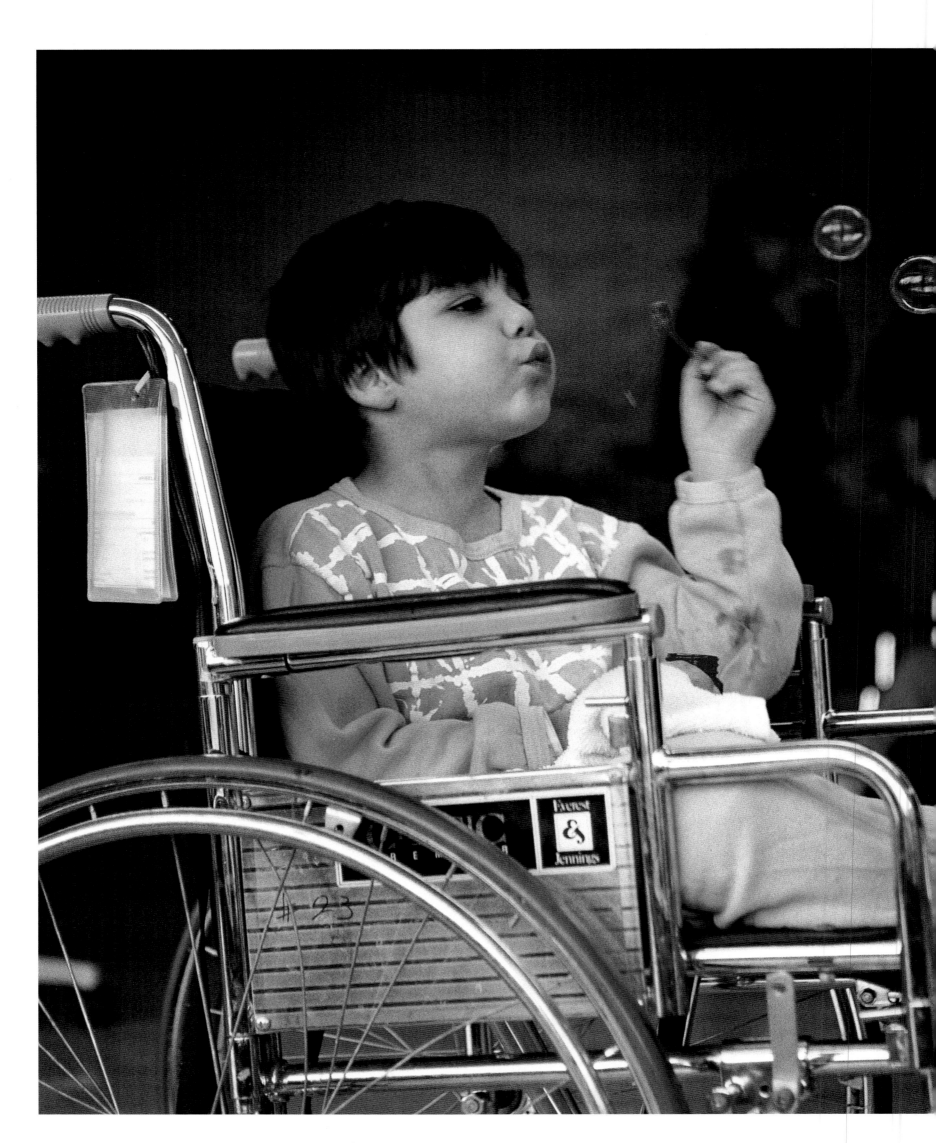

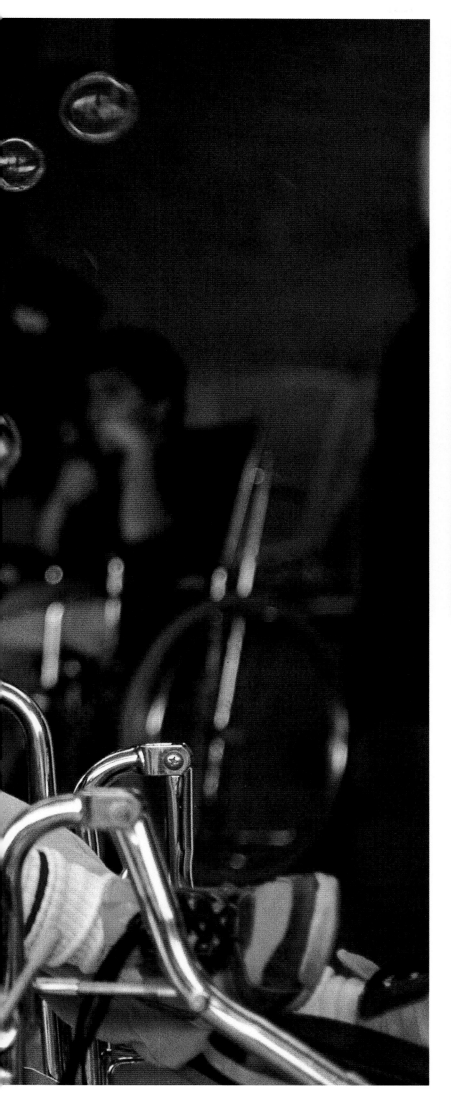

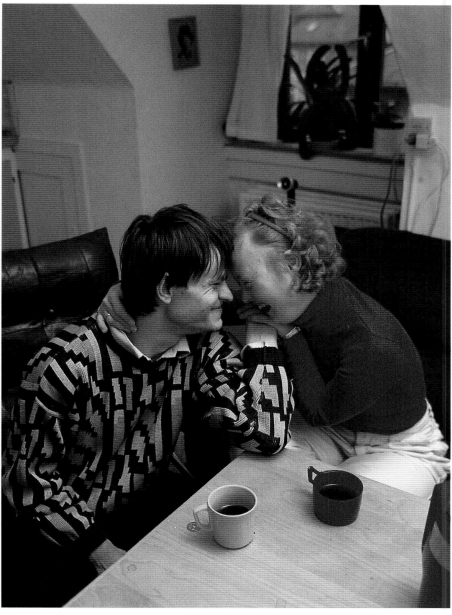

◄ **Far from the war that cost him much of his right leg,** six-year-old Mohamed Beydoun recuperates at the Chicago Unit of the Shriners Hospital for Crippled Children, where he arrived soon after an artillery shell tore through his family's Beirut living room in 1986. Mohamed now walks with the help of an artificial leg. The costs of his treatment and hospital stay, like that of children at the twenty-one other Shriners Hospitals in the United States, Canada, and Mexico, were covered entirely by the Shrine of North America. The Shriners spend about $200 million annually to operate their network of hospitals.
Photo by Gary S. Chapman

▲ **Young love flourishes at a halfway house** for mentally retarded adults in Frederiksberg, Denmark. Both thirty-year-old Rubin Alsted and his twenty-four-year-old fiancée, Bende Svensson, had been institutionalized before moving to this group house on the outskirts of Copenhagen, where they will learn the skills they need to function in their own apartment. Danish mental health officals encourage the integration of mentally retarded adults into everyday society.
Photo by Stephanie Maze

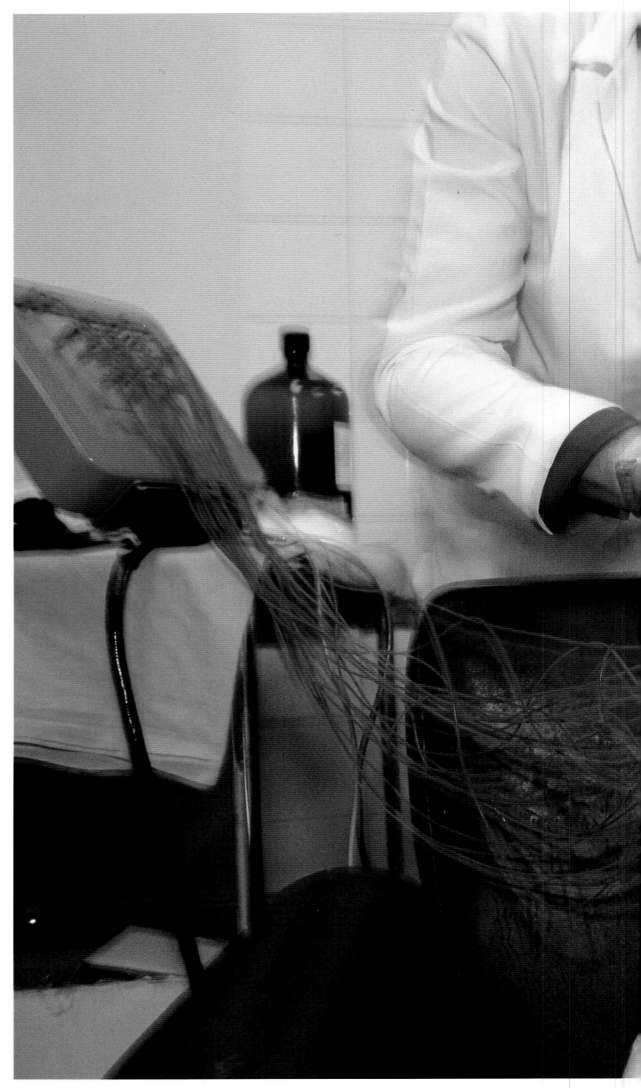

▶ **Measuring the brain's electrical impulses,** a technician at King Hussein Hospital in Amman, Jordan, runs an electroencephalograph, or EEG, on a young epileptic. The EEG, which came into widespread use in the 1940s, allows doctors to monitor brain activity in comatose patients, and serves as an aid in diagnosing strokes and brain tumors. In the case of the approximately two percent of the world's population that suffers from epilepsy — a condition characterized by brief periods of time when brain cells misfire, often causing seizures — the EEG will show a sudden abnormal electrical discharge. "It's as if," says Dr. Barry Tharp of Stanford University, past president of the American EEG Society, "you'd put an electrode to the head and shot electricity through it." Famous epileptics in history include Socrates, Alexander the Great, Fyodor Dostoyevsky, Harriet Tubman, and Richard Burton.
Photo by George Y.F. Chan

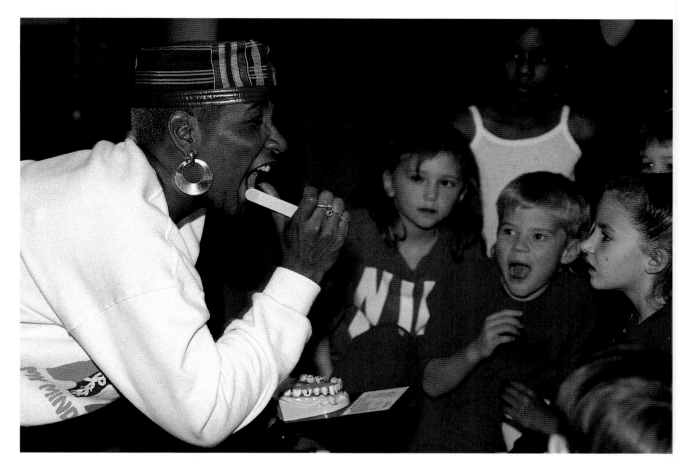

▲ **With the help of "Mr. Gross Mouth," the model of a mouth with yellow teeth,** health educator Bambi Sumpter of the South Carolina Department of Education explains the effects of chewing tobacco to her young audience at Seven Oaks Elementary School in Columbia. Sumpter, here showing the children what her own healthy palate looks like, holds a doctorate in public health and travels throughout South Carolina in a health education van. Besides visiting classrooms to talk directly with children, she consults with teachers on how best to give students information on nutrition, human sexuality, and drugs. "We start talking about alcohol and drugs," says Sumpter, "in kindergarten."
Photo by Annie Griffiths Belt

◀ **Nosing around at the Scitech Discovery Center** in Perth, Australia, schoolchildren Caroline and Andrew Motteram learn how the senses of taste and smell work. Lights go on in various parts of the model's huge brain when objects, like the bottle here, are placed on the lips and under the nose. "The exhibit shows children that it's the brain that tells the taste and smell of things," says the Discovery Center's Ann Ghisalberti, "not the tongue and nose."
Photo by John Marmaras

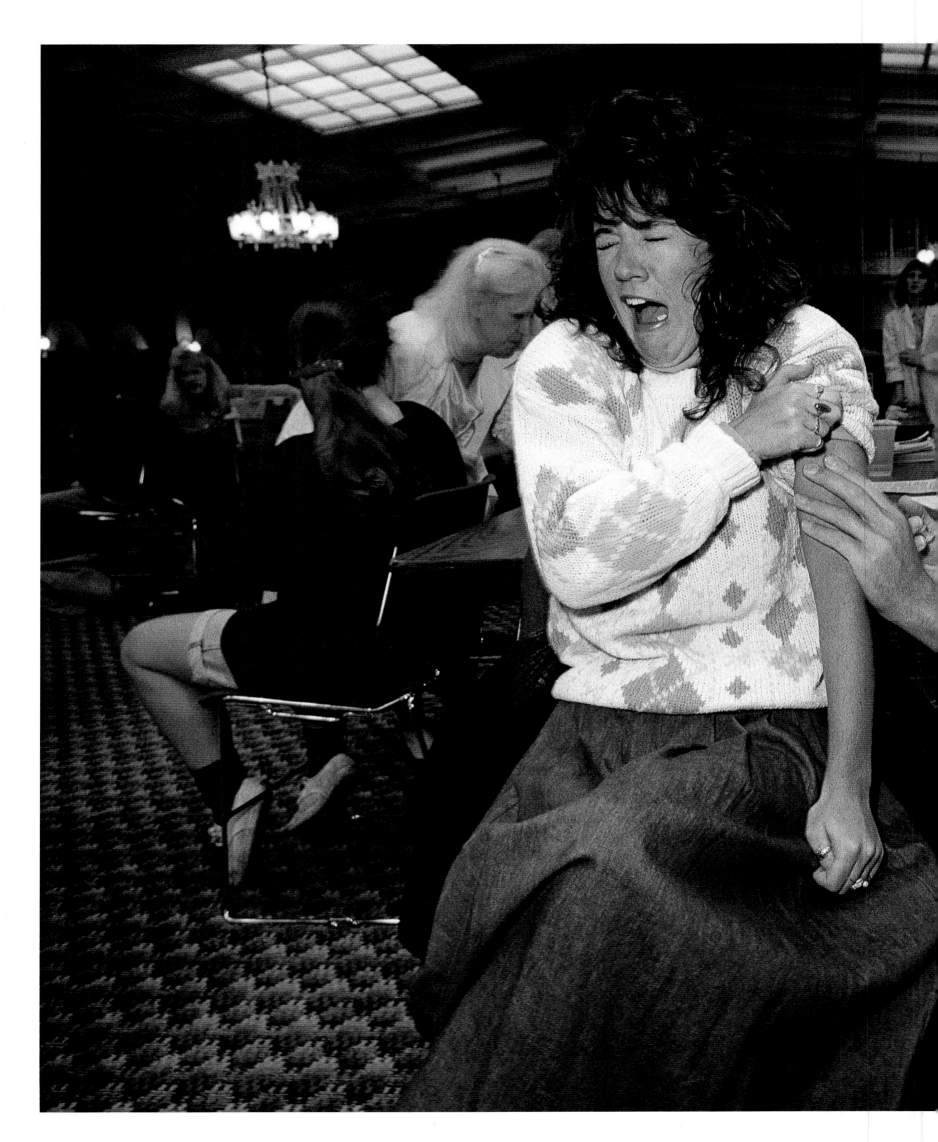

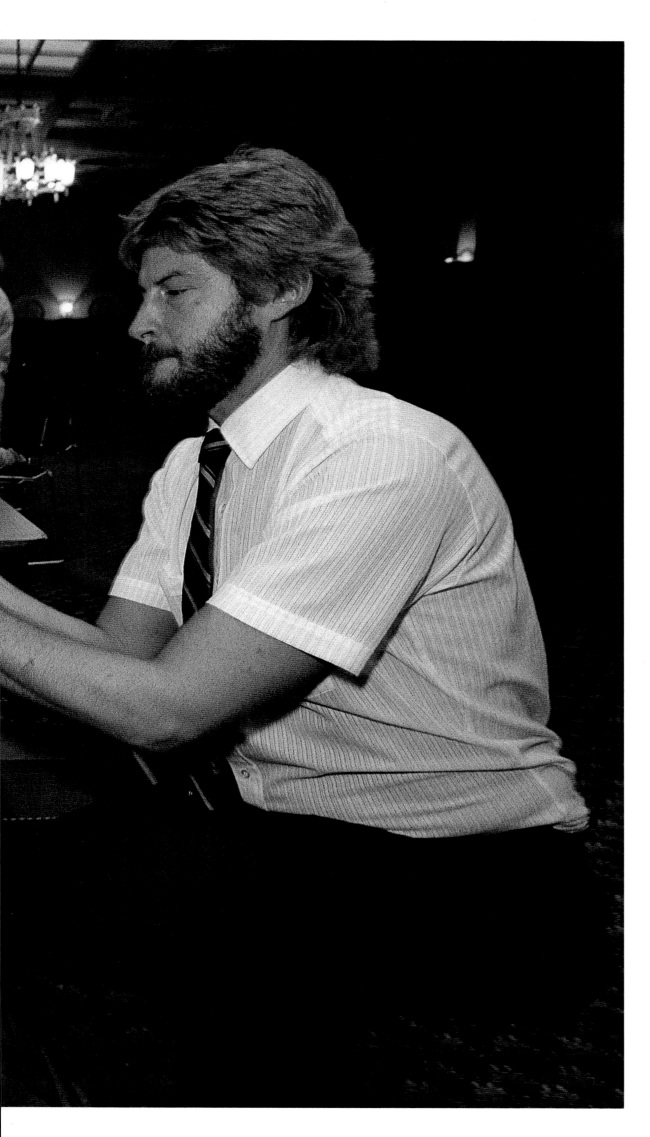

◄ Measles isn't just for kids, as college administrators around the country are discovering, so the University of Iowa now requires students who haven't had a measles shot since 1980 to roll up their sleeves before they enroll for classes. The American Academy of Pediatrics recommends that all educational institutions beyond high school require students to prove they've had two doses of measles vaccine — one as an infant and one as a teenager.

Public health officials had hoped to wipe out the disease — which in adults can lead to pneumonia, miscarriage, encephalitis, or even death — by 1982, but now say there's no end in sight. Many Americans vaccinated as children in the 1960s were either inoculated too young or given a vaccine that has faded in effectiveness, leaving an estimated seven million adults vulnerable to the disease. Here, James Goodrich of the Iowa Department of Public Health vaccinates twenty-one-year-old senior Juliann Maren, a communications major. *Photo by Kim Komenich*

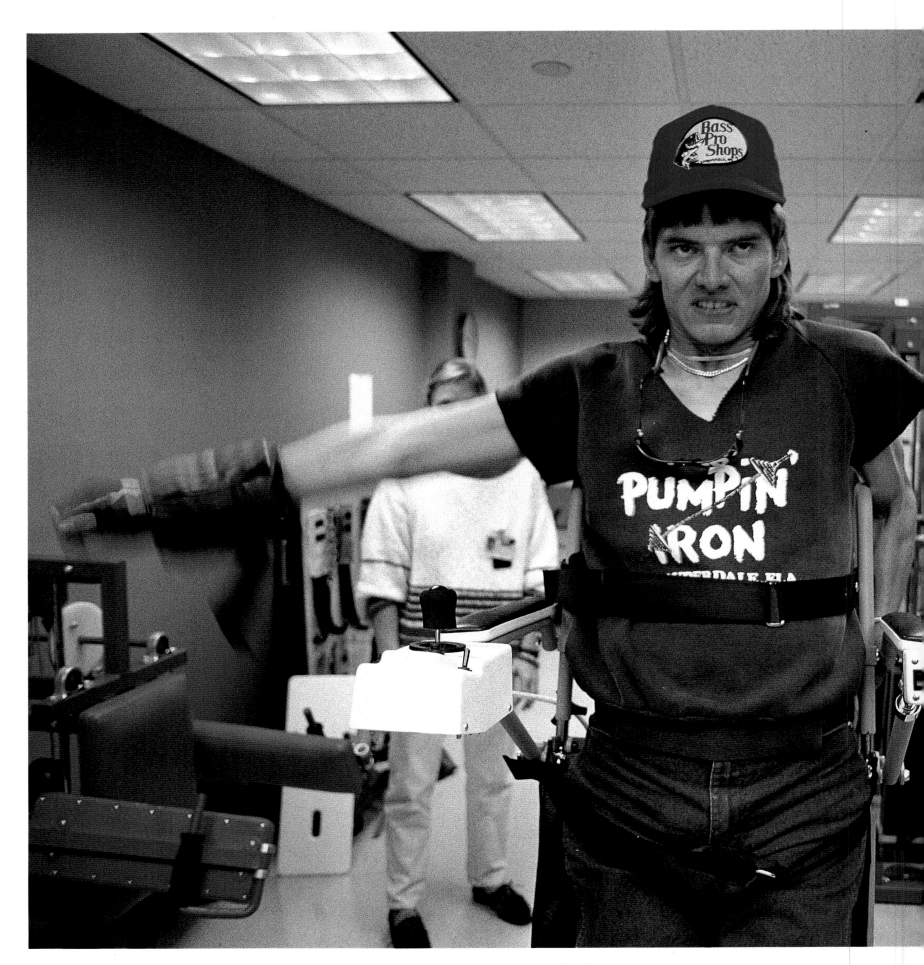

▲ **Strengthening arm muscles he once thought were dead,** quadriplegic Eric Mann lifts weights while strapped into a stand-up wheelchair at the Miami Project to Cure Paralysis. The center, which is affiliated with the University of Miami School of Medicine, is the most comprehensive spinal cord injury research facility in the world, and features biofeedback devices to identify muscles that still generate electrical impulses. Therapists then work with volunteers like Mann, who are treated free of charge in exchange for serving as research subjects, to build up muscles that show some rehabilitation potential. "When you're working out and getting stronger," says Mann three years after hitting his head on the bottom of a friend's swimming pool, "you don't want to leave." *Photo by Randy Olson*

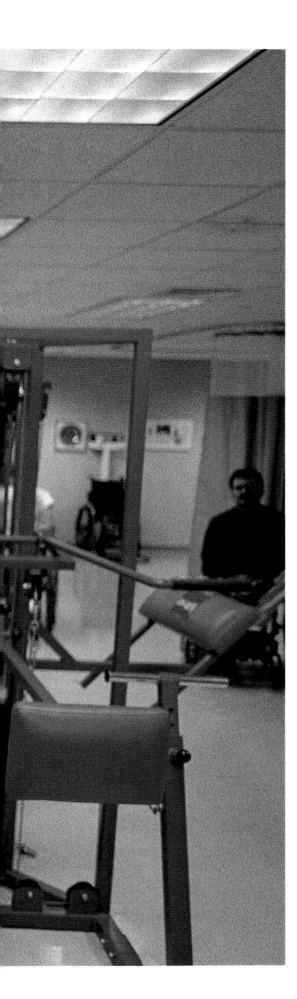

After My Stroke, A New World

JOSEPH CHAIKIN
WITH JEAN-CLAUDE VAN ITALLIE

WHEN I WOKE UP FROM MY HEART OPERATION IN MAY 1984, I FOUND I HAD suffered a stroke. I couldn't find any words, except the word yes. Whether I wanted to say I love you, or I hate you, or no, I could only say yes. I woke up aphasic. I couldn't even say my name. And I couldn't understand anyone. Everyone seemed to be speaking in a foreign language.

I have worked in theatre all my life as an actor and a director. So speaking is paramount for my work. I must understand and be understood.

Before my stroke, I was a babbler. I talked a lot, I enjoyed talking, and I was articulate. I spoke clearly, and my words were well formed. Now I make mistakes when I talk. But that's okay. Even when I sound awkward, it can be funny.

A few weeks after my stroke I became depressed. I felt imprisoned. I wanted to stop talking completely, to hide in silence and watch faces.

But what's the point of being depressed constantly? The universe is vast with possibilities. You must be generous and speak even if it is hard. Sometimes now I even feel ecstatic. But mostly I just do my work.

Talking to a friend is more important to me now. Every word I hear, every moment I share, matters more. I feel more. I feel words now—they carry more sensual meaning. I cry and laugh more easily. How do I convey feelings? Hello, I say to my friend on the telephone. I must sing out the word, Hellloooo! The sound of voices speaking is music.

As I am constantly learning words, I live with passionate questions about words. I wonder all the time: what is the meaning of that word, what is between words, what is under words? What is the meaning that I hear in the voice that is not words? These questions are rich for me.

Other changes have come with the stroke: logistics, directions are difficult. And time has become abstract. A day—it's a page in my date book. A day can be as long as a century, or as quick as a walk down the block.

I heal through work. I work hard every day. My work includes push-ups, speech, music, reading, directing, learning and speaking about aphasia, telling the taxi driver where I need to go, and ordering a meal in a restaurant. Aphasia has made me a pupil of everyday life.

Healing is not to learn again what I knew before. Healing is to learn something new, to be constantly surprised. Healing is like a gate opening.

Millions of people around the world live with aphasia, but most people don't even know the word. Aphasia—it's not only my disability, but the vehicle for my continuing to open, deepen, and grow.

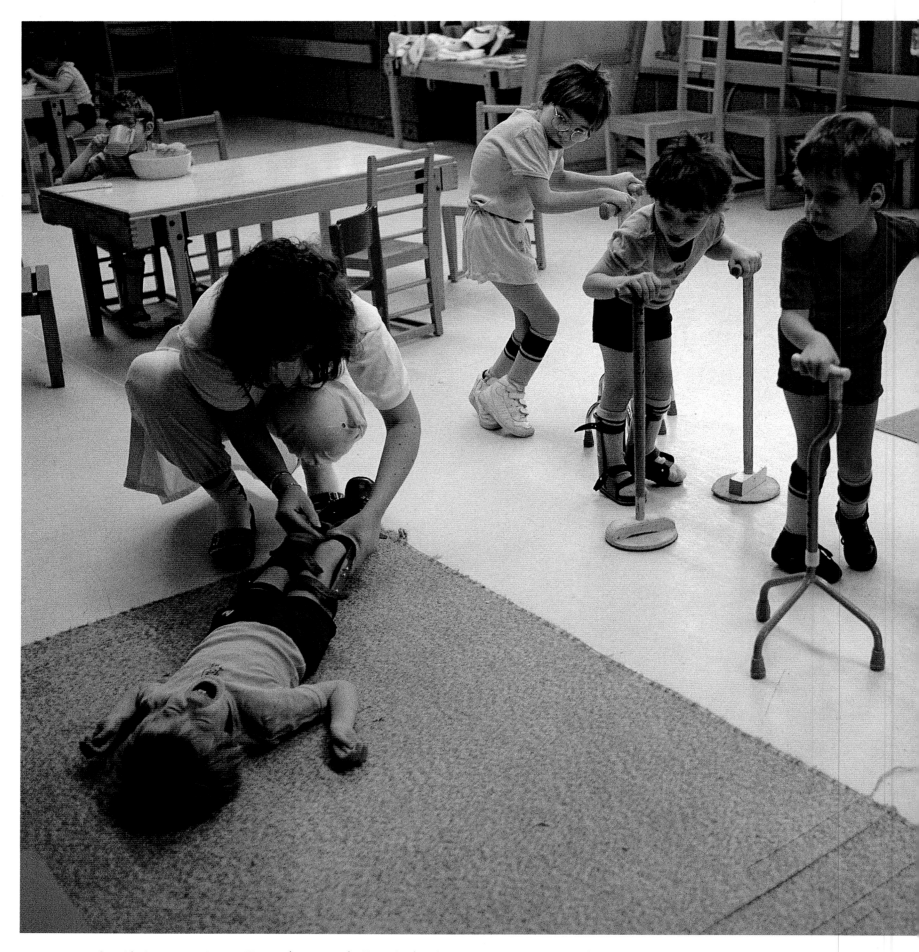

▲ **In a kindergarten class unlike most others,** children at the Petö András Institute in Budapest learn the determination it takes to live normal lives despite their disabilities. Parents around the world send their offspring to the Hungarian facility, officially known as the Petö András State Institute for Conductive Education of the Motor Disabled and Conductors College. The institute's guiding philosophy is that motor problems are essentially learning disorders that many children can overcome with the proper training. The teachers, or conductors, function as physical therapists, psychologists, and speech therapists as they work to help disabled children become more independent. The conductors, who undergo a comprehensive four-year program before they begin working with the children, stress individual solutions for individual problems, working closely with each child at the institute.

Photo by Péter Korniss

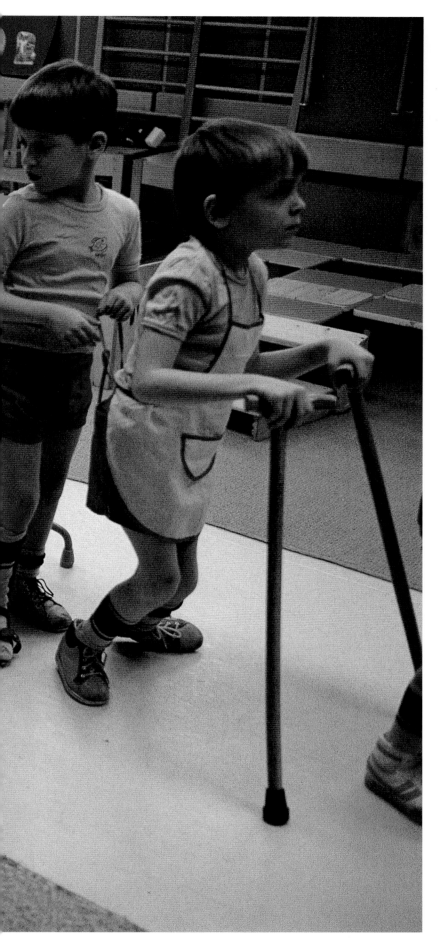

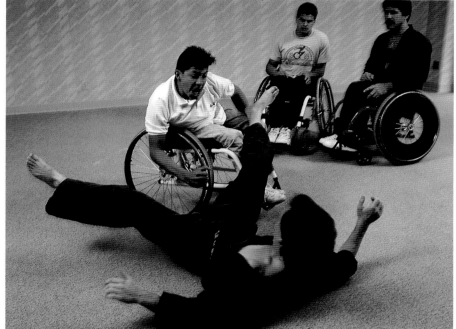

▲ **Paraplegic Tony Lara uses a quick *kung fu san soo* move** to deck Ben Smith during a martial arts course at Casa Colina, a southern California rehabilitation center noted for its wheelchair athletes. Instructor Ron Scanlon, far right, is an eighth-degree black belt in the ancient self-defense art of *kung fu san soo*, using his wheelchair as a weapon where the able-bodied might use their legs. Scanlon, who was paralyzed from the waist down in a car accident at the age of nine, says that "being in a wheelchair gave me confidence as an individual." Marvels fellow *kung fu san soo* master Bill Lasiter: "Ron is the first handicapped person I've ever seen who can teach upright people how to kick."
Photo by Alon Reininger

PHOTO ESSAY | Portrait of a Healer

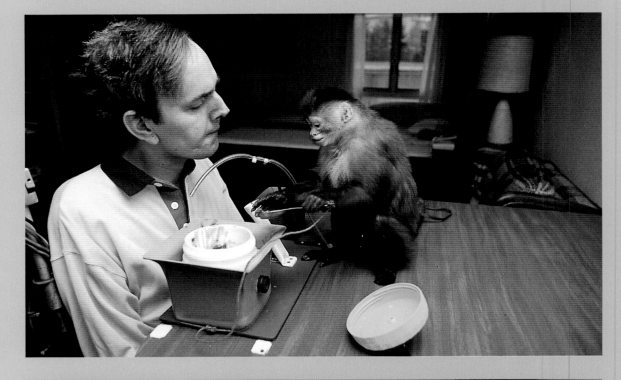

"She's a good friend," says quadriplegic Robert Foster of his roommate Hellion, a six-pound capuchin monkey. But the amazing Hellion is more than that: since 1979 she has fed Foster, run a sweeper over his hardwood floors, turned pages in books for him, changed the tapes in his cassette player, and brought a seemingly endless supply of cheer to the pair's apartment in Watertown, just outside Boston.

Hellion understands about a dozen voice commands, and Foster also gets her attention with a laser beam that he controls from the chin rest on his wheelchair. He rewards her with a gulp of fruit juice for a job well done, and he can jolt her with a low-level shock if she gets too rambunctious. Since Hellion first moved in with Foster as an experiment, three years after he was paralyzed from the neck down in a car accident, the Boston-based organization Helping Hands has placed more than a dozen monkeys with quadriplegics. The cost of training and maintaining the animal is borne by Helping Hands.

"Robert's patience and tolerance are fantastic," says the organization's founder, Mary Joan Willard. As the first Helping Hands participant, "he sacrificed two years to help us develop this program." But for Foster, the sacrifice was well worth it: he has a loyal, affectionate, and playful helper who should live about eighteen more years, until the age of thirty—a helper who, he says with affection, "thinks she's a person."
Photos by David H. Wells

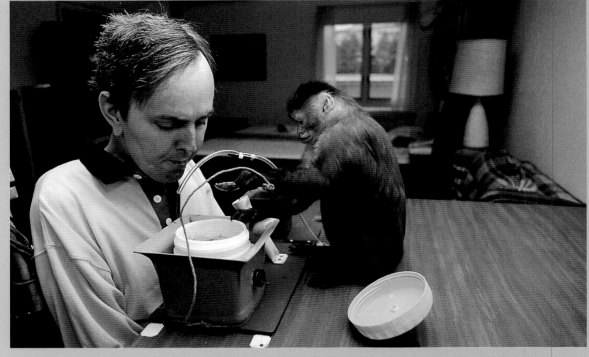

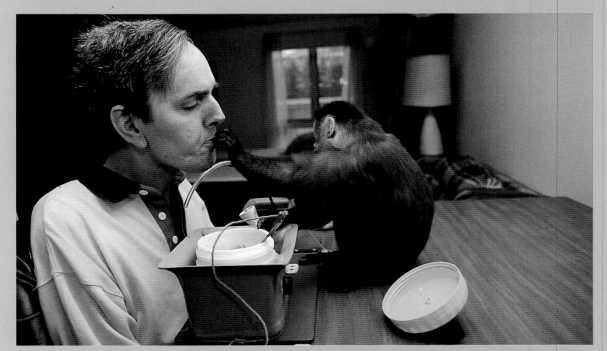

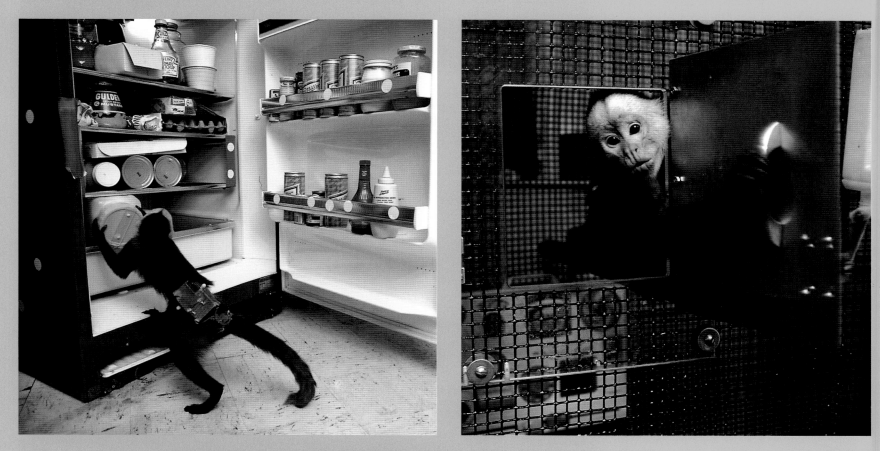

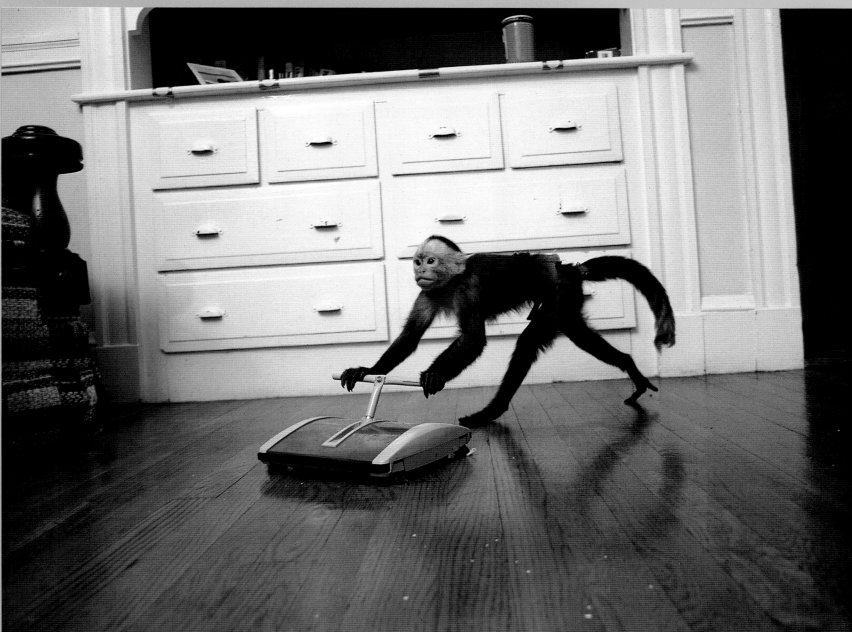

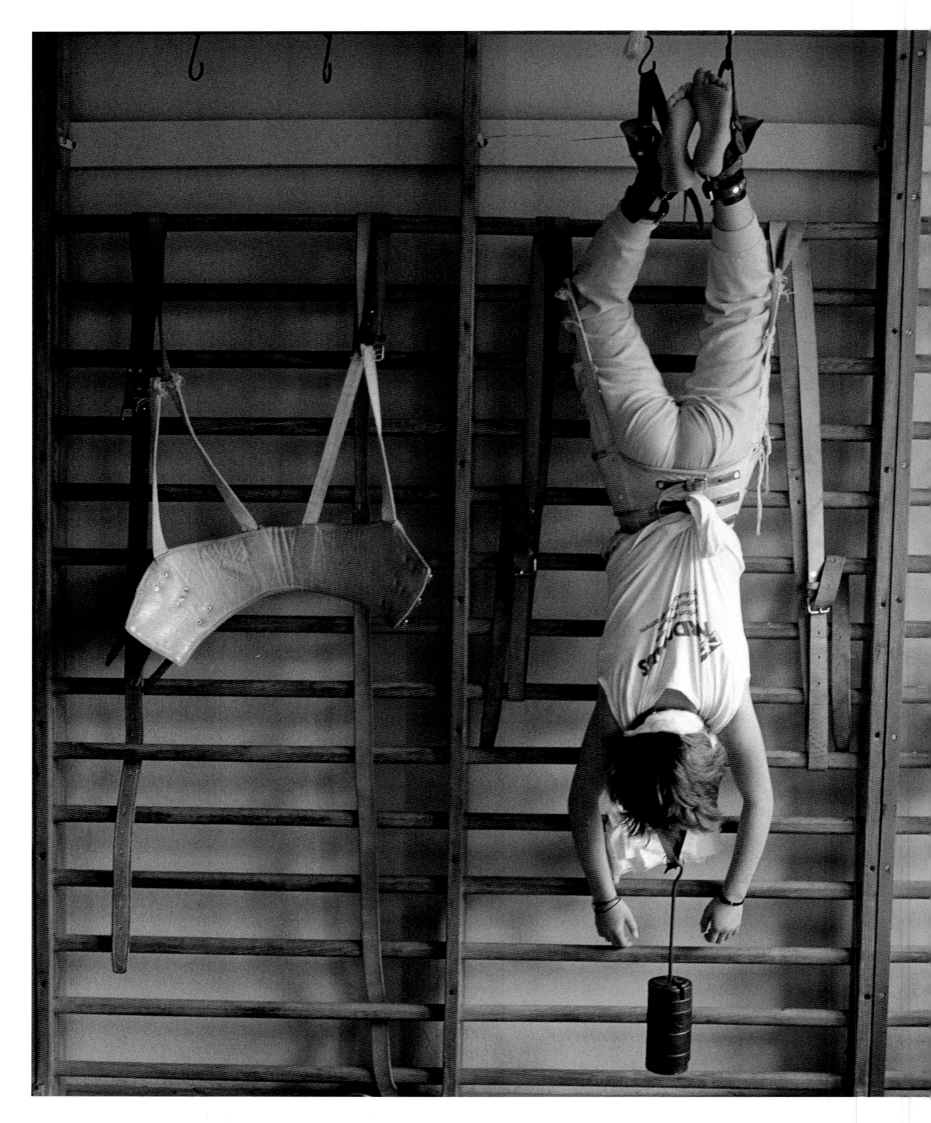

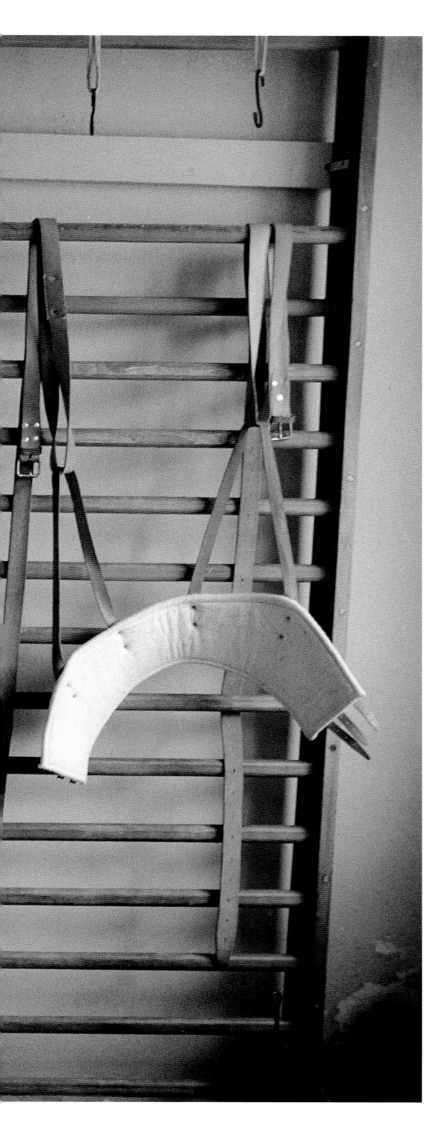

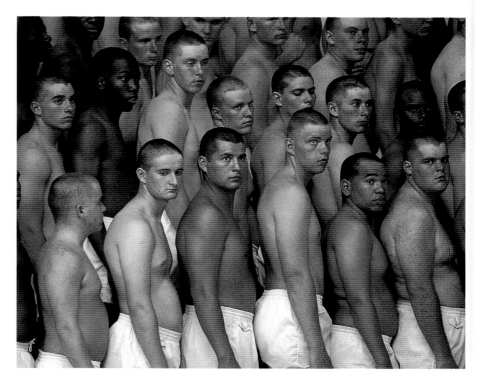

◄ **In a technique rare in the United States but commonly used in Europe,** a thirteen-year-old girl's painful back condition is treated with inverted traction at the Metropolitan Center for Rehabilitation in the Polish city of Konstancin. The weight of the upper body and the weight hanging from the neck produce traction, a procedure that may be uncomfortable — the younger patients call the Metropolitan Center's traction room "the torture chamber" — but is not dangerous. A patient can hang in this position for up to fifteen minutes at a time.
Photo by Tomasz Tomaszewski

▲ **It's the second day of boot camp for these prospective sailors** at the San Diego Naval Training Center, where some 33,000 recruits are whipped into shape each year. The eight-week session features about five hours a week of intense physical training for the recruits, who usually "are not in peak physical condition when they arrive from civilian life," according to Navy spokesman Paul Versailles. The recruits march to and from the classrooms where they spend most of their day, and by the end of their training are required to run three miles in twenty-one minutes.
Photo by Karen Kasmauski

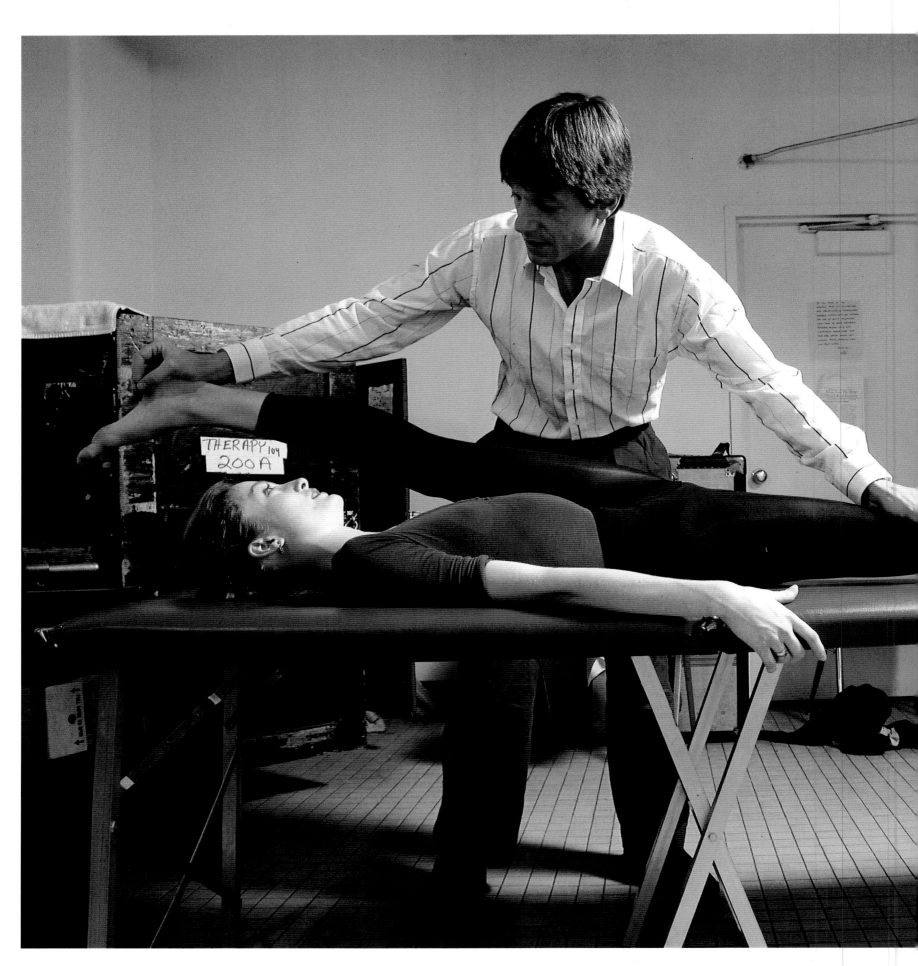

▲ **Peter Marshall insists that ballet dancer Julie Kent has tight hamstrings,** even as he stretches her into a position that "would snap every tendon in my body if I tried it." Physical therapist Marshall treats twenty-five to thirty-five members of the American Ballet Theater each day, both in the company's home base of New York and on the road. Ballet, he says, is "a very healthy activity. Though dancers suffer many sprains and minor ailments, they don't really have a high incidence of serious, long-term injuries."
Photo by Jim Mendenhall

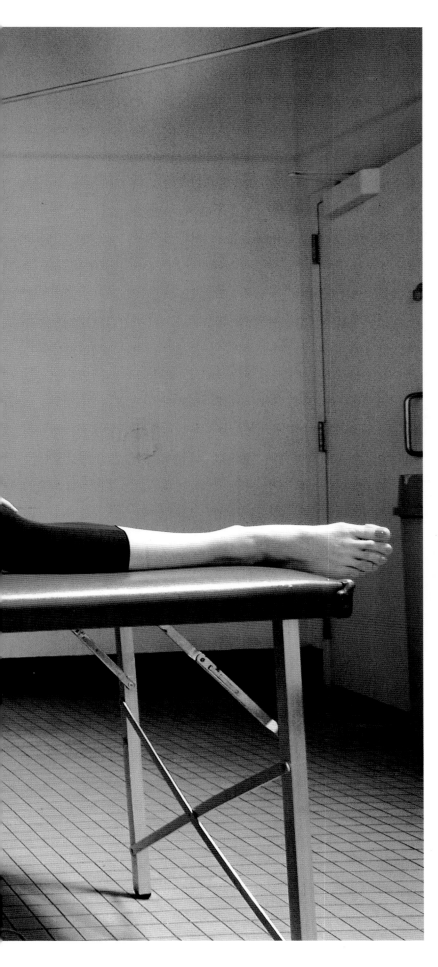

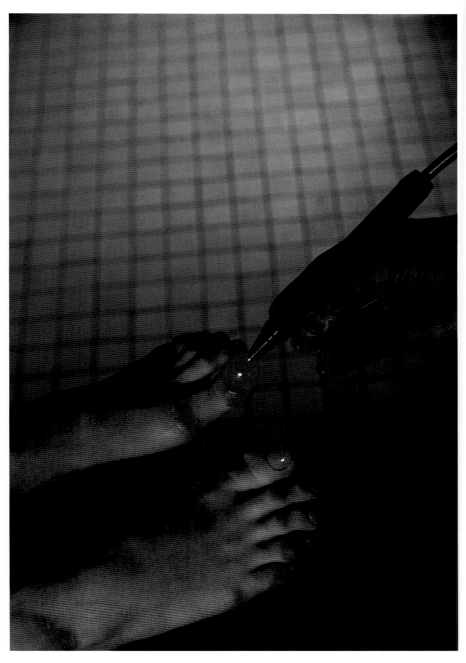

▲ **A low-power cold laser relieves the pain under a ballet dancer's toenail** caused by standing "on point" in shoes that are little more than cardboard and glue covered in silk. In contrast to conventional medical lasers, which are used to burn or cut tissue, the low-power laser used by American Ballet Theater physical therapist Peter Marshall appears to be beneficial in the treatment of ailments such as tendinitis and stress fractures. Says dancer Julie Kent, "When Peter's using the laser, you don't feel a thing." *Photo by Jim Mendenhall*

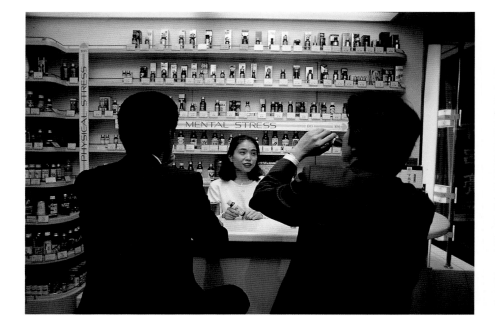

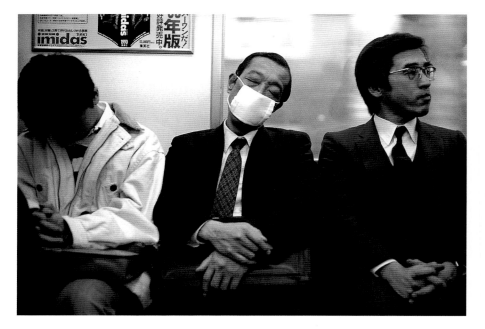

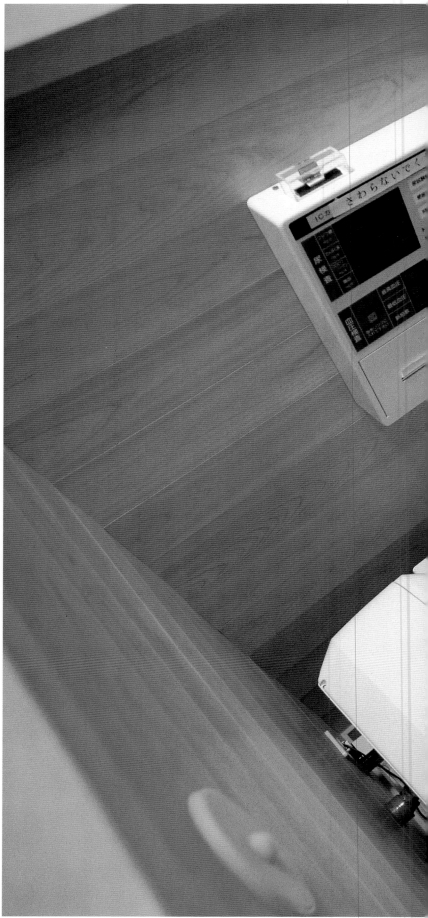

▲ **Designed to keep the sick from infecting the healthy and the healthy from picking up stray germs,** the *masuku,* here worn by a commuter on Tokyo's Yamanote train line, came into vogue in Japan following the devastating world flu pandemic of 1918, which killed about twenty million people — more people than died in battle in World War I, World War II, and the Korea and Vietnam conflicts combined. Although doctors now believe that hand-to-hand contact plays a bigger role in spreading colds and flus than do sneezing and coughing, the *masuku* is still worn by some Japanese as a polite precaution during cold and flu season.
Photo by Torin Boyd

▲▲ **Squeezing their concern for health into a busy schedule,** commuters at a Tokyo train station make a quick stop at a vitamin bar. The bartender, who is also a trained vitamin adviser, offers more than 200 types of drinks; the big seller among the 900 or so customers who stop in daily is a mix of vitamins B-1, C, and E, which goes for about a dollar.
Photo by Torin Boyd

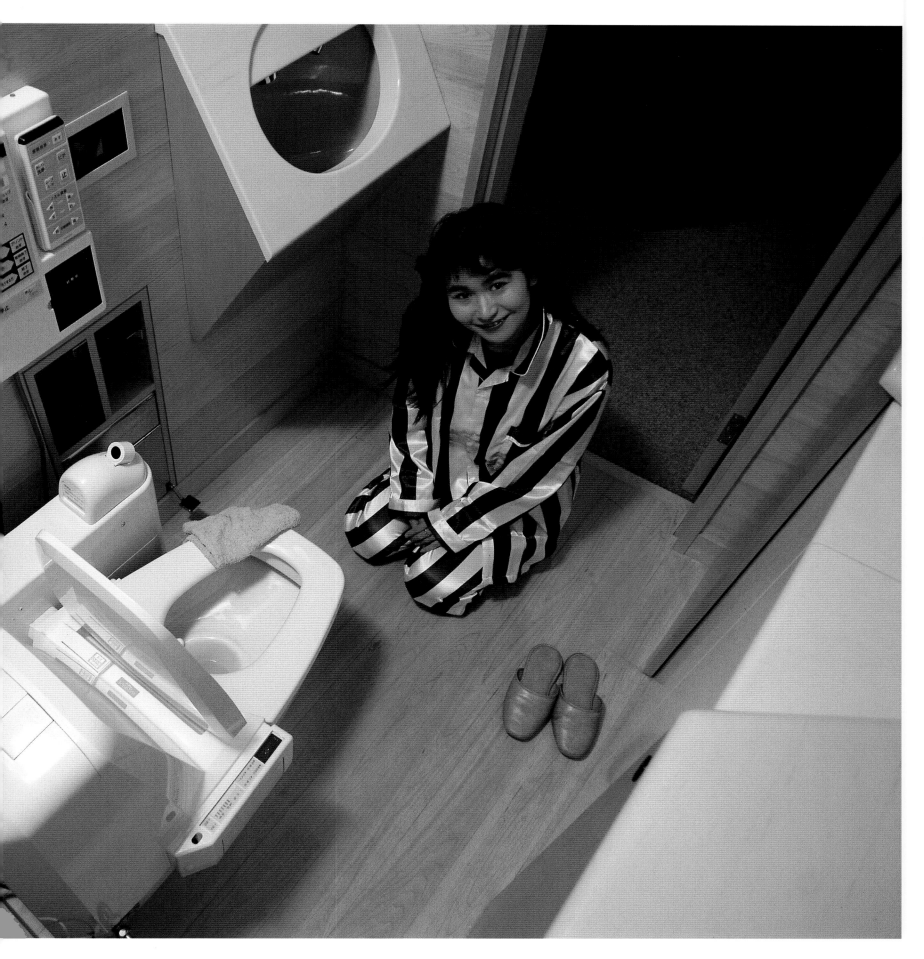

▲ **Hygiene goes high-tech with this Japanese toilet,** capable of taking a user's blood pressure and temperature as well as measuring urine for glucose, albumin, urobilinogen, and blood. And it's comfortable too, with a heated seat, several washing functions, and a drying fan — all with wireless remote control. But don't throw out the old toilet just yet: the Health Management Toilet System is still in the test phase, and the price tag is likely to be high enough that most of the toilets will end up in hospitals.
Photo by Torin Boyd

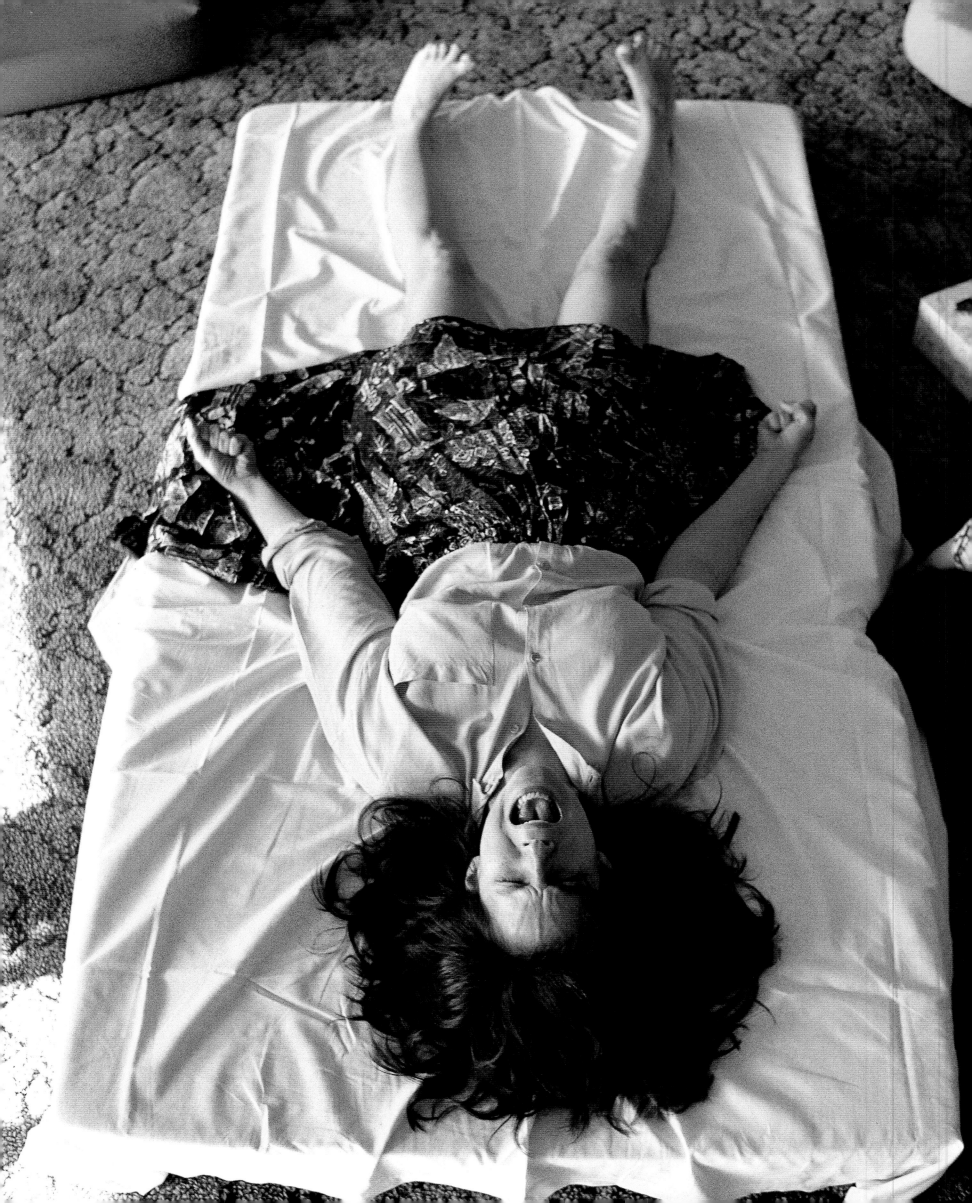

Finding the
Healer Within

NORMAN COUSINS

WHAT CAN WE LEARN FROM PATIENTS WHO HAVE RECOVERED FROM supposedly irreversible illnesses, including malignancies, cardiac infirmities, and diseases of the joints and muscles? Is there anything in these recoveries that might be useful to others similarly afflicted?

For the past ten years, I've had the opportunity to meet with a significant number of such patients. In talking with them, I was reminded that Hippocrates viewed the treatment of disease as a dual process. One part was represented by systematic medicine; the other part was the full activation of the patient's own healing system. In the centuries since the great physician taught his students under the sycamore tree on the Greek island of Kos, there has been a shift away from the concept of the patient as the center of the healing process. The physician has come increasingly to the fore as the dominant force.

The patients I studied, however, were not content to be passive participants in their own illnesses. Most of them were told, when the diagnosis of illness was made, that the chances for recovery were slim. Unfortunately, a significant number of these patients experienced a severe downturn following the diagnosis. Some of them suffered from panic and depression, not uncommon reactions to serious disease. Many cancer patients, for instance, report difficulty sleeping—a difficulty that stems as much from their fear as from their pain.

Similarly, some heart attack patients never reach the hospital alive, not just because of the condition itself, but because panic may cause further constriction of the blood vessels, imposing an intolerable additional burden. Brain research is now turning up evidence that attitudes of defeat or panic not only constrict the blood vessels, but create emotional stresses that have a debilitating effect on the endocrine and immune systems. Conversely, attitudes of confidence and determination activate benevolent and therapeutic secretions in the brain.

One patient I worked with briefly, whom I'll call Sheila, provided a dramatic example of the importance of the mind in the recovery process. When I first met her, she was a thirty-four-year-old woman facing a mastectomy for life-threatening breast cancer. She was reluctant to have the operation, feeling that male doctors are too casual in suggesting that women have their breasts removed. Based on what I knew of her case, I urged her to have the surgery, and spoke to her about the importance of having high expectations going into the operating room—of seeing the surgery as a chance to free her body from an offender, rather than the beginning of a downward spiral

◄ **Three years after her young husband died of lung cancer,** Lisa Bresnahan demonstrates for cancer patients the power of emotion in coping with illness. Bresnahan became a cancer support group leader after joining a group with her late husband, and says she still screams out her pain in stressful moments. *Photo by Steve Ringman*

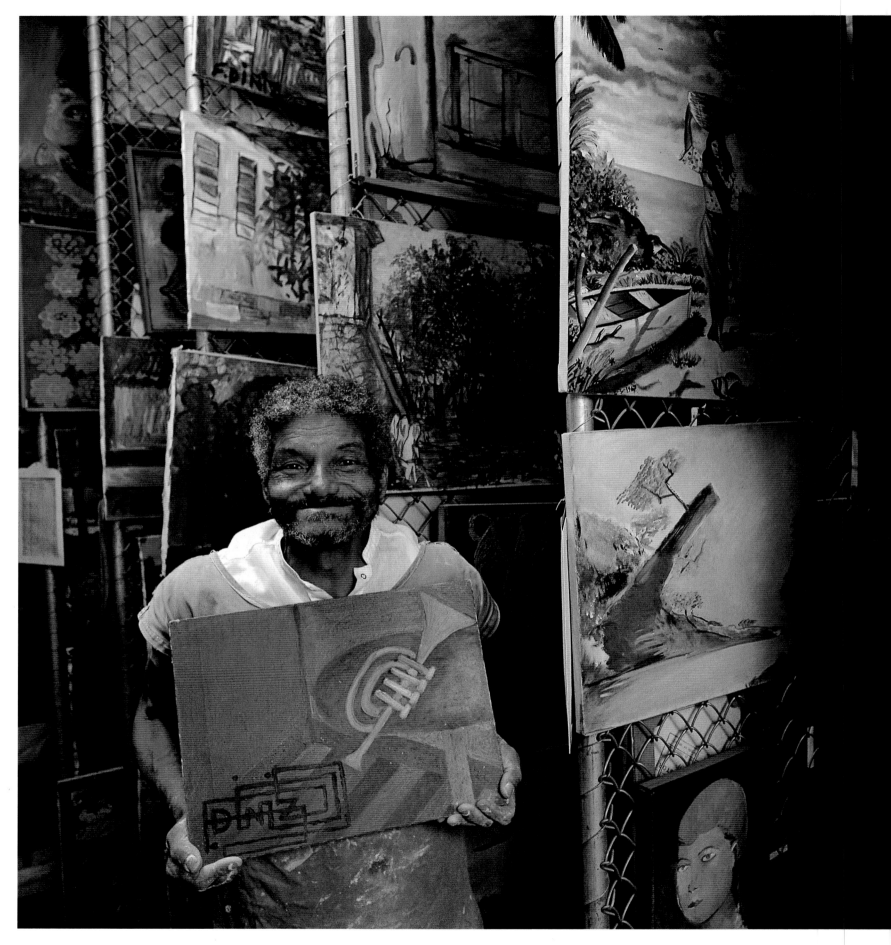

▲ **Therapy for mental patient Fernando Diniz becomes art** for the rest of us at Rio de Janeiro's Museum of Images from the Unconscious. Art critics and psychotherapists from around the world make pilgrimages to the Pedro II Psychiatric Center, which houses the museum's 250,000 pieces of patient-produced art — and where Diniz, whose work is often singled out by visiting curators, has spent forty of his seventy-one years. Psychiatrists have long recognized the healing attributes of creating art, and the Museum of Images from the Unconscious helps scholars as well. Said the late British psychiatrist R.D. Laing, "This museum represents a major contribution to the scientific study of the psychotic process." *Photo by Claus C. Meyer*

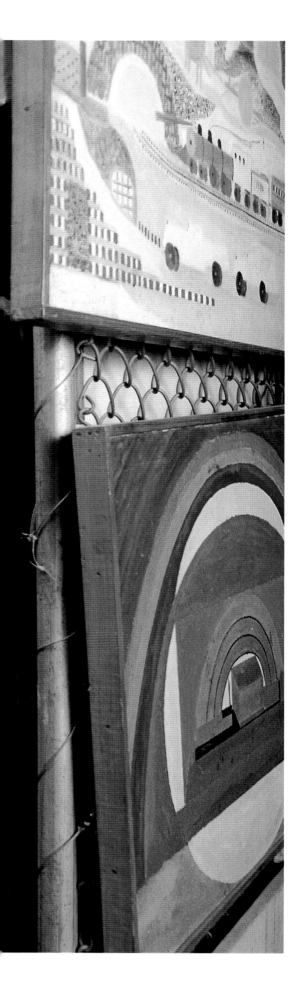

toward death. We talked for a while about the studies that have given a scientific basis to the anecdotal stories of the mind's power in fighting illness, and she thanked me and left.

She decided to go ahead with the surgery, but a week or so later her physician called me to say the operation had been canceled. The tumor, which the doctor had described to me earlier as "a hand grenade," had disappeared entirely. Sheila was taking no medication at the time; the only explanation is that her own cancer-fighting capability had risen to the occasion, with the full array of immune cells that produce the body's own chemotherapy and infuse it into the cancer cells.

While not every story is as remarkable as Sheila's, most of the patients I studied made a conscious decision, when their spiraling panic and illness reached a point of desperation, to reject all notions of inevitability. They became determined not to rely exclusively on treatment provided by others, but to take an active part in the quest for recovery. They accepted the physician's diagnosis and the unfavorable odds that came along with it, but refused to be deterred by the accompanying prediction of doom.

All of them were, in their own way, living out an ancient idea that is coming back into favor through current medical research—the idea that the healing system is connected to a belief system, that attitudes play a vital part in the recovery process. The medical community has acknowledged the human brain's ability to exercise a measure of control over the autonomic nervous system, and as a result is paying renewed attention to the patient's role in overcoming disease and maintaining good health.

Clearly, in our modern age, treatment for any disease requires the best that medical science has to offer; all the emotional determination in the world usually falls short without prompt and consistent medical intervention. But just as clearly, treating physical illness without paying corresponding attention to emotional needs can have only a partial effect.

More than 2,000 years after the death of Hippocrates, we are coming back to the original Hippocratic ideal of the patient not as a passive vessel into which the physician pours therapeutic skills and medicaments, but as a sovereign human being capable of generating powerful responses to disease. These powerful responses won't reverse every incidence of disease or illness; otherwise, we would live forever. But by beginning to recognize these powers, we are enhancing vital elements of the recovery process.

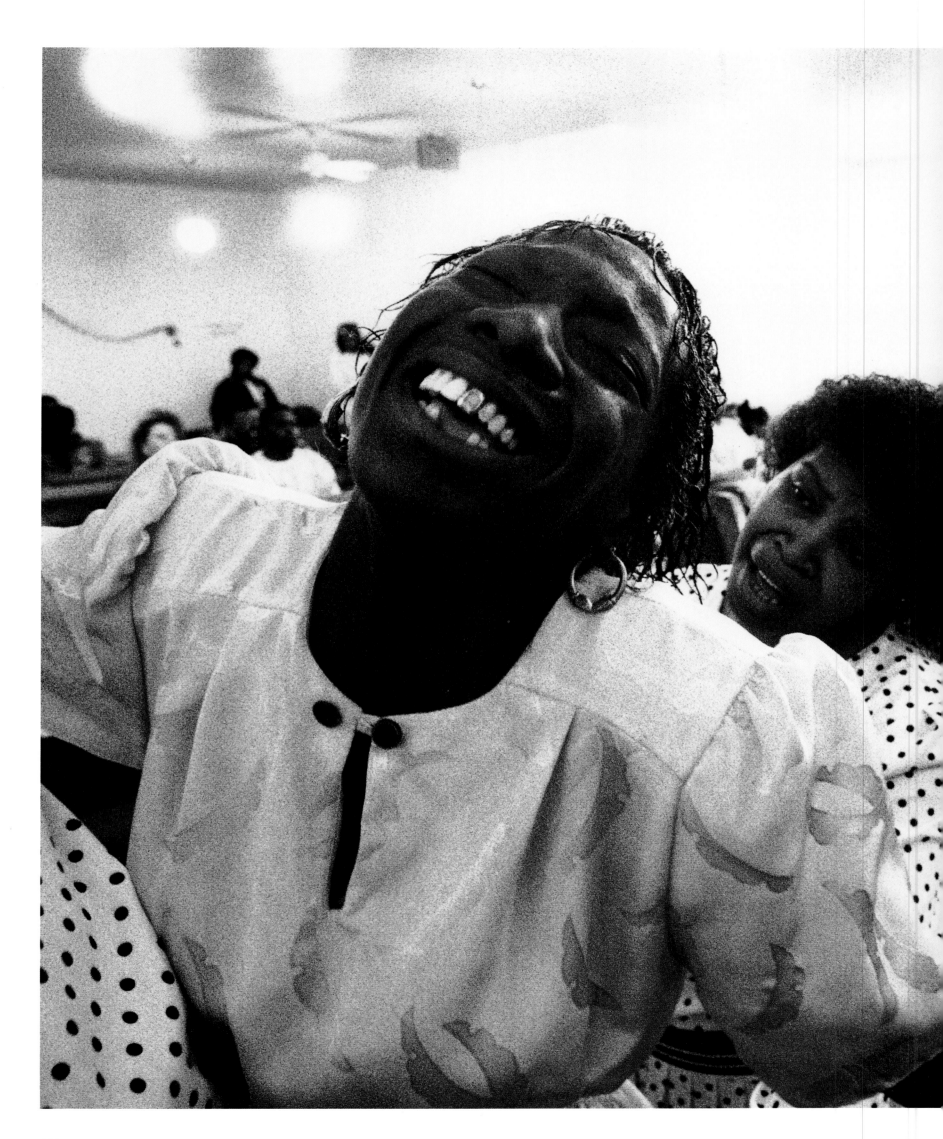

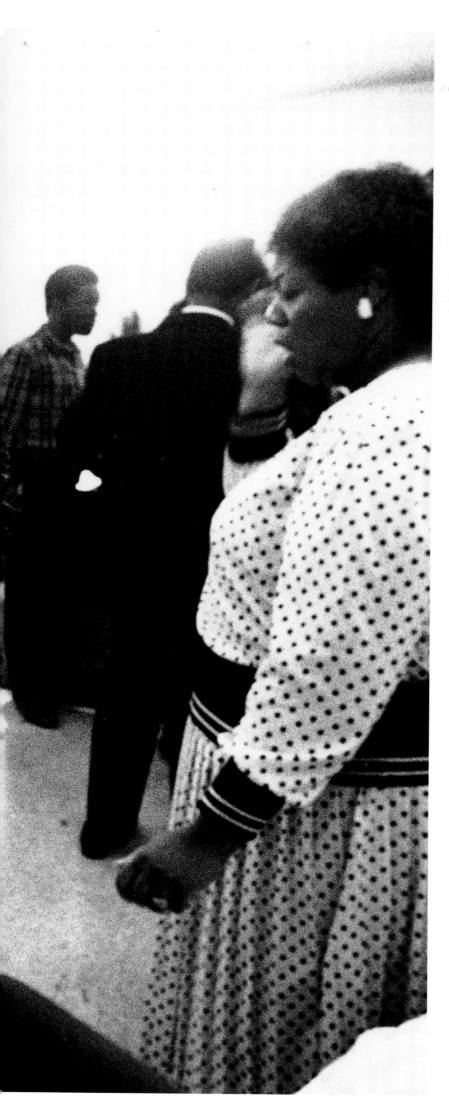

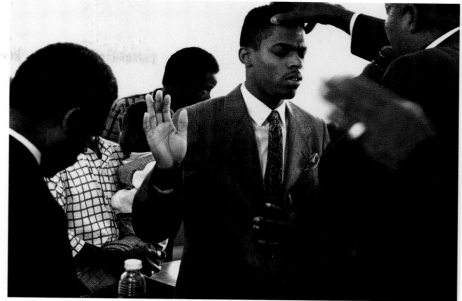

◄ **Moving with the spirit, a Texas woman looks to religious ecstasy** to heal her at the Deliverance Tabernacle Church of God in Christ. With an organist, guitarist, pianist, drummer, and saxophonist providing musical accompaniment, members of the Dallas church reach such a pitch of religious fervor that they speak in tongues — a sure sign, they say, of salvation.
Photo by J.W. Fry

▲"**We heal people through Jesus. We say special prayers for the ill.** You have to believe, and then we pray for you. That's all you need," says Sherman Mannor, Jr., the assistant pastor of the Deliverance Tabernacle Church of God in Christ. Here, pastor Ozell Byrd blesses Mannor's son Terry.
Photo by J.W. Fry

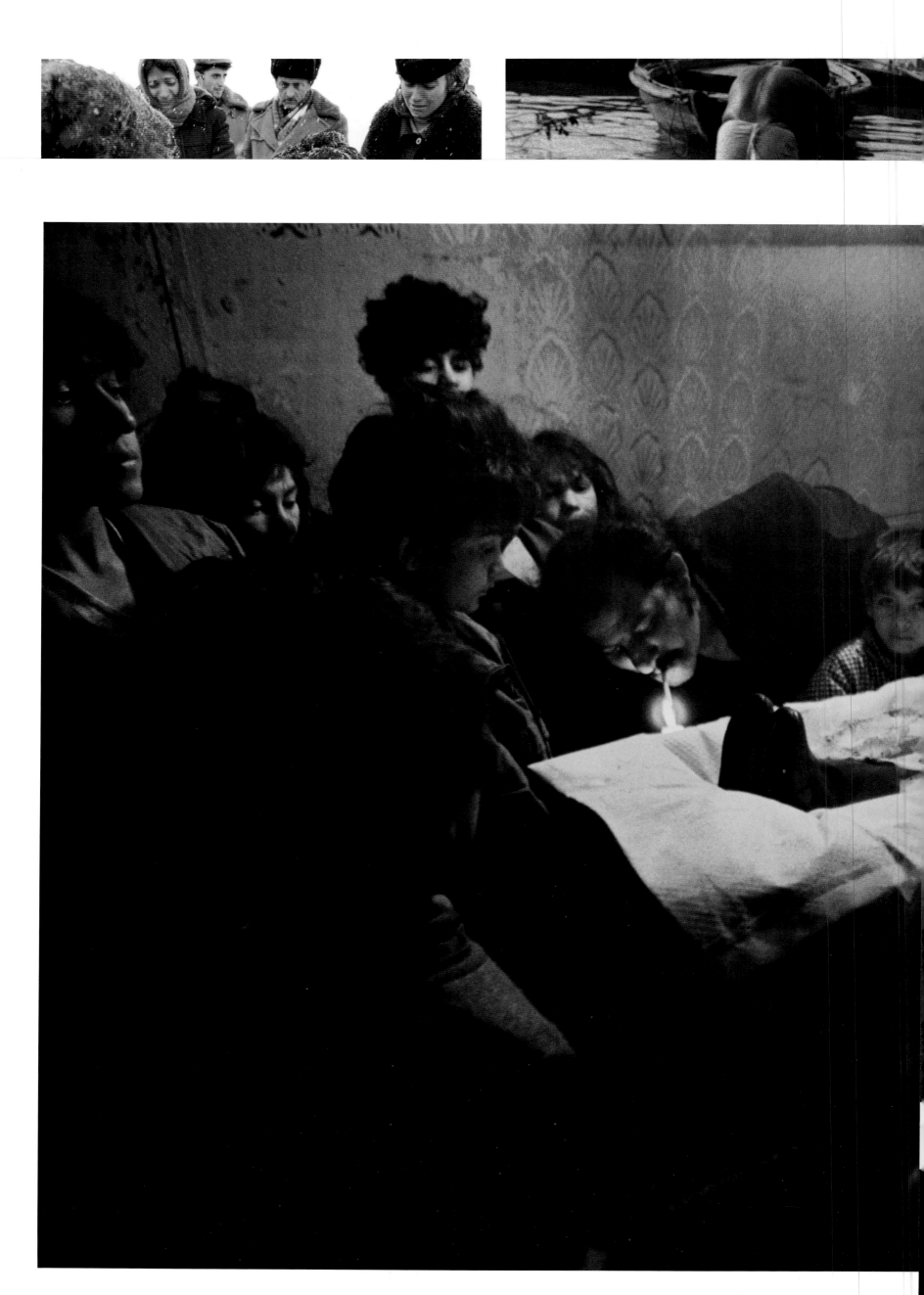

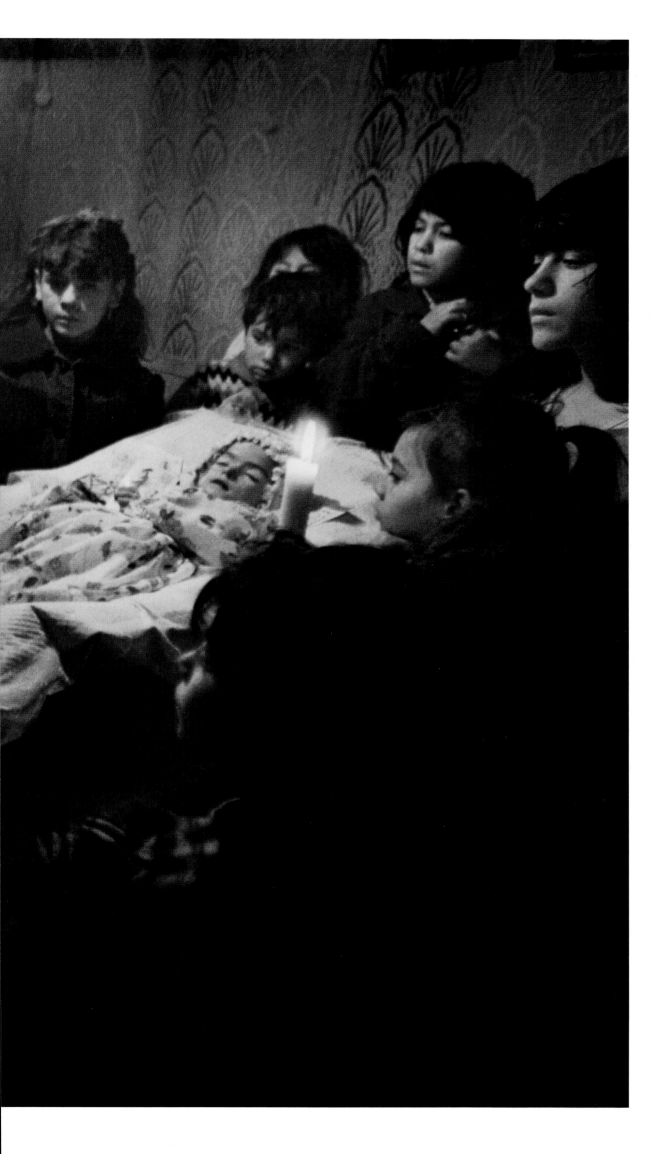

◄ **On the last night of a three-day Gypsy wake** in Bystrany, Czechoslovakia, friends and relatives gather around the body of a four-year-old girl. By custom, the body is never left unattended during the wake, which is followed by a burial ceremony. "This was a moment before the late evening," says photographer Mišo Suchý, "when all the kids of the community came by. It was absolutely silent. That's what I remember most — the silence."
Photo by Mišo Suchý

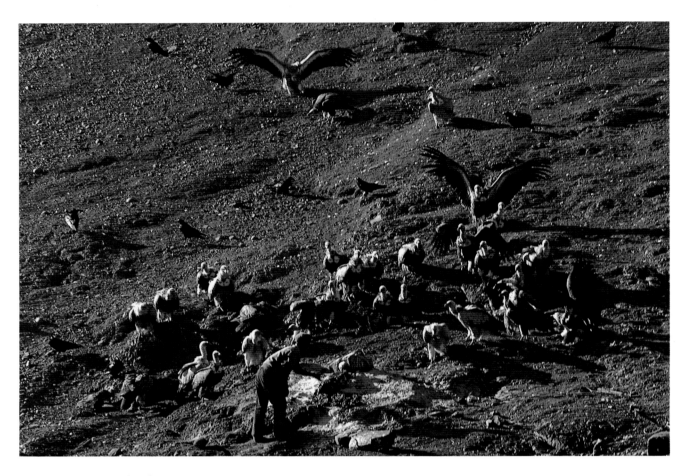

▲ **Bodies fly up to heaven more quickly when vultures carry them,** say the people of Tibet, where "sky burials" are a common occurrence. In a land so hard and rocky that digging a deep grave is impractical, corpses are ritually chopped up and left on boulders for the birds. There are some exceptions: holy men are usually cremated, victims of murder or execution get shallow earth graves, and the bodies of petty criminals and people who die of serious disease are dumped into rivers.
Photo by Leong Ka Tai

▶ **A chance at immortality awaits the frozen residents** of Trans Time, Inc., in Oakland, California. In the hope that medical science will one day find a cure for the disease that killed them, each of the seven people suspended upside down in one of Art Quaife's full-length capsules set aside at least $135,000 for the privilege of being frozen in liquid nitrogen at minus 320 degrees Fahrenheit within a few hours after death. "Every year," says company president Quaife, "millions of people are cremated or begin rotting underground. They're giving up their ability to survive. My message is that life is a bowl of cherries, and it's better to be alive than dead."
Photo by Nina Barnett

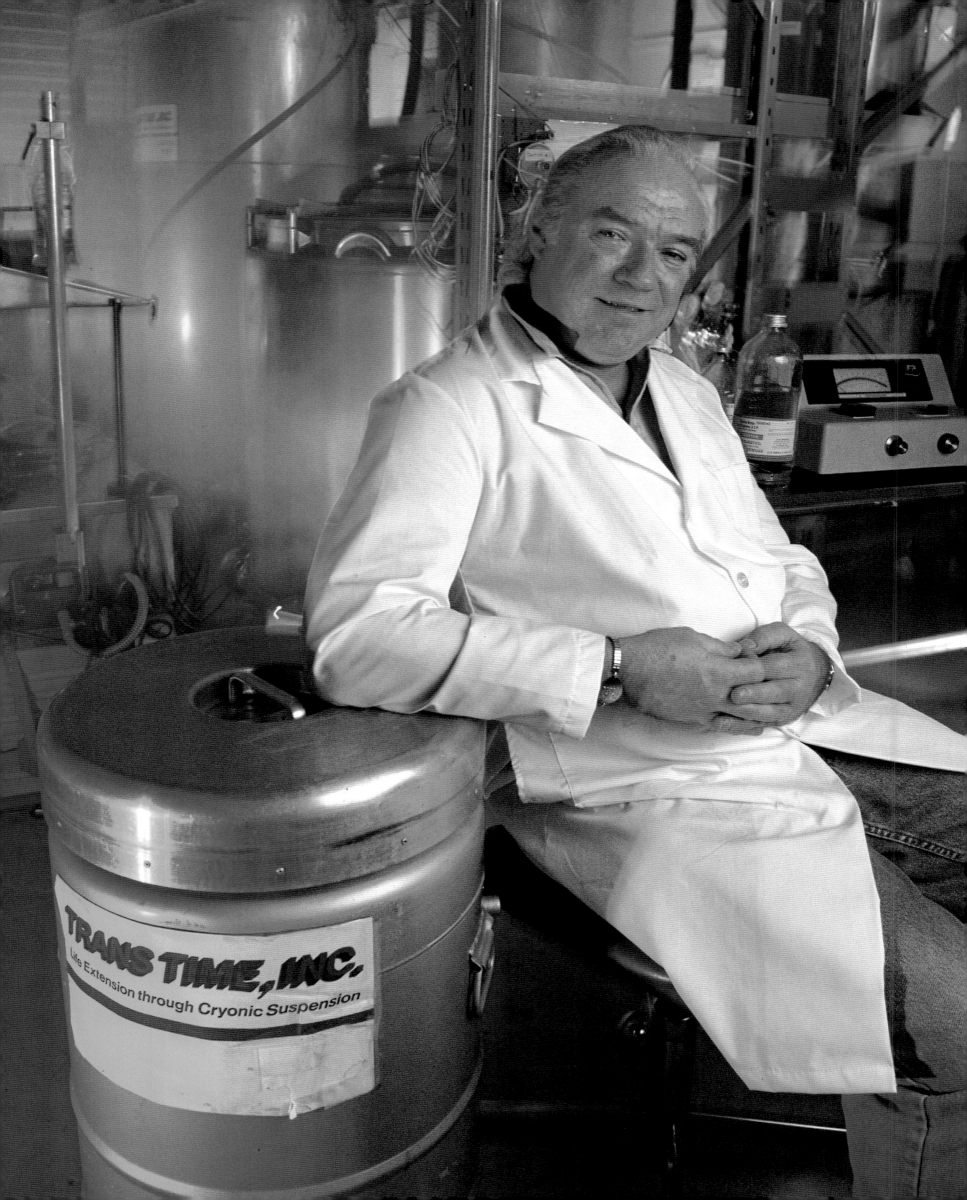

TRANS TIME, INC.
Life Extension through Cryonic Suspension

Combining t'ai chi and Western-style aerobics, residents of Harbin loosen up on the frozen banks of the Songhua River in northeastern China. *Photo by Robin Moyer*

DAWN OF THE MILLENNIUM

*As the century draws to a close, I think many of us are
surprised and impressed by the paradox that we are
still alive, and that we are still mortal. So is our planet, under
siege from industrial pollutants that have impaired
the ability of the skies, oceans, streams, forests, and wildlife
to regenerate themselves.*

—Judith Thurman

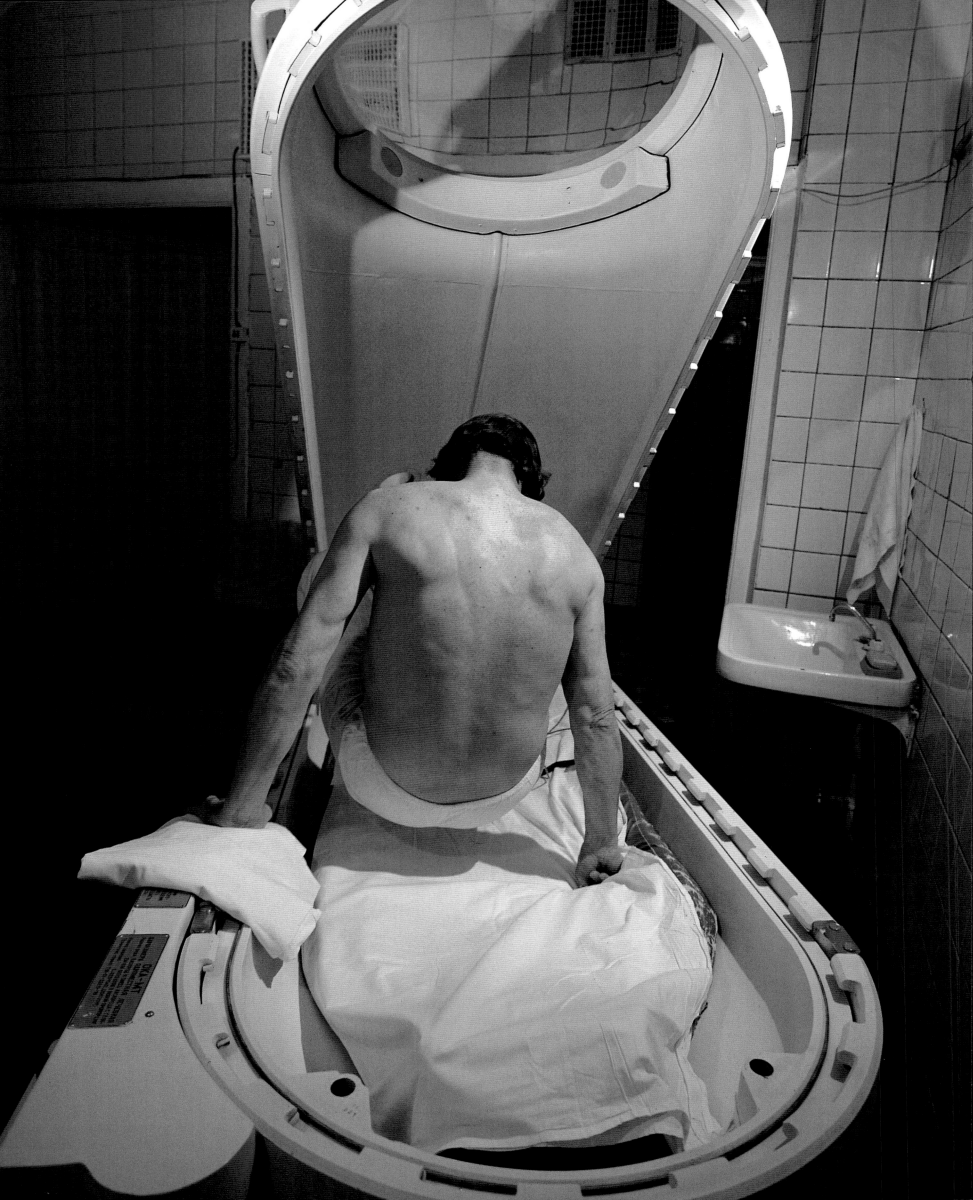

Reflections on the Twenty-First Century

JUDITH THURMAN

I GREW UP IN A POST-WAR HOUSING DEVELOPMENT BUILT ON LANDFILL that I have to assume was clean. The little garden apartments were rented by "intact" families: hopeful, hard-working young couples and their 2.5 children. The sidewalks hadn't been poured yet; the trees were saplings. And the sky overhead was of a gleaming, featureless blue that no longer exists in American cities except, perhaps, over a cemetery, on the last day of a four-day weekend. It was Technicolor blue: too pure and too untroubled to seem real. It is a color that has since been blurred, along with so many other certainties, and notions of order and purity, from that era.

The kids who grew up in the pristine suburbs of the fifties learned to fear death in their own way. From kindergarten on, we practiced taking shelter from the Russians' H-bombs by crawling under plywood desks in classrooms with glass walls. With the advent of warm weather, we began to worry about iron lungs. Swimming pools were off-limits to us, and we were strictly forbidden by our anxious parents to share a cup, or to let our lips touch the spout of a drinking fountain. The photographs from Hiroshima haunted our dreams. But more intimately frightening was the image of the March of Dimes poster child in her ruffled pinafore and her leg braces.

One afternoon in 1959, the fourth grade of my elementary school was summoned to the gym, where we were lined up to receive a sugar cube steeped in the Sabin polio vaccine, or—we didn't know which—a placebo. The vaccine had been approved for testing among schoolchildren, and I remember how proud, daring, and euphoric I felt to be participating in the experiment, and in history. The euphoria, I think, was a child's first vicarious taste of power, a taste of victory—not only over polio, but over all of life's oppressive and uncontrollable forces. When I opened my mouth to receive my dose (of placebo, as it turned out), I felt the kind of awe and fervor that believers bring to Communion. But in many ways, that lump of sugar—so mundane yet so transforming—was the emblem of the faith that an entire generation would place in medicine's magic powers to heal.

Our faith may have been naive, but in its historical context, it wasn't misplaced. I have a son now. He was born in 1989. His life expectancy, at birth, was seventy-two. The life expectancy of my mother, born before the First World War, was forty-seven. The life expectancy of her father, born in 1871—the year of the Paris Commune—was somewhere around thirty-five. Until the discovery of sulfa drugs in 1932, the greatest of medical specialists was virtually helpless to cure the simplest infectious disease, and the humblest country doctor of today seems omnipotent by comparison.

◄ **Pure oxygen under pressure awaits this user of a hyperbaric chamber** in Moscow's Botkin Hospital. Although documented medical uses of the hyperbaric chamber are relatively few, the allure of pure oxygen under pressure continues to entice researchers in the United States and the Soviet Union. The chamber is most commonly used in the United States to treat sufferers of carbon monoxide poisoning and the bends, but the National Aeronautic and Space Administration (NASA) is sponsoring secret research involving other possible uses. In the Soviet Union, doctors use the chamber to treat a variety of health problems — including trauma, chronic alcoholism, gastric ulcers, and cancer — a practice most American doctors do not condone.
Photo by Sam Garcia

But even a well-inoculated child frets deeply about survival. I was anguished for weeks when my science teacher explained that the sun was a slowly cooling star that eventually would burn out. At the same time, I was elated to learn that penicillin had been discovered attacking the bacteria in a petri dish of common mold. I figured that in the aftermath of a nuclear war, when my family had regrouped with blankets, flashlights, and lunch boxes at the nearest subway station, I could grow my own supply on stale bread. Such thinking was probably typical of a generation that believed the end of the world was just as imminent as the discovery of a panacea for its ills.

As the century draws to a close, I think many of us are surprised and impressed by the paradox that we are still alive, and that we are still mortal. So is our planet, under siege from industrial pollutants that have impaired the ability of the skies, oceans, streams, forests, and wildlife to regenerate themselves. Smallpox has been exterminated, but development is killing the rainforest, which has been a living laboratory for modern pharmaceuticals. By the year 2000, public health officials hope to announce the worldwide eradication of polio. But when can we hope for such an announcement about dysentery, which kills more than three million children every year? And when can we expect such an announcement about AIDS?

The great Danish storyteller, Isak Dinesen, suffered from another infectious disease that once spread death and hopelessness, one that is now treatable with antibiotics: syphilis. Alluding to it in a tale, she wrote: "There exists a true humanity, which will ever remain a gift, and is to be accepted by one human being as it is given to him by a fellow human. The one who gives has himself been a receiver. In this way, link by link, a chain is made from land to land and from generation to generation. Rank, wealth, nationality in this matter all go for nothing.... Strange and wonderful to consider how in such community we are bound to foreigners whom we have never seen and to dead men and women whose names we have never heard."

It's time that we accepted Dinesen's moral challenge to consider the real meaning of the word immunity. Not until the beginning of this century did it have the sense, "exempt from disease." Its original definition was exempt from service, duty, or liability—an unfair freedom or privilege. In that light, perhaps, we should reframe our goals for medical research and progress in the next century. We need activism and vigilance on environmental issues, and the abolition of the inequities in the delivery of health care. We need preventive medicine that discourages our bad habits and fortifies our resistance. We need tireless research on and dedication to a cure for the diseases of modern life. But materially and spiritually, we can no longer afford "immunity."

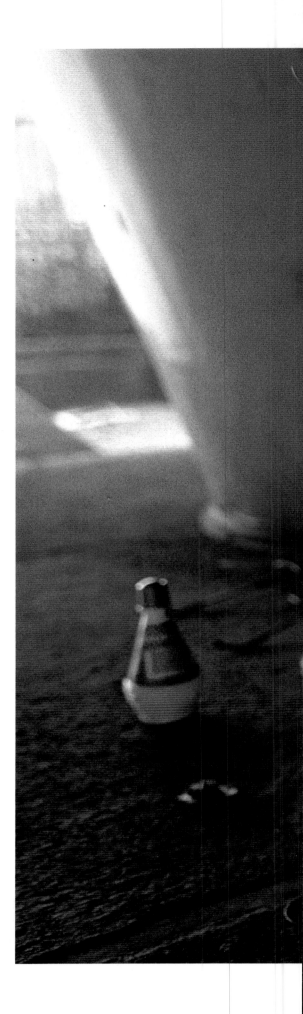

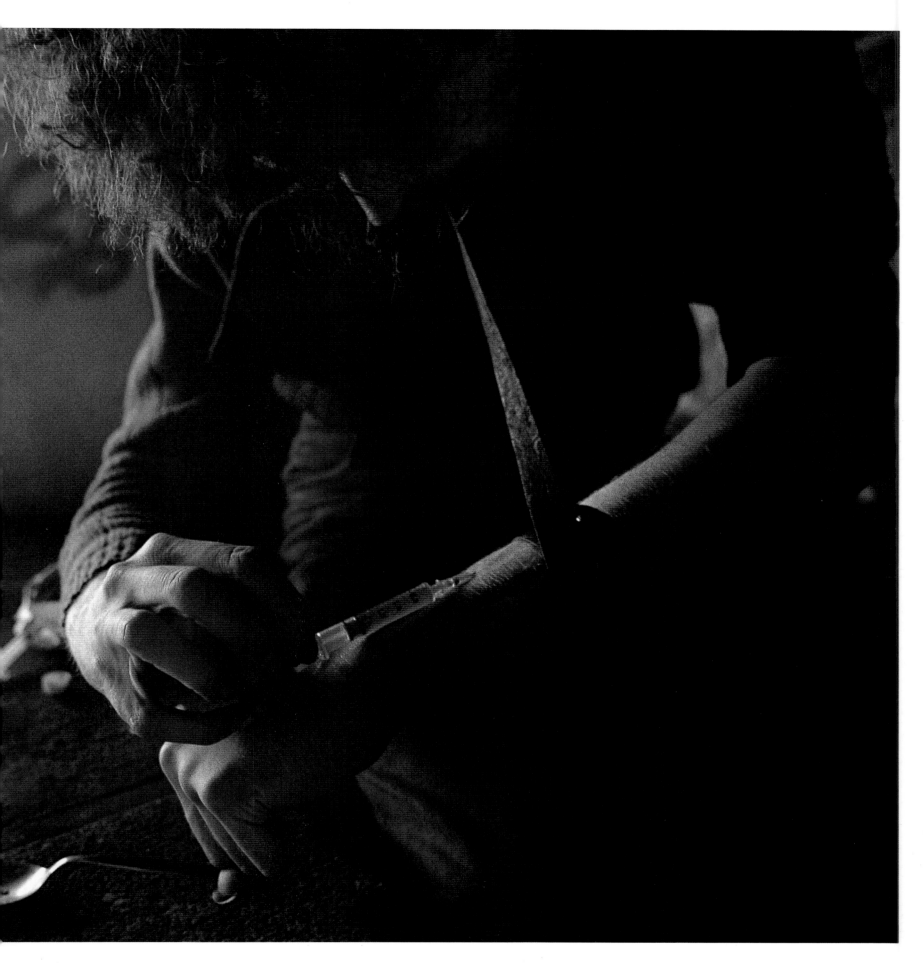

▲ **One of the millions of people around the world addicted to drugs,** a Dutch heroin addict known as "The Professor" finds refuge under a bridge in Amsterdam. In the United States, heroin, a derivative of the opium poppy, has been challenged by crack cocaine in recent years as the illegal addictive drug of choice. An estimated half-million Americans are addicted to heroin; a like number are presumed to be addicted to crack. Many more are addicted to legal drugs such as alcohol and tobacco. *Photo by Barry Lewis*

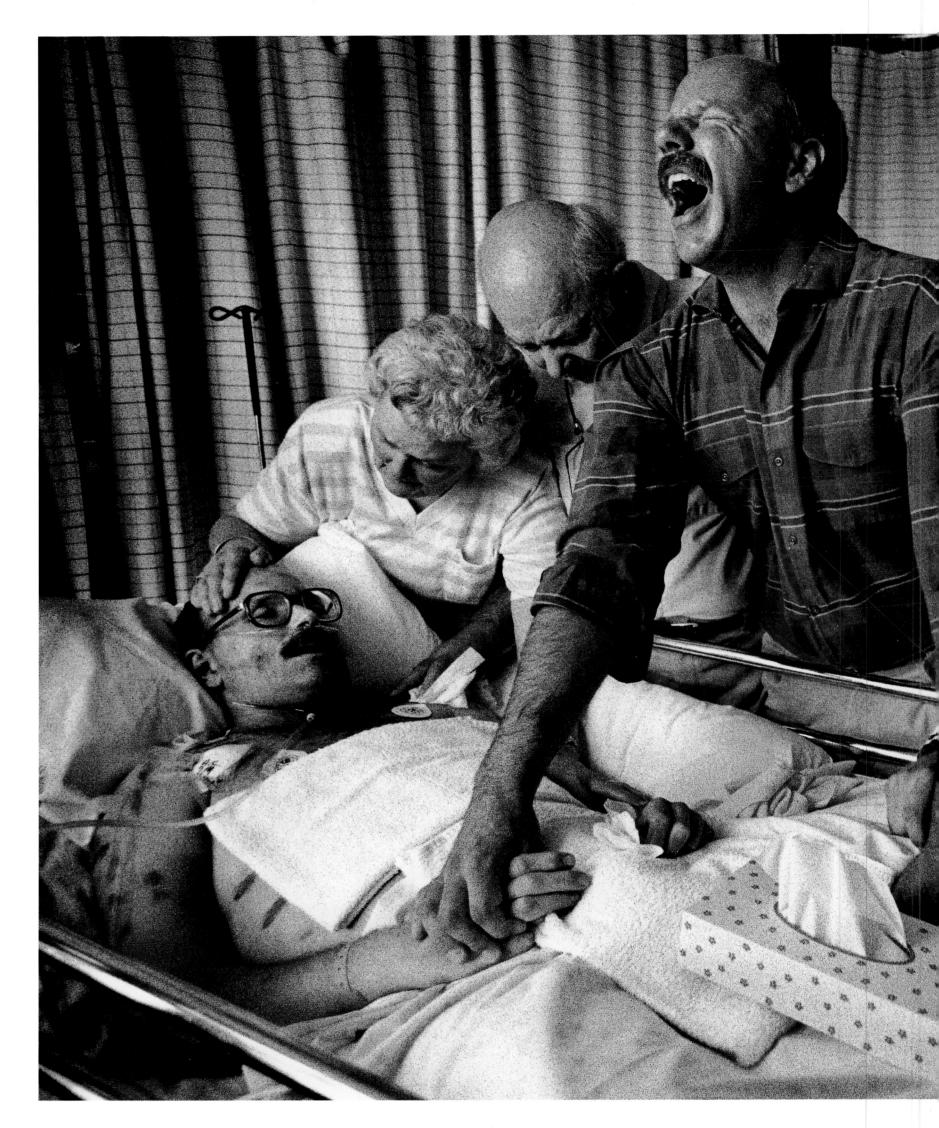

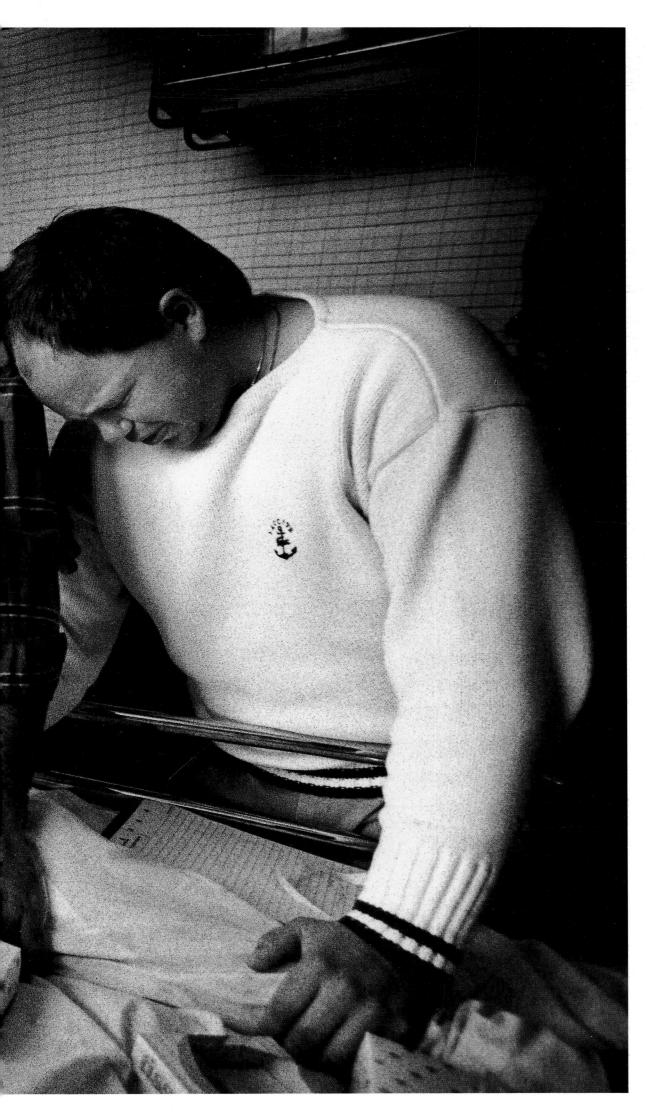

◄ **The killer virus of the 1980s claims another victim,** as the family of thirty-three-year-old Tom Fox mourns at his bedside in his final moments of life. "I love you so much, son," says Doris Fox, moments after Tom has told her and his father Bob, his older brother, Bob Jr., and his younger brother, John, that he could no longer breathe. "Just relax and let it go. You're almost there." On Tom's request, moments earlier, a doctor had withdrawn the ventilator that was forcing pure oxygen into his starving lungs.

By the end of the 1980s, more than 300,000 people, including 70,000 Americans, had died of diseases associated with acquired immune deficiency syndrome; as many as ten million more were infected with the human immunodeficiency virus, or HIV, which causes AIDS. Some progress has been made in the development of drugs that treat the symptoms of AIDS, thus prolonging the lives of many patients, but health officials say that a cure is still many years away. Currently, the most optimistic hope for the near future is that AIDS will become a manageable chronic condition, similar to diabetes.

"Good night, Tom," says Bob, Jr. "He's letting go," adds his father. Then, ten minutes after the removal of the ventilator, Tom dies.
Photo by Michael A. Schwarz

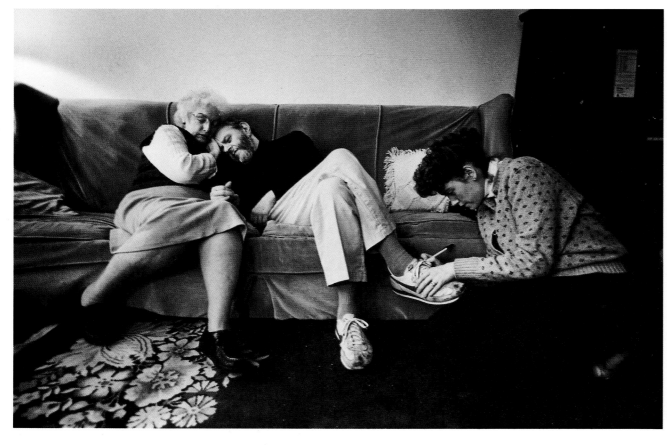

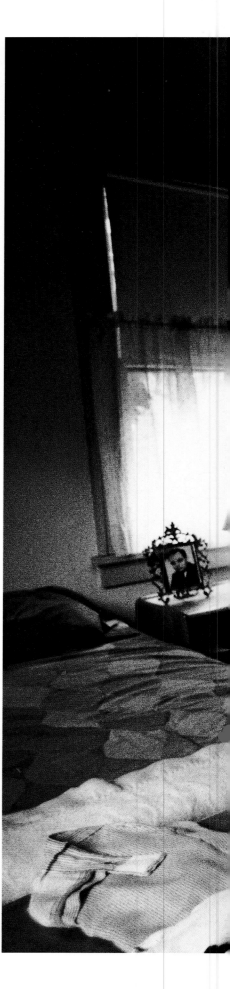

▲ **"There are two sets of victims: the patients and their families,"** says John Jaeger, executive director of the New York City chapter of the Alzheimer's Association.

About ten percent of people over the age of sixty suffer from Alzheimer's, a disease marked by brain lesions that cause forgetfulness, disorientation, confusion, sleep disorders, wandering, incontinence, and eventually death. Ellen Berliner of Mt. Lebanon, Pennsylvania, watched her husband, Art, deteriorate for six years before she made the decision to institutionalize him. "It was an agonizing time," says Ellen *(right, with Nanci Keefe of the Alzheimer's research clinic at the University of Pittsburgh Medical School)*. Art was fifty-seven years old, and a successful marketing executive, when diagnosed with the disease, which is named after the German neurophysicist who identified it in 1907.

There is no known way to prevent or treat Alzheimer's, and in fact no way to diagnose it. "Right now," Jaeger says, "it's a diagnosis of elimination. If it isn't anything else, it's Alzheimer's."

Ellen comforts Art *(above)*, as their daughter Lauren writes his name on his shoes as a prelude to

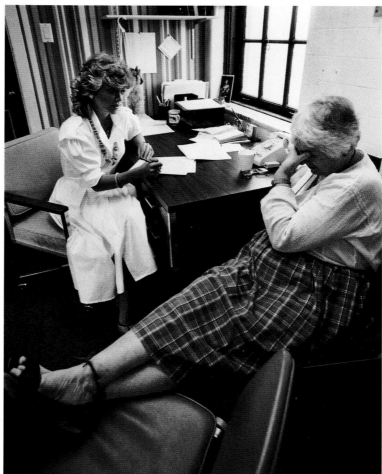

his institutionalization. Now, Art can no longer speak, and doesn't recognize Ellen *(right)*, although "he does know that I'm this nifty person who comes and hugs him and kisses him."

Adds Ellen: "I don't laugh and

have fun like I used to. I miss him in my life. Nearly everyone in this situation goes through a similar thing — they're not married, they're not single, they're just in limbo."
Photos by Lynn Johnson

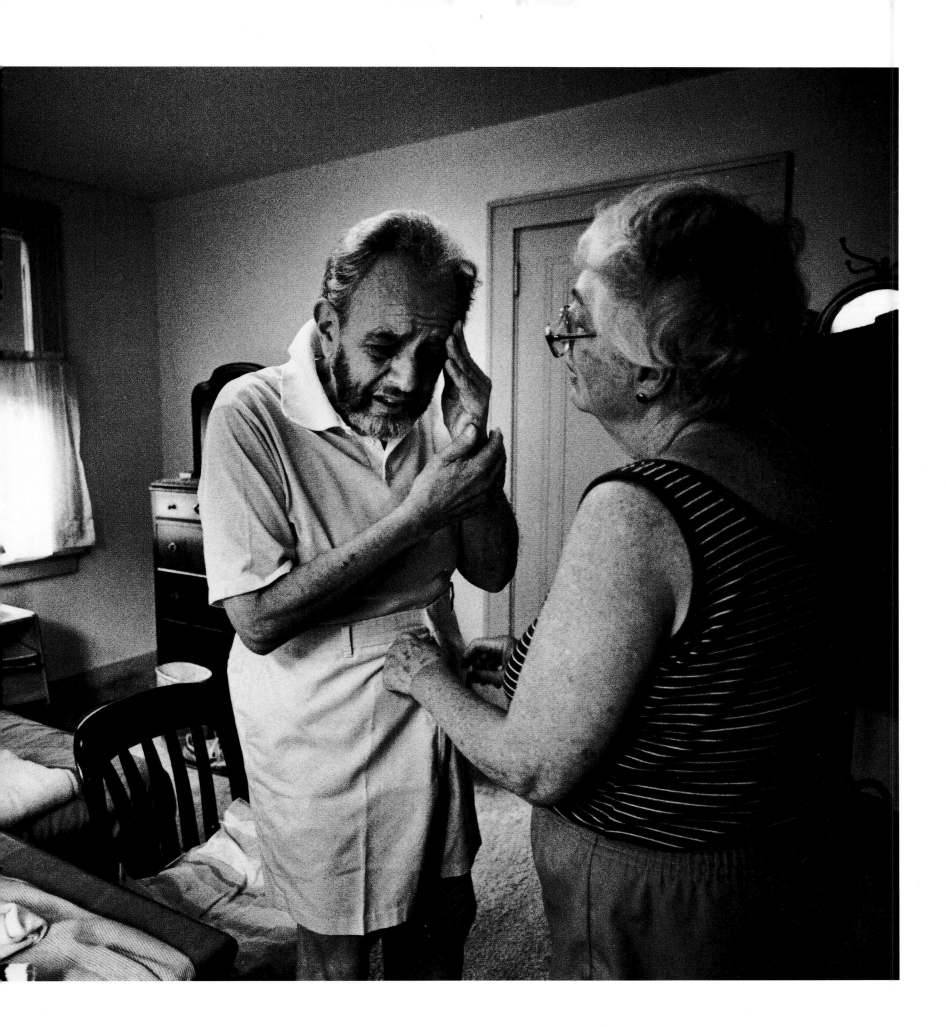

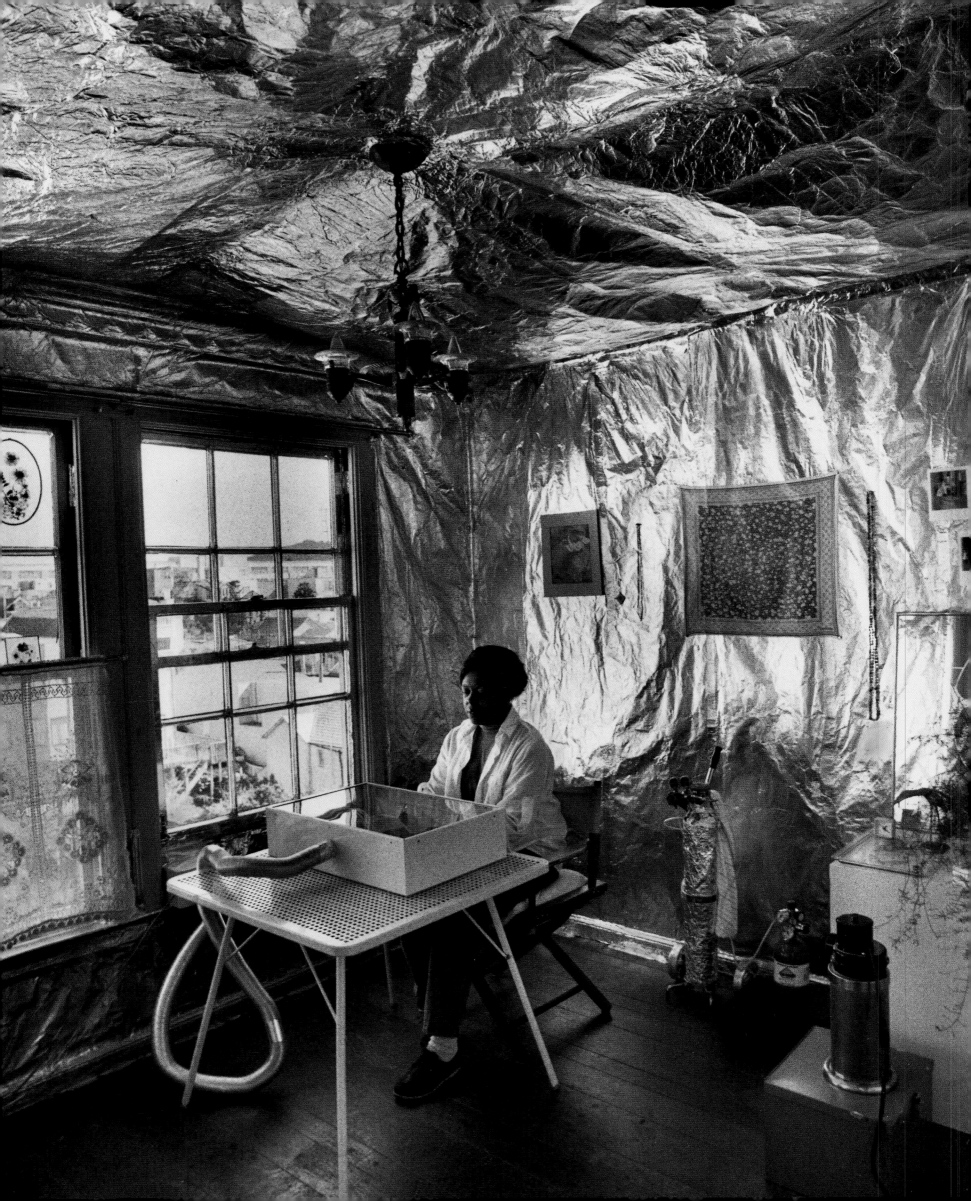

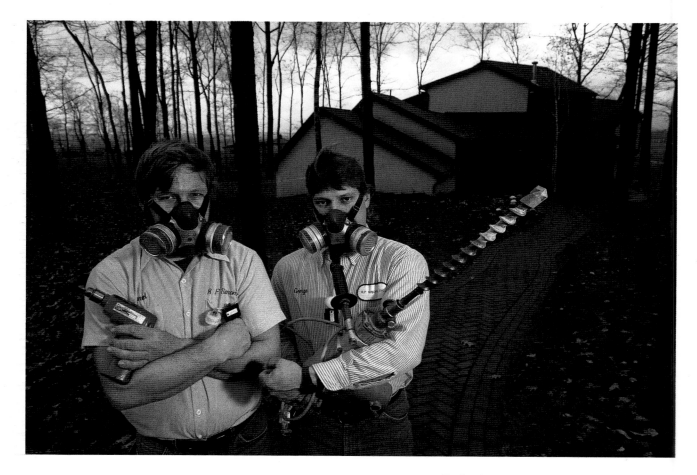

◄ **Victim of a strange and frightening twentieth-century syndrome,** Anita Hill lives in a world devoid of comforts that most Americans take for granted. The highly allergic Hill suffers from what has come to be known as environmental illness. Her house is draped in foil, and she uses a specially designed box to read books so she doesn't have to touch or smell the pages.

Some epidemiologists say environmental illness is psychological in nature, but a National Academy of Sciences commission disagrees, saying that fifteen percent of the U.S. population has "an increased allergic sensitivity to chemicals commonly found in household products." The syndrome is most commonly marked by the inability to tolerate fumes from paint, copy machines, fabric stores, cigarettes, and detergents. Symptoms can include seizures, headaches, nausea, irregular heartbeat, and muscle aches.
Photo by Frederic Larson

▲ **Radon-busters prepare to root out the potentially dangerous gas** from a house in Barto, Pennsylvania. The colorless, odorless, and tasteless radon, which comes from the natural breakdown of uranium, is usually harmless in outdoor air. It can, however, occasionally reach dangerous levels in enclosed spaces, increasing the risk of lung cancer for those who breathe it. Radon remedial specialists, like Daniel Dise and George Russell, typically try to create a pressure field outside or underneath a house to draw the gas out.
Photo by Michael J. Bryant

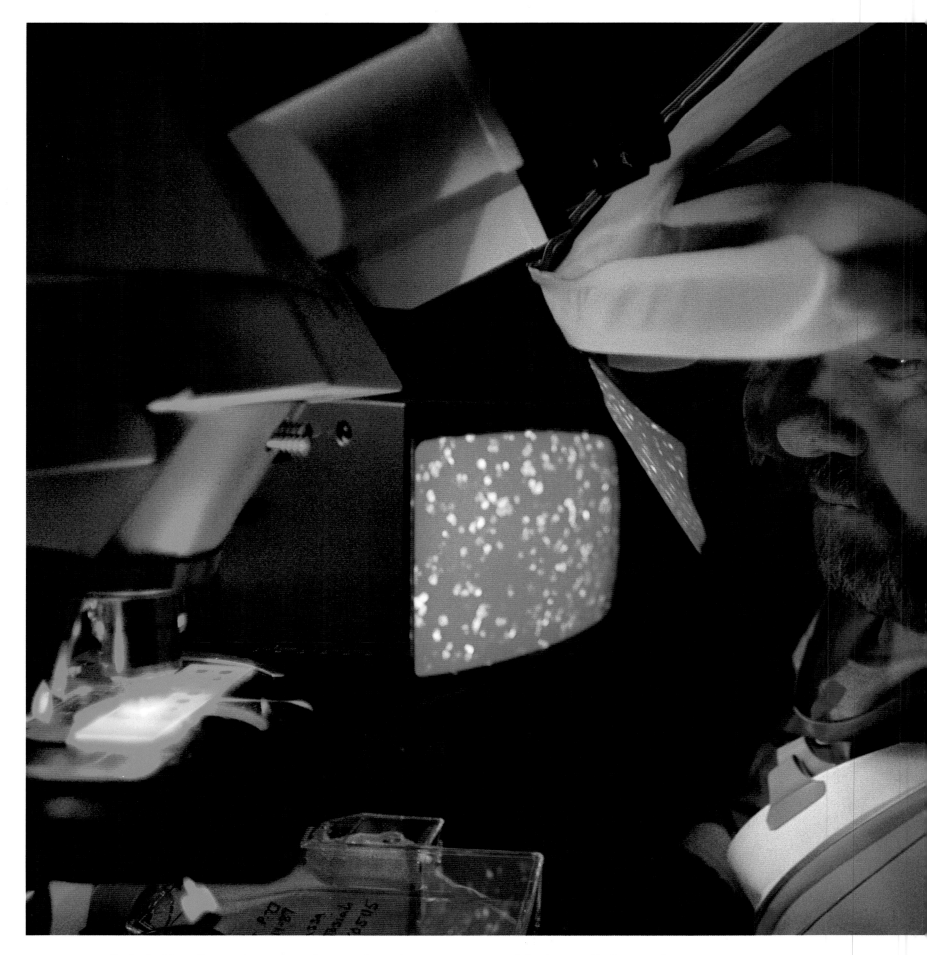

▲ **Protected from the most lethal viruses known,** Dr. Michael Kiley of the Centers for Disease Control in Atlanta watches a television monitor hooked up to a microscope in order to look for cells infected with deadly Lassa fever. Before entering the laboratory, one of only two such maximum-containment facilities in the United States, Kiley and his fellow researchers don full-body, pressurized suits that are connected by hoses to a breathing air system. Inside the lab, where the researchers study a variety of deadly viruses, the air is filtered, and the doors, walls, floors, and ceilings are sealed airtight. As the researchers leave, their suits are chemically decontaminated in a special chamber. "It's normal work," says Kiley, "once you get used to the suit." *Photo by Matthew Naythons, M.D., with Bill Pierce*

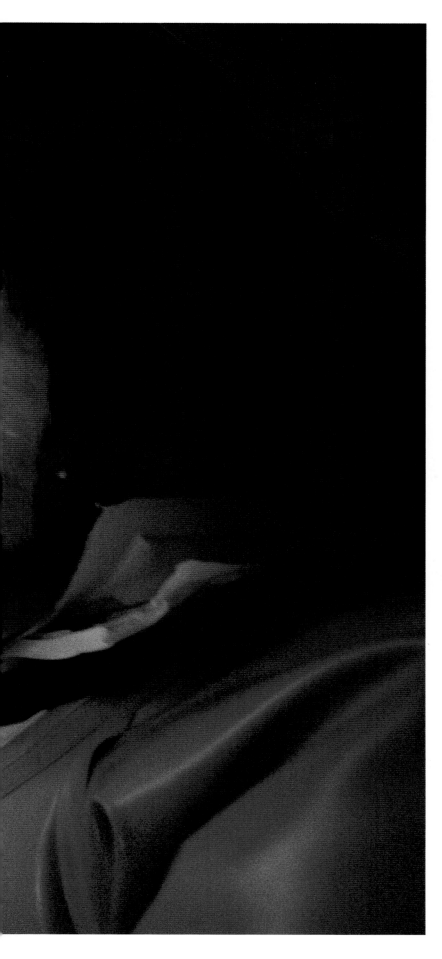

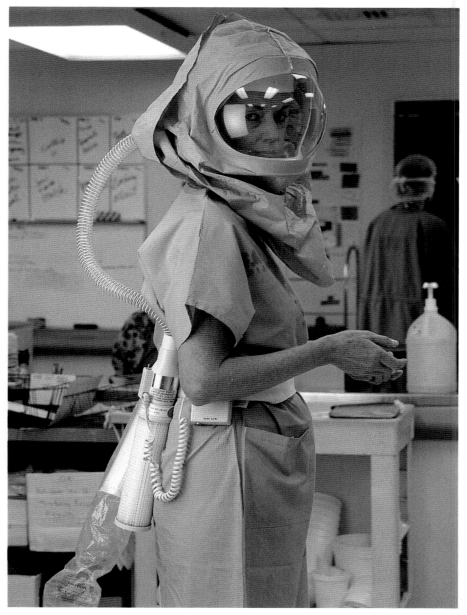

▲ **Shrouded in controversy as well as in her protective suit,** San Francisco orthopedic surgeon Lorraine Day models the operating room garb that she claims protects her from exposure to the AIDS virus. Twenty-seven U.S. health workers were accidentally infected with the virus in the 1980s, but most medical experts say that suits like Day's, which is designed to keep her from breathing aerosolized blood particles, don't solve the problem — and may contribute to misconceptions about how AIDS is spread. "It's very difficult to get infected," says Dr. Laurens White, a past president of the California Medical Association, "even in the operating room. And there's no proof that inhaling infected blood will give you AIDS."
Photo by Nina Barnett

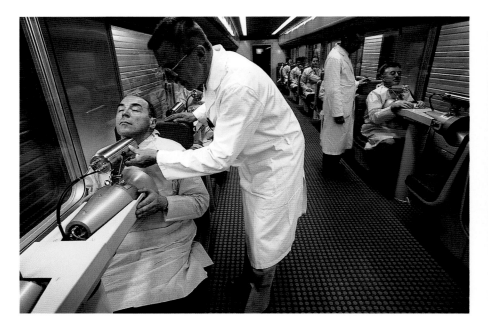

▲ **This traveling radiation-detection lab is one innovation** the French hope they never have to use. The high-speed railroad car can reach the site of a nuclear accident anywhere in Europe within twenty-four hours, and is capable of measuring human radiation poisoning as well as environmental samples. After the Chernobyl accident in 1986, the French sent a similarly equipped truck to the Soviet Union. France has one of the world's most ambitious nuclear power programs, with more than fifty plants in operation.
Photo by Karen Kasmauski

▶ **Transfixed by the horror of human destruction,** schoolchildren at the Hiroshima Peace Memorial Museum look at a wax re-creation of the aftermath of the atomic bomb dropped on the Japanese city by the United States on August 6, 1945. Official estimates are that 80,000 people were killed in the bomb blast, and that another 60,000 died from its effects within a year. The man-made plague of weaponry has become exponentially more powerful in the years since atomic bombs were dropped on Hiroshima and, three days later, Nagasaki. One MX missile has more than 200 times the power of the Hiroshima bomb, and one Trident submarine carries about 1,000 times the power.
Photo by Karen Kasmauski

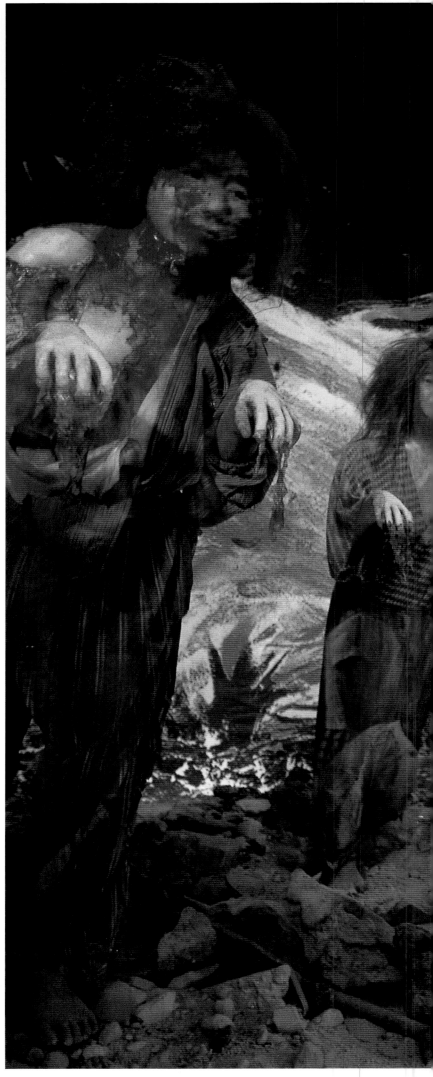

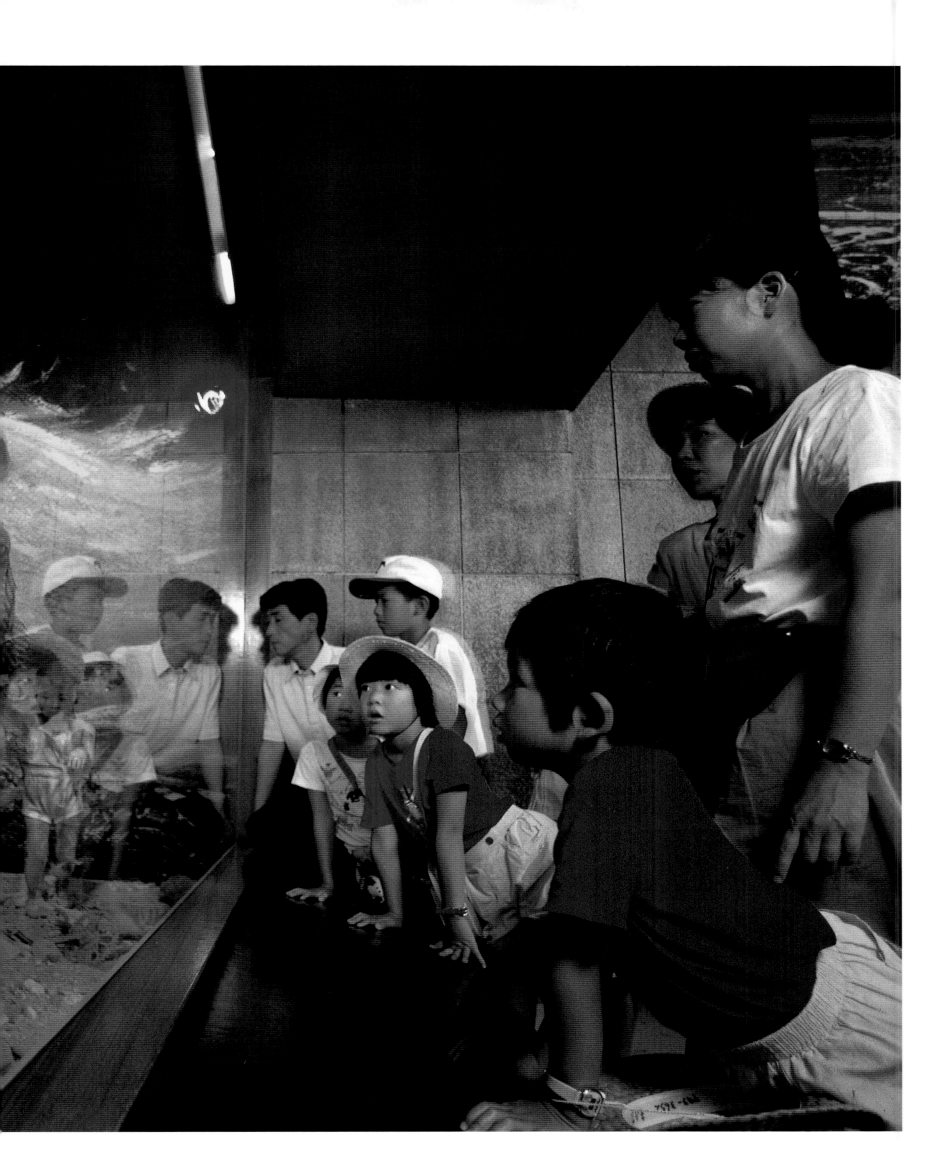

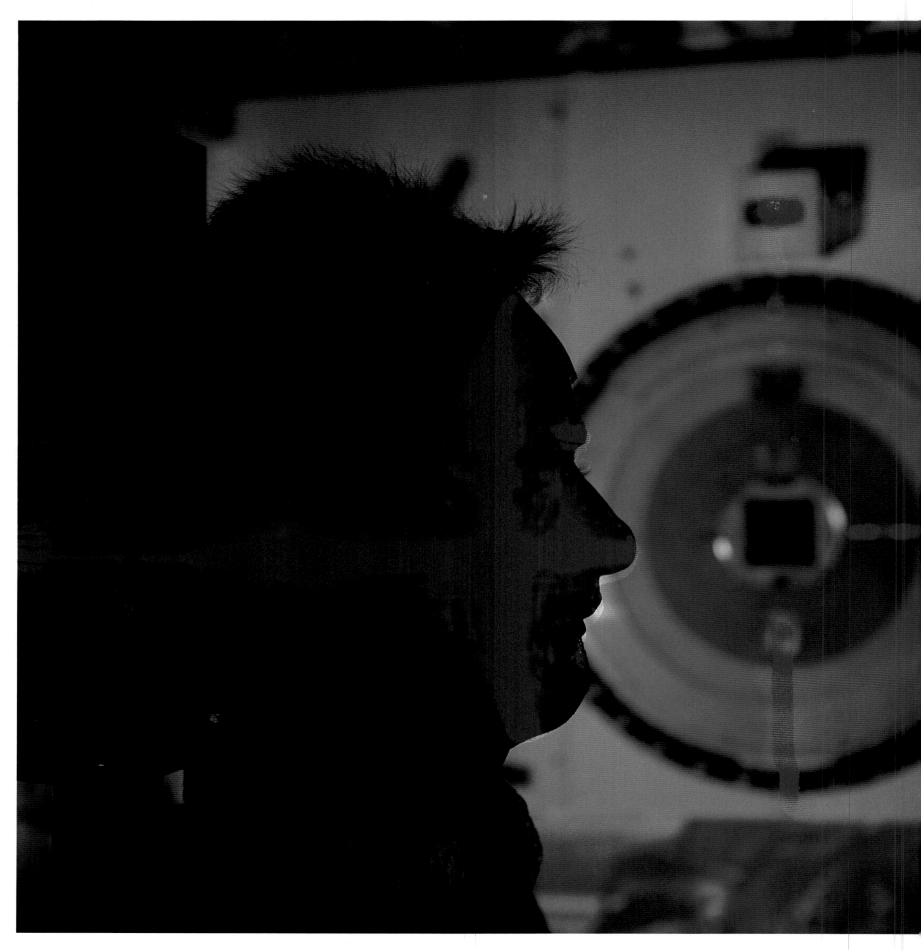

▲ **A neon laser beam glows red in preparation for neutron therapy for cancer patients** at the Fermi National Accelerator Laboratory in Batavia, Illinois. The low-power neon laser is used to align the patient with the neutron beam, which then attacks the tumor. Patients whose tumors may resist conventional radiation therapy come to Fermi as often as three times a week for treatment with the colorless neutron beam, which goes through the patient in a procedure as painless as an X ray. The side effects are no worse than those of other forms of radiation therapy, leading Fermi's Dr. Arlene Lennox to say, "I'd like to bring the technology we have here into hospitals." The cost, she adds, would be about fifteen million dollars per hospital.
Photo by Gary S. Chapman

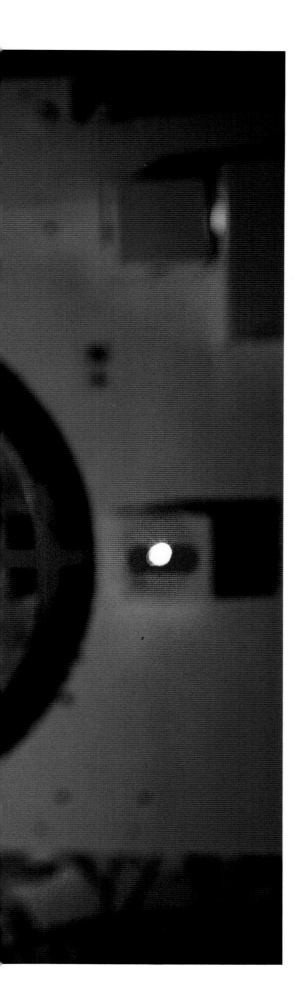

The Brain and Its Mysteries

R I C H A R D   R E S T A K ,   M . D .

At every moment, the miraculous, wonderful brain operates on three interconnected, interdependent levels of ever-bustling activity. At the behavioral level, ideas and thoughts originate in the cerebral cortex and are expressed in spoken and written language, in gesture—even in the thoughtful employment of silence.

At the microscopic level, untold numbers of the brain's 200 billion nerve cells or neurons are activated in intricate weblike patterns that one neuroscientist once whimsically compared to an enchanted loom. With each cell communicating with between 1,000 and 10,000 other cells, the total number of possible interactions exceeds the number of particles in the universe.

And even further down, on the molecular level of brain organization, around sixty neurotransmitters, the brain's chemical messengers, stimulate, inhibit, or modulate communication. In addition, information is conveyed by means of the living brain's biochemical, bioelectric, and magnetic field forces.

Each of the three levels is related to and reflects each of the other two levels in ways that we cannot explain. It's unlikely that any fully convincing explanation is even possible, since thoughts, neuronal activity patterns, and neurotransmitter interactions involve separate and distinct methods of discourse and understanding. For instance, no matter how much we learn about the brain, it's unlikely that a sentence such as "I love you" will ever be precisely correlated with the swirling of neurotransmitters or the kaleidoscopic interplay of several million neurons. That's because love and neurons and neurotransmitters, like stars and starlings and starlets, cannot be meaningfully equated.

Of course, the brain is not as mysterious to us as it once was; we've learned more about the brain in the past 50 years than we did in the previous 500. The scope of this accomplishment tempts us to believe that one day we will fully understand the brain. But it's helpful to remember the ancient Asian proverb, "The eye that can see all things cannot see itself." Can the brain that knows all things know itself? Are our attempts to understand the brain, in other words, limited by the brain itself? So far, no fully satisfying response to that intriguing philosophical inquiry has been forthcoming.

Nevertheless, fruitful explorations into the brain's mysteries will continue. And, as additional discoveries occur, even more tantalizing insights into the brain's functioning arise. Because of the intimate connections between the brain and the mind, discoveries about the brain provide information about the intriguing and mysterious creatures that are likely to remain more fascinating to us than anything else in the universe—ourselves.

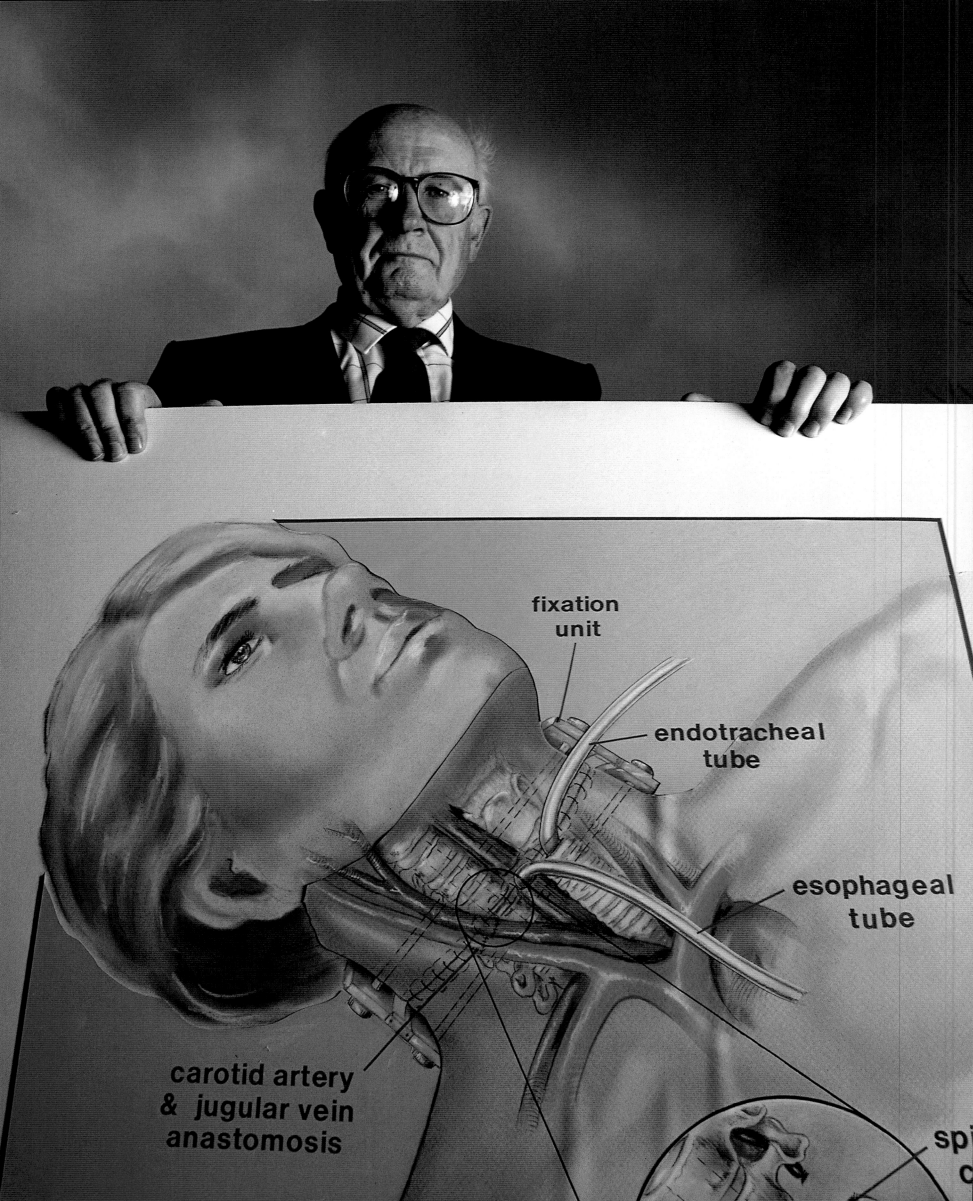

fixation
unit

endotracheal
tube

esophageal
tube

carotid artery
& jugular vein
anastomosis

sp

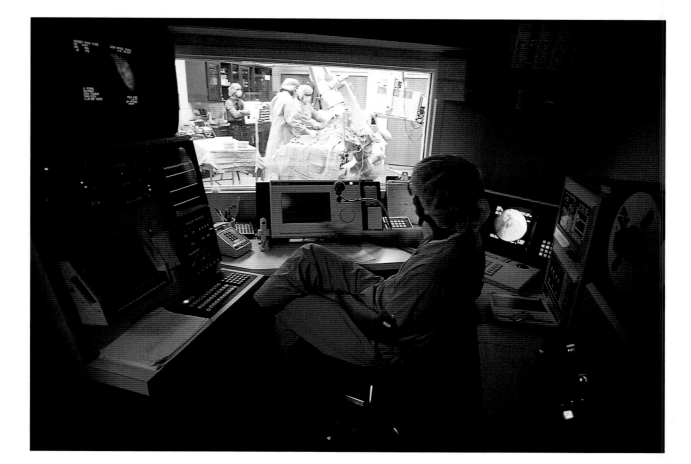

◀ **Head transplants may seem like science fiction,** but Dr. Robert White is perfectly serious: he says the day is coming when he'll be able to perform what he prefers to call a "body transplant," in which a healthy human head is taken from a diseased body and placed onto a healthier one. White, the director of neuro-surgery and of the brain research laboratory at Cleveland Metro-politan General/Highland View Hospital, performed a head transplant operation on a monkey in 1970, and says the major barrier to human head transplants is that "we don't yet have a way of growing the spinal cord back together again so that the brain could regain function of the body." White, who also works as an adviser to the Pope on medical ethics, remains committed to the idea, but adds, "We'd want to do a study to see how long a person could be expected to live before we did the operation."
Photo by Patrick Tehan

▲ **Computers make diagnosis and patient evaluation easier for X-ray technologist David Cain,** in a control room at Enloe Hospital in Chico, California. More than a million dollars worth of equipment lines the walls where Cain monitors a patient's electrocardiogram, or EKG, and blood pressure as the patient undergoes a digital subtraction angiography to evaluate the state of the heart's arteries.
Photo by Steve Ringman

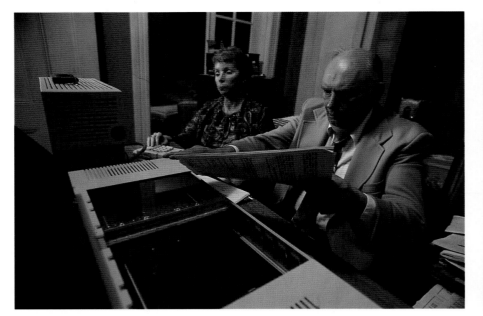

▲ **The printed word comes magically to life** for blind couple Jean and Richard Agnew of Bloomfield, New Jersey. The Kurzweil Personal Reader uses nine different voices to read aloud almost any printed text the Agnews place on it. The fifty-two-pound unit, which has been on the market since 1987, also includes a carrying case for portable use, a talking calculator, and a speed monitor to modulate the pace of the reading. "We used to have someone come in and read to us every week," says Richard. "The problem was, we had to hold the mail until somebody read it for us, and we often missed events. This machine has changed our lives."
Photo by Jim Mendenhall

▶ **Simultaneous eye operations are monitored from a viewing room** above the operating theater at the Institute of Eye Microsurgery in Moscow. More than 200,000 patients come annually to the institute — also known as "Fyodorov's clinic" after its flamboyant founder, Svyatoslav Fyodorov — most of them in the hopes that a laser-aided operation known as radial keratotomy will cure their myopia, or nearsightedness. The operation, in which several doctors work on each patient in an assembly-line fashion, calls for small incisions to be made in the cornea. Although the procedure has been performed in the United States since 1978, it is not officially endorsed by the American Academy of Ophthalmology. The procedure helps some patients, the Academy says, but in some cases might go too far in the other direction, leaving the patient farsighted.
Photo by Sam Garcia

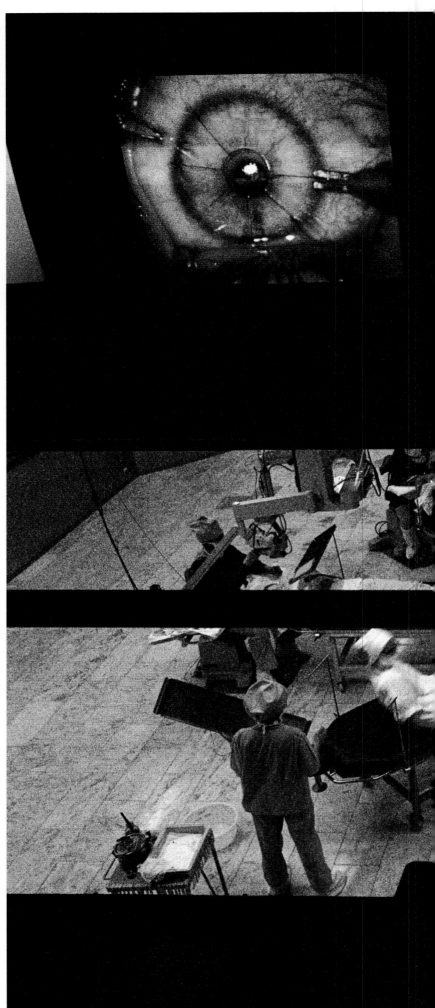

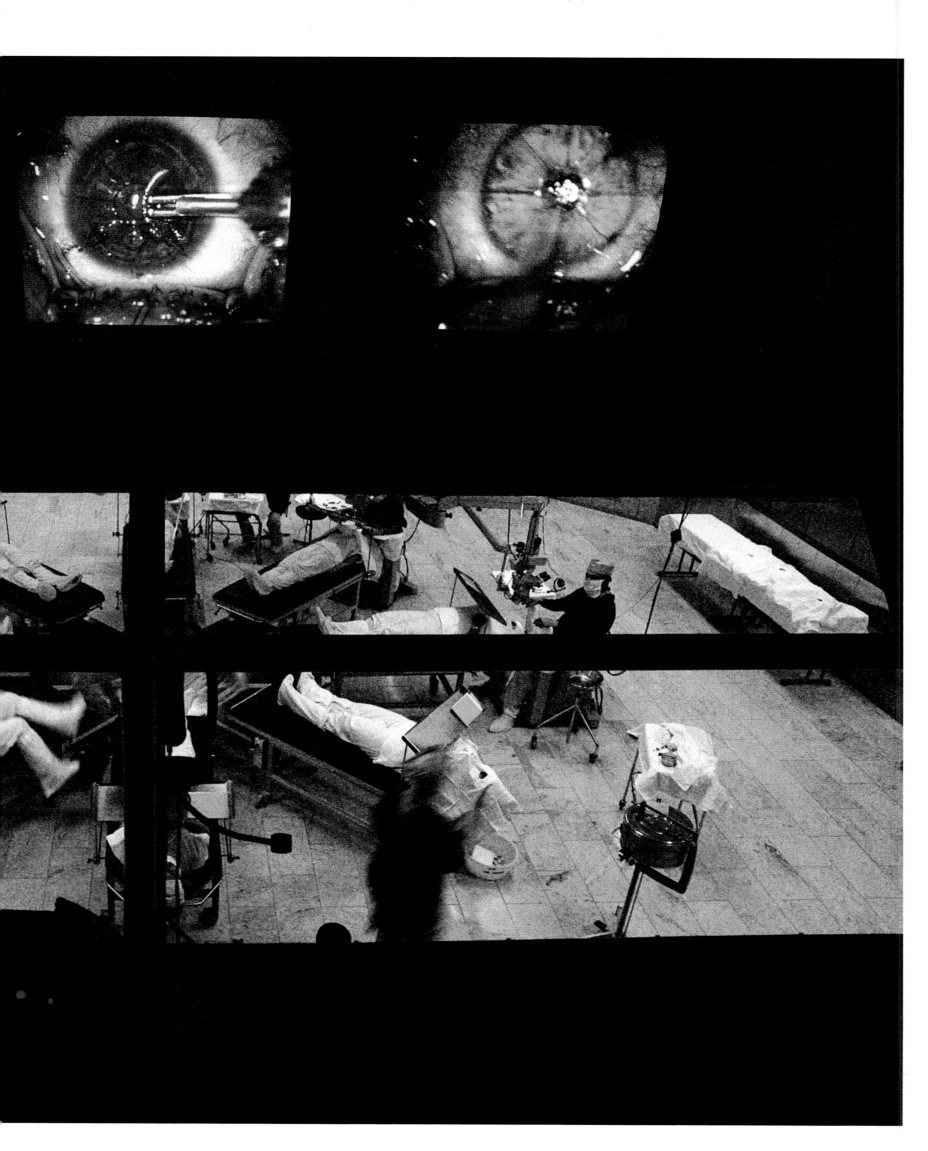

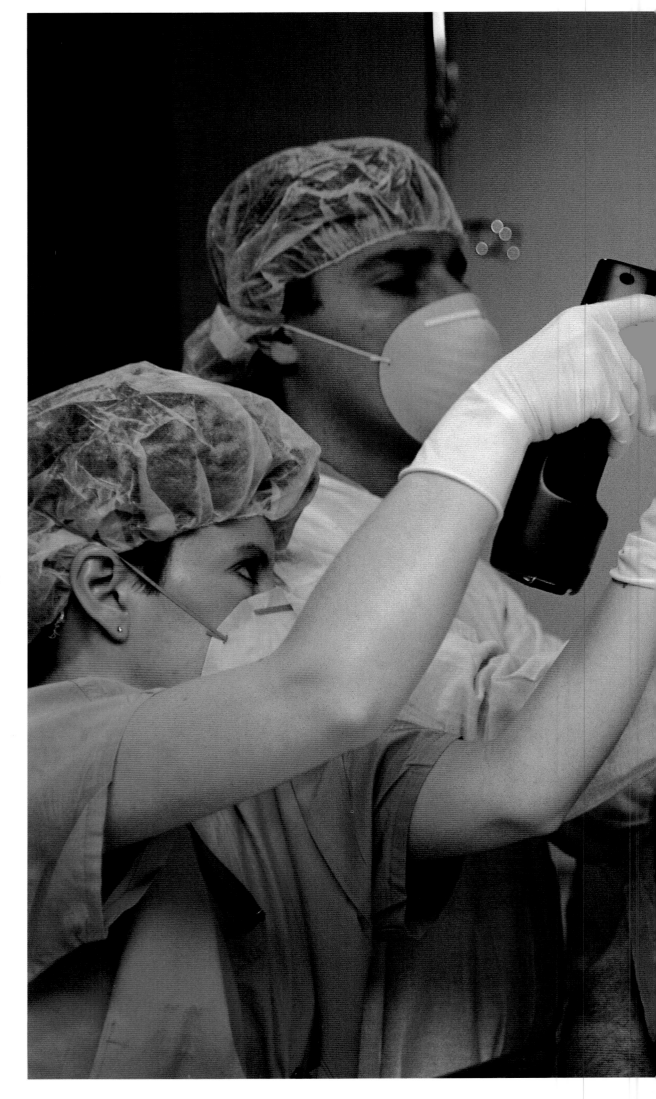

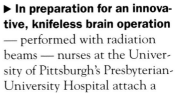

▶ **In preparation for an innovative, knifeless brain operation** — performed with radiation beams — nurses at the University of Pittsburgh's Presbyterian-University Hospital attach a stereotactic head frame to forty-seven-year-old Martin Randal. Once the nurses have tightened the frame, designed to keep the mildly sedated Randal from moving his head, doctors will use one of the world's fifteen gamma-ray "knives" to focus radiation beams on an arteriovenous malformation, or series of tangled and weakened blood vessels, in Randal's brain. A single gamma knife treatment of about twenty minutes begins the process of scarring the weakened vessels, which will prevent them from rupturing. Randal will walk out of the hospital the next day, but the healing process will continue for several months.
Photo by Wally McNamee

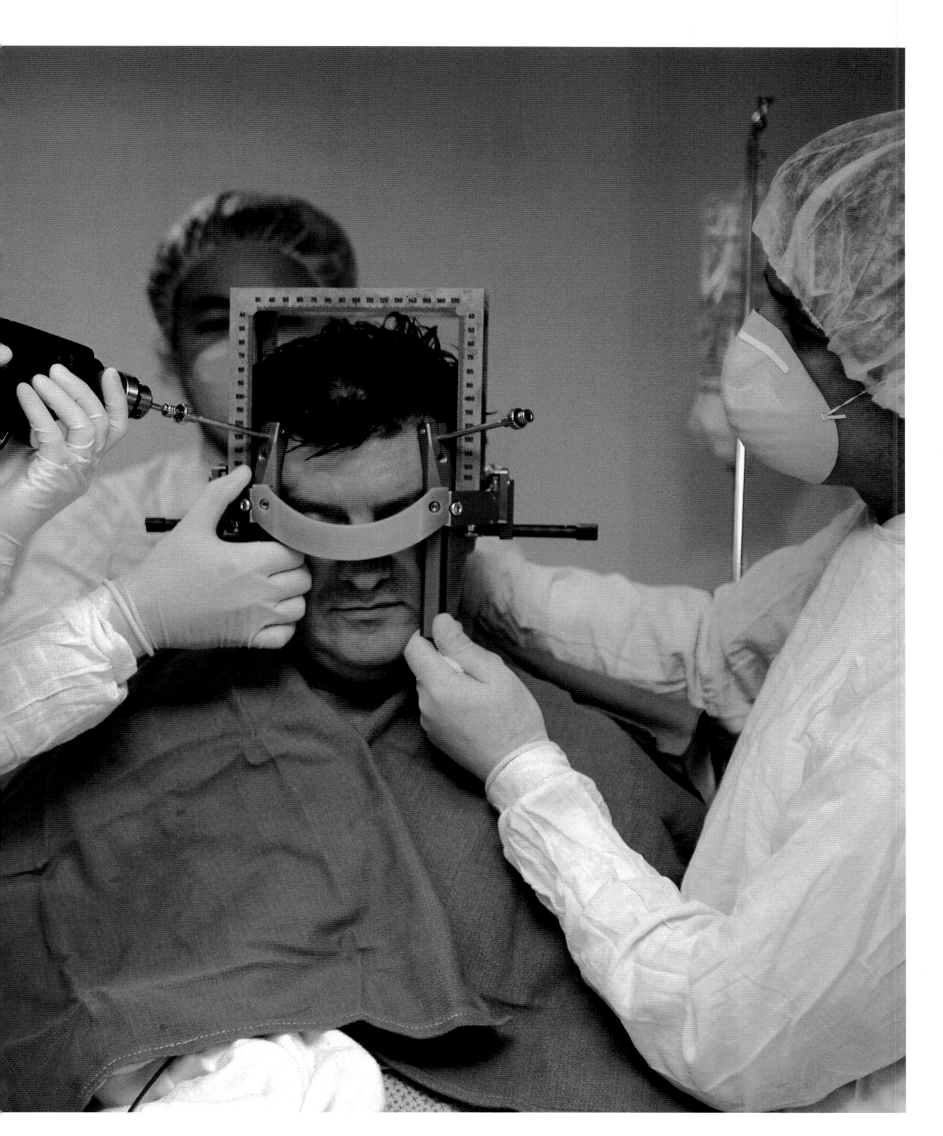

In Search of Nature's Secrets

RICK WEISS

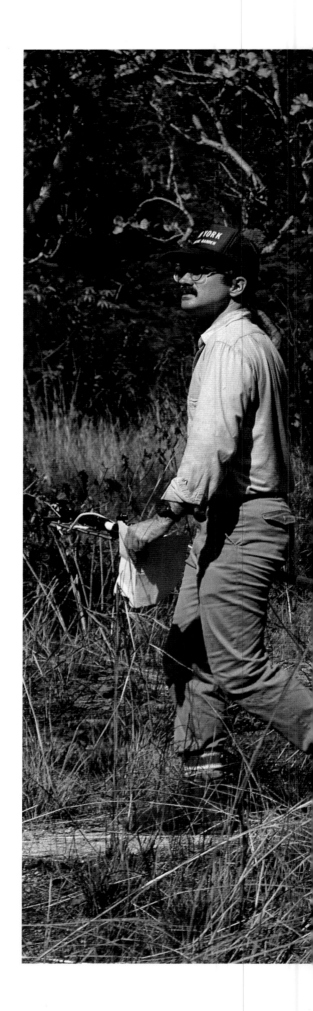

CHINESE PEASANTS GAIN RELIEF FROM A COLD OR COUGH BY SIPPING A tea made from tough, green twigs of the shrub ephedra. They have done so for at least 5,000 years, without the benefit of clinical trials and with little insight into the biochemistry of the plant's active ingredient, ephedrine.

Halfway around the globe, sniffling Americans consume a purified version of the same ingredient in their over-the-counter cold and flu remedies. By reading the insert that comes with their foil-lined bubble-packs, they may learn that ephedrine stimulates the central nervous system, raises blood pressure, and dilates the tiny air sacs deep within the lungs. But few have a clue that their patented pill has botanical origins.

With our fixation on tablets and caplets, syrups and shots, we often forget that the Earth is a living apothecary, and that its residents have for millennia engaged in a painstaking apprenticeship aimed at mastering the secrets of its stockroom shelves.

Prescriptions inscribed upon baked clay tablets and Egyptian papyruses document humanity's early preoccupation with naturally occurring drugs. Countless numbers of our ancestors died nibbling on poisonous mushrooms or neurotoxic shellfish in their search for medicine. Informed at first by trial, error, and observation of animals—many of which appear to be remarkably savvy in their recognition of plants with antibiotic, purgative, or other properties—humans gradually have evolved to the point where pharmaceutical drugs are virtually a staple of life in industrialized countries.

Yet for all their sophistication, the modern drugs so common today in the developed world are not far removed from the plants that were relied on by our ancestors—and are relied on still in much of the world. Many antibiotics are produced by soil-dwelling microorganisms; blood-thinning anticoagulants come from marine plankton; and the bark of willow trees produces salicylic acid, a precursor of common aspirin with similar pain-relieving properties.

Thousands of plant and animal species may harbor compounds with some medicinal value. Unfortunately, many of them are on the verge of extinction before ever having divulged their critical secrets. With modern technologies capable of screening 40,000 raw compounds every year for their potential value in fighting cancer, AIDS, or other diseases, researchers are working feverishly to identify these organisms before it's too late.

And even as some scientists race to learn what they can from disappearing species, others are creating entirely new ones. Biologists are learning

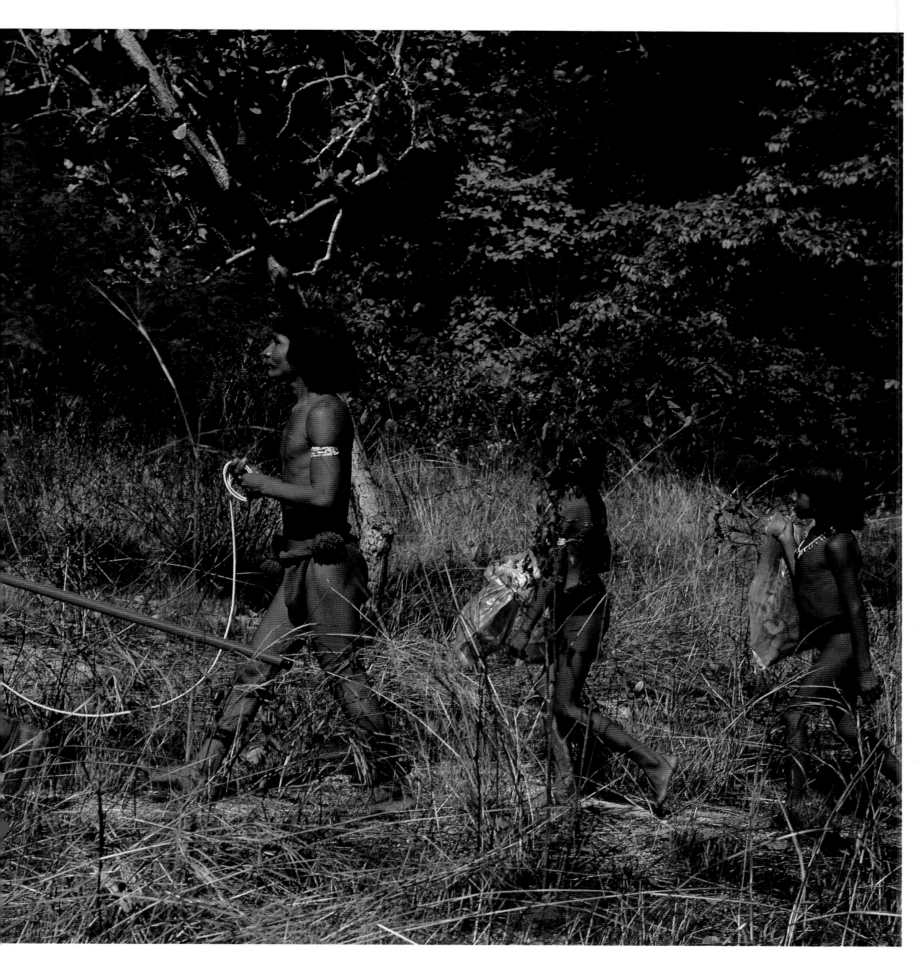

▲ **Racing against time to find plant species that could save millions of lives,** Brian Boom of the New York Botanical Garden and three local residents survey the fast-disappearing tropical rainforest in Venezuela for uncataloged plants. Boom uses the orange pole to snag branches and leaves from a distance of thirty feet; the man behind Boom, from the Panare tribe, carries the cord that Boom uses to close the pincers at the end of the pole.

Less than one percent of the plants in the world's tropical rainforests have been examined for their potential medicinal properties; those tested have yielded drugs used to treat leukemia, tetanus, strychnine poisoning, and other diseases. The New York Botanical Garden is among several institutions under contract with the National Cancer Institute to collect tropical plants in the hopes that more cancer treatments may be found in the world's rainforests — which are being destroyed by humans at the rate of about 150 acres per minute.
Photo by Diego Goldberg

how to harness the power of living cells by genetically engineering them to produce drugs that are more potent and more specific than anything found in nature. There is some fear that these gene-altered microorganisms, plants, and animals—untrained in the etiquette of ecological restraint—could someday become environmental bullies, disrupting the Earth's delicate biological balance. It's too soon to tell, but the early returns on the potential benefits of genetic manipulation are encouraging.

Already, scientists have tinkered with tobacco plants, coercing them to make monoclonal antibodies with vast therapeutic and diagnostic potential. And experimental, gene-altered sheep and mice now produce in their milk therapeutic enzymes and hormones not usually found there. Once scientists perfect the technologies for extracting designer drugs from engineered tobacco leaves and milk, they hope to raise these plants and animals as living biofactories to produce medicines more cheaply than can be achieved in the laboratory.

Ultimately, gene therapists hope to implant genetically engineered cells within our bodies, eliminating the need for some traditional drugs. Hemophiliacs, for example, who lack the blood-clotting protein called factor VIII and who today must receive periodic infusions of this compound, might get permanent implants of factor VIII-producing cells that would secrete, within their bodies, the lacking protein in therapeutic quantities.

Despite the humbling fact that almost nothing is known about how medicines perform their physical and spiritual alchemy, we have moved successfully from plants to chemicals to gene-altered animals in our quest for drugs. But even the most creative drug designer acknowledges the value of Mother Nature's arboretum as a starting point from which to create new compounds. With record numbers of plants becoming extinct every year, it is crucial to preserve at least some tissues or seeds from as many of these as possible—if not to grow them again, then at least to decode their hidden genetic messages, which may someday spell the cures for diseases that are yet to arrive. And in the long run, perhaps we will recognize that even these exquisitely encoded biological secrets represent only the veneer behind which lies the true essence of medicine—that enigmatic mediator between health and disease.

▶ **Success in treating childhood leukemia comes from the rosy periwinkle plant,** held here by a young girl on the tropical island of Madagascar, off the African coast. The plant is the source of the chemical compounds vincristine and vinblastine, which aid in the treatment of leukemia, Hodgkin's disease, and other cancers. Just forty plant species provide ingredients for one-fourth of the prescription drugs sold in the United States today. *Photo by Frans Lanting*

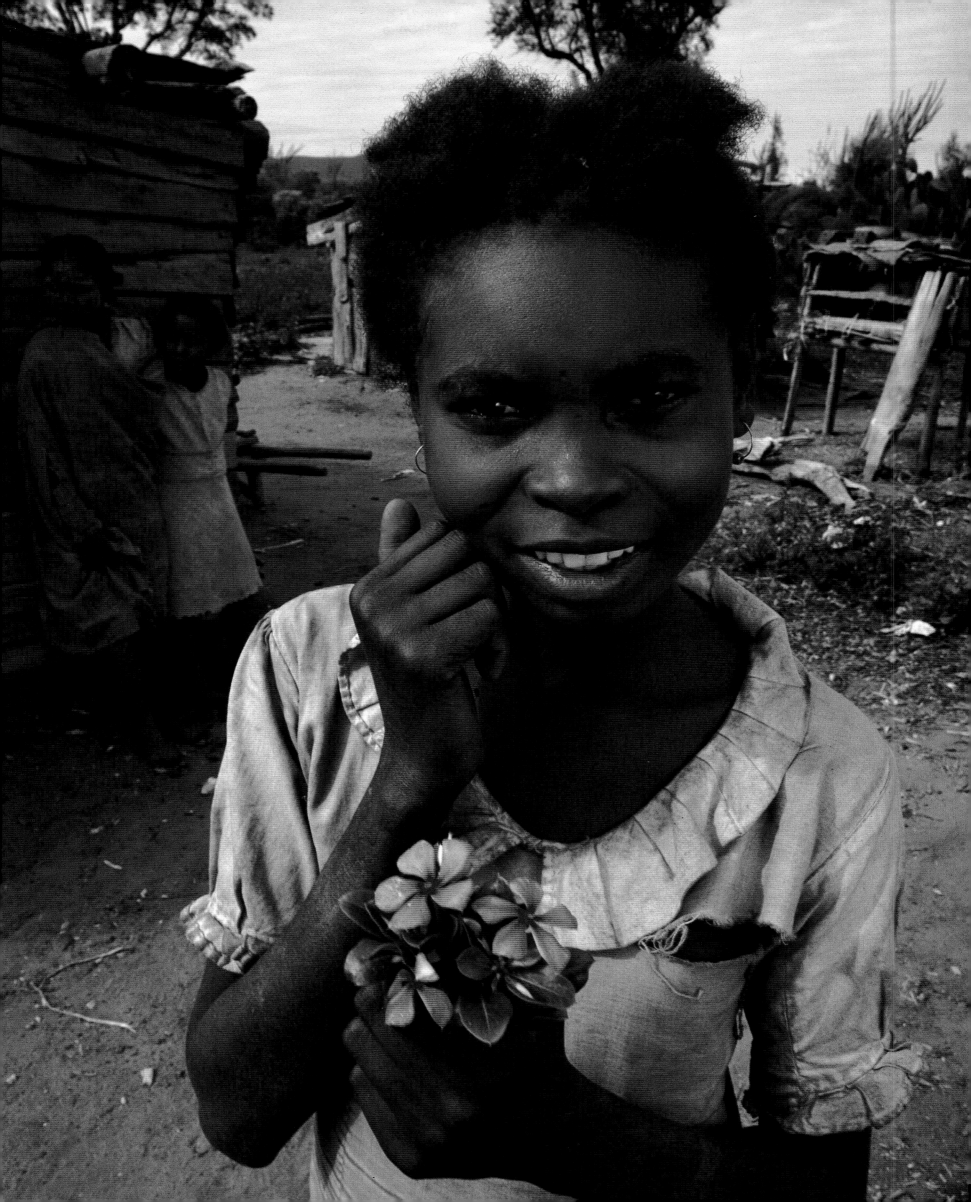

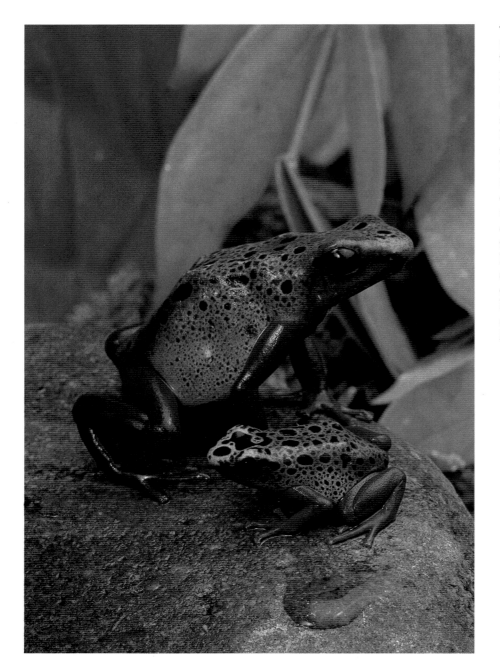

◄ **Beautiful, poisonous, and possibly the source of important drugs,** these tiny dart-poison frogs are native to the tropical rainforests of Central and South America. The toxic sweat from several of the 120 known species of dart-poison frogs has long been used by hunters, who dip their arrows in it. The toxin from one family of dart-poison frogs is so deadly that a frog less than an inch long can provide enough sweat to kill fifty humans. Researchers are hoping to use the same toxic sweat, in some form, to create drugs that will stimulate the heart and brain, control pain, and relieve muscle spasms.
Photo by George Grall

► **Technicians prepare dangerous scorpions for their twice-monthly milking** at Brazil's Instituto Butantan — the world's only hospital and research center that specializes in the treatment of poisonous bites. The institute turns poison into treatment by manufacturing antivenin from the venom of scores of scorpions and snakes. More than one million people worldwide are bitten by snakes every year. In the United States, says Dr. Howard McKinney of the Poison Control Center in San Francisco, the person statistically most likely to be bitten is a white male between the ages of eighteen and thirty-five who has been drinking.
Photo by Claus C. Meyer

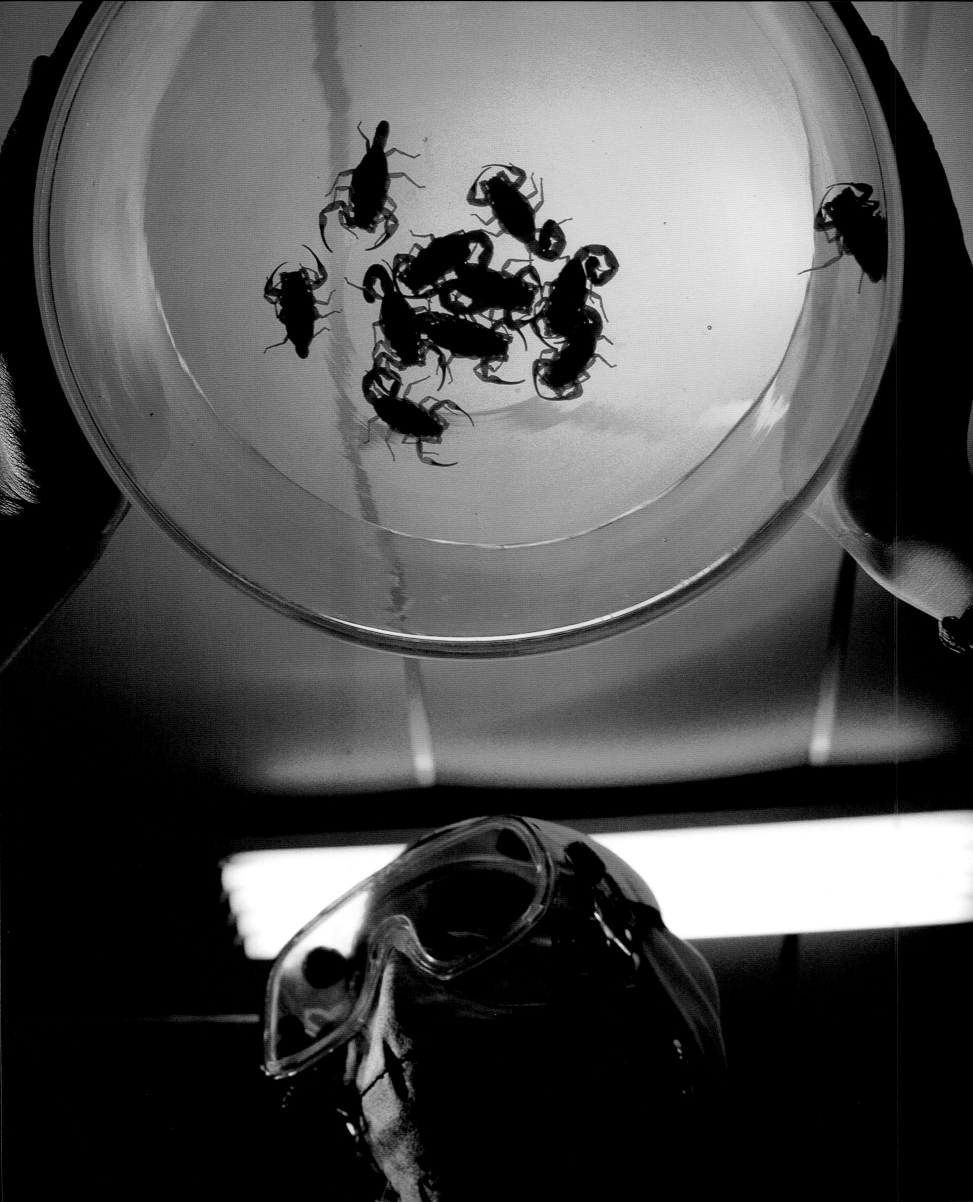

PHOTO ESSAY | *The Power of Light*

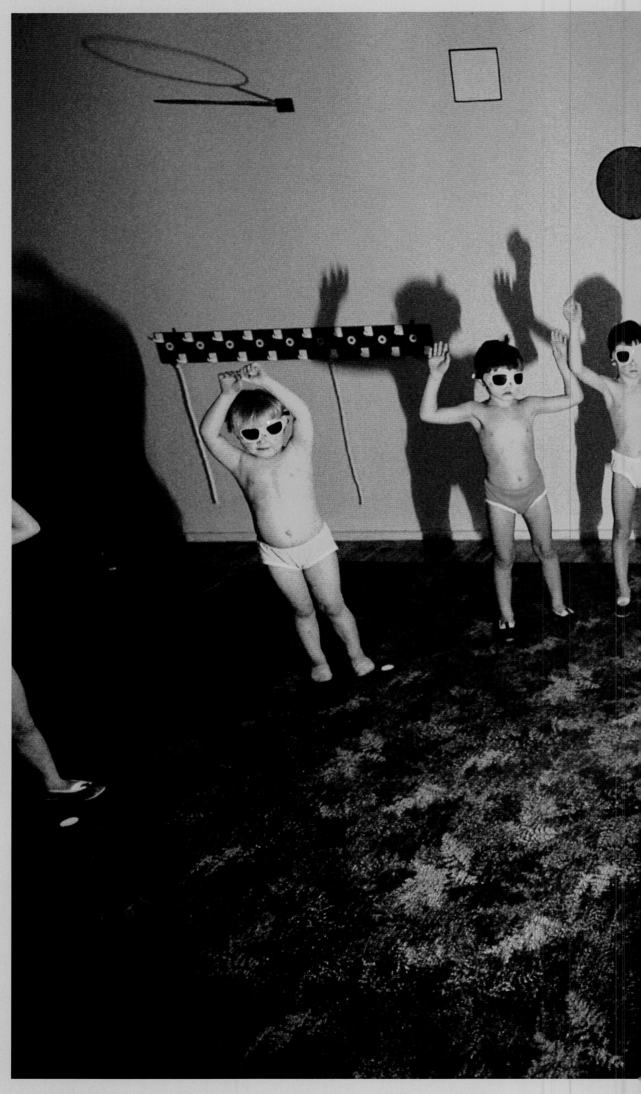

Healing power is all around us in the form of sunlight, which contains energy vital to both plant and animal life and intimately affects human mental and physical well-being. Without sunlight, for instance, some people suffer from seasonal affective disorder, or SAD, a depression that deepens as winter's shadows lengthen.

Nowhere is light's life-sustaining power more evident than in the earth's polar regions. In the Soviet Union's far northeastern village of Ostrounoye, in the Bilibino region some 200 miles north of the Arctic Circle, kindergarten students receive a daily dose of ultraviolet light (right and below) to compensate for the lack of sun, which

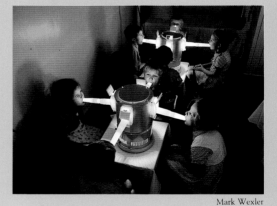

Mark Wexler

peeks over the southern mountain ridges for just minutes a day in mid-winter. Ultraviolet light, absorbed by the skin, is a major source of the body's vitamin D; without it, the children would suffer bone diseases and malformation, rickets, and tooth decay.

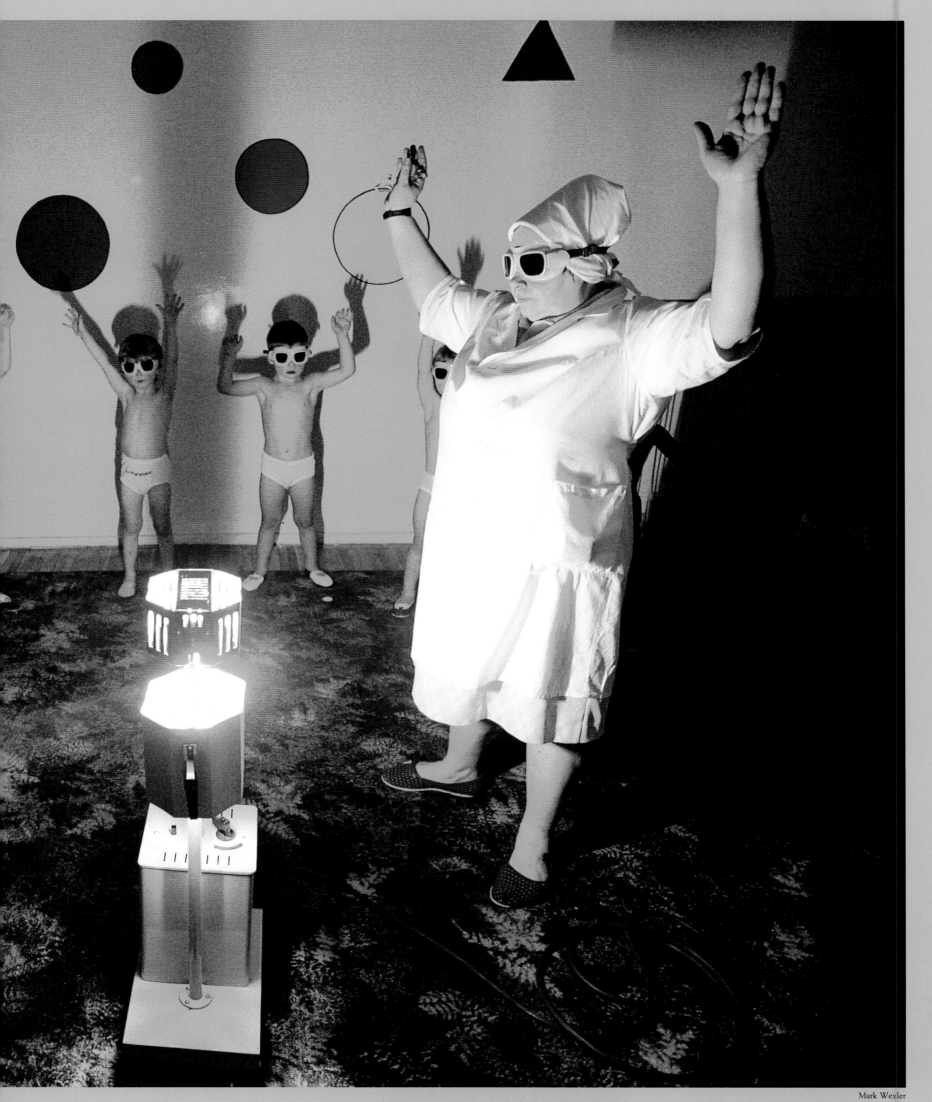

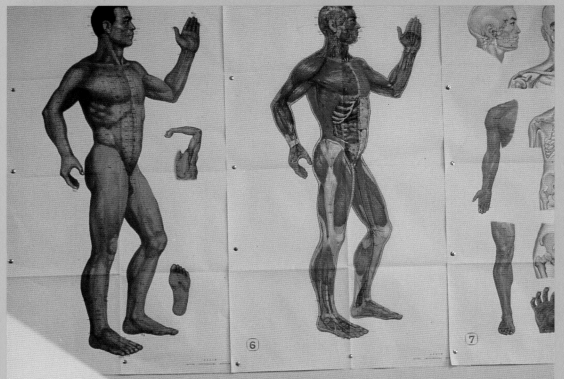

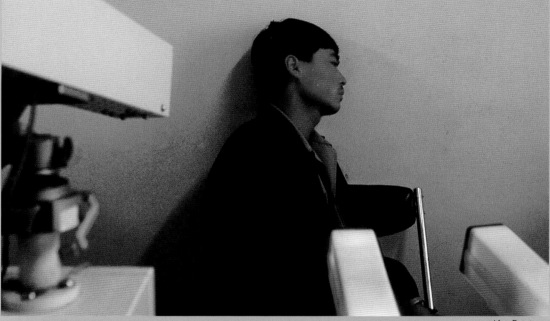

Alon Reininger

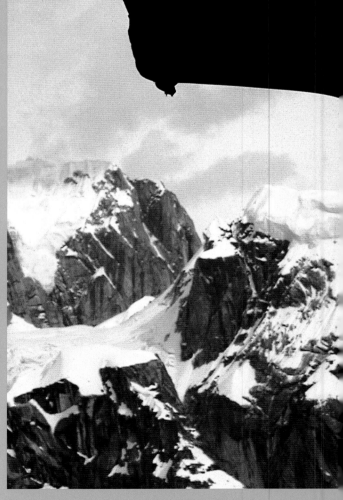

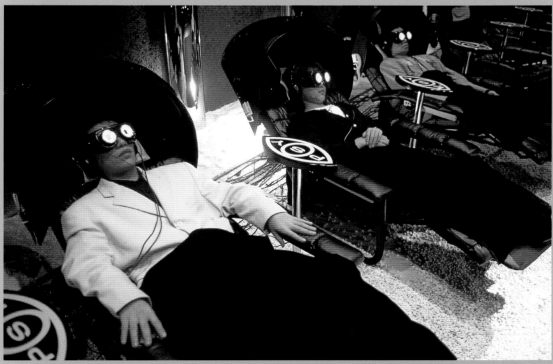

Torin Boyd

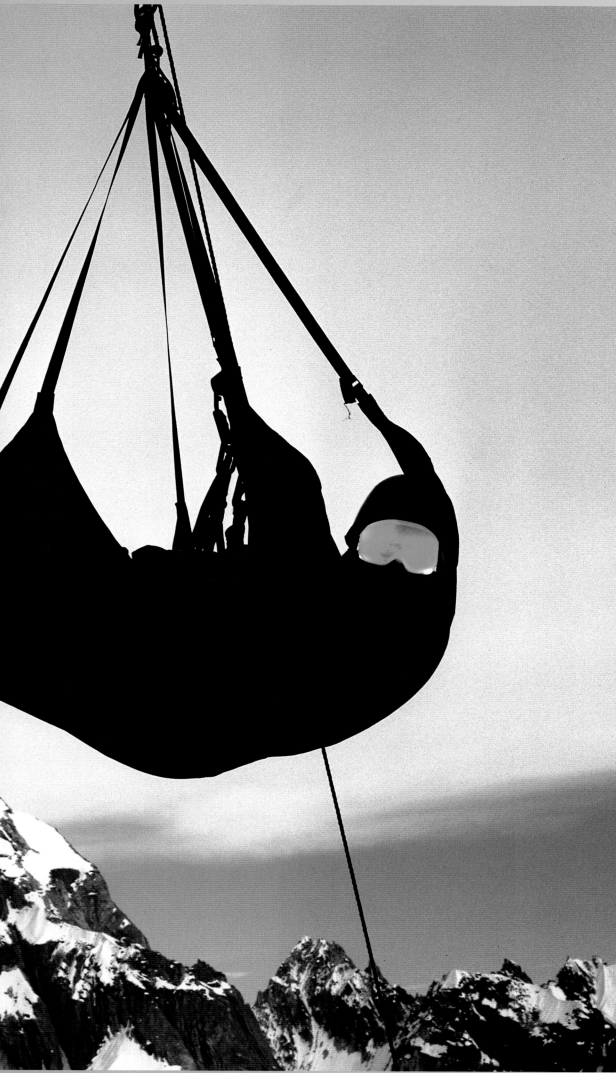

Louie Psihoyos

Laser light is used instead of acupuncture needles at the Traditional Medicine Hospital in Beijing (upper left). Low-powered lasers—extremely narrow, pulsating red beams of light that can penetrate the skin up to ten millimeters—are shot into one of the body's 700 meridian points, stimulating energy pathways just as the traditional needle does. Laser acupuncture is gaining acceptance in the United States, where practitioners offer the treatment to patients fearful of needles.

At Tokyo's Brain Mind Gym, overworked business executives are soothed by synchronized pulsations of light and sound emitted by goggles and headphones (lower far left). The light and sound combat stress by lulling the brain into a state of deep relaxation, called a theta wave state. The facility opened in March 1989 and claims 2,500 members.

Mountain climbers, too, use light with sound to relax. With the body continuously struggling for air, insomnia is common at high altitudes. Dangling from a ledge on Alaska's Mount Barrille (left) may not be the easiest place to sleep, but climbers say Tranquilite glasses help them drift off. A static blue light in the goggles accompanies the sound of a waterfall in the headphones, allowing the brain to subconsciously order a slowdown in heart rate, blood pressure, and breathing.

Expectations of
a New Era

M I C H A E L   C R I C H T O N ,   M . D .

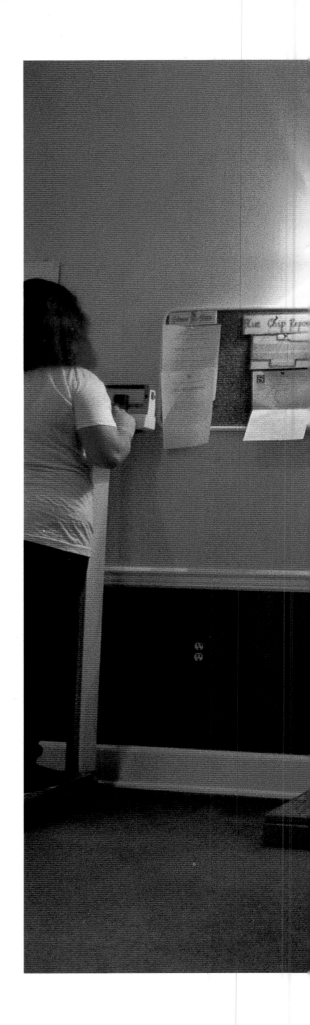

I N THE FIRST FEW YEARS OF THE TWENTY-FIRST CENTURY, A CLIMBER more than sixty-five years old will stand on the summit of Mount Everest. Absurd as such an idea might have seemed twenty-five years ago, mountaineers are now so sure it will happen that they speculate about who it will be, not if it will be.

The image of an exultant senior citizen atop the highest peak in the world points up the changing perceptions of age in industrialized societies. We are doing everything to a later point in life than we did a few decades ago, and Americans now expect to compete at sports, to be sexually vigorous, to bear children, and to raise families at a much older age than ever before. It's been said that the current generation of younger Americans isn't trying to hold off the ravages of age—it expects to.

These new expectations represent a major transformative force in future medical care. Throughout the twentieth century, medicine has advanced primarily by improving high-technology curative care: intensive-care units, bypass and transplant surgery, antibiotics and chemotherapy. But curative care has its limits, and nothing makes that clearer than the image of a sixty-five-year-old atop Everest, or a forty-five-year-old woman bearing down in childbirth, or a fifty-year-old astronaut. To maintain a high level of fitness we must avoid physical decline, not repair it: open heart surgery, even at its most effective, will never make you as good as new, especially if you intend to climb Mount Everest. And for the major killers of American society—heart disease and cancer—the most effective preventive measures involve changes in lifestyle.

The physician as lifestyle expert, as wellness adviser, has already begun to appear. And increasingly, as medicine develops predictive procedures and genetic profiles, the doctor will be able to use technology as a preventive rather than a curative measure: to administer tests, for example, and then tailor preventive measures for individual patients with the same specificity with which he or she now dispenses medications for diseases.

Advances in medical technology will also extend the current trend toward non-invasive diagnostic procedures, such as nuclear magnetic resonance imaging and ultrasound. Treatment will change along similar lines. Surgery will be less common, and hospitalization much rarer. As patients, we will expect more procedures to be done quickly, painlessly (and inexpensively) on an outpatient basis. Microtechnology will revolutionize medicine with a whole

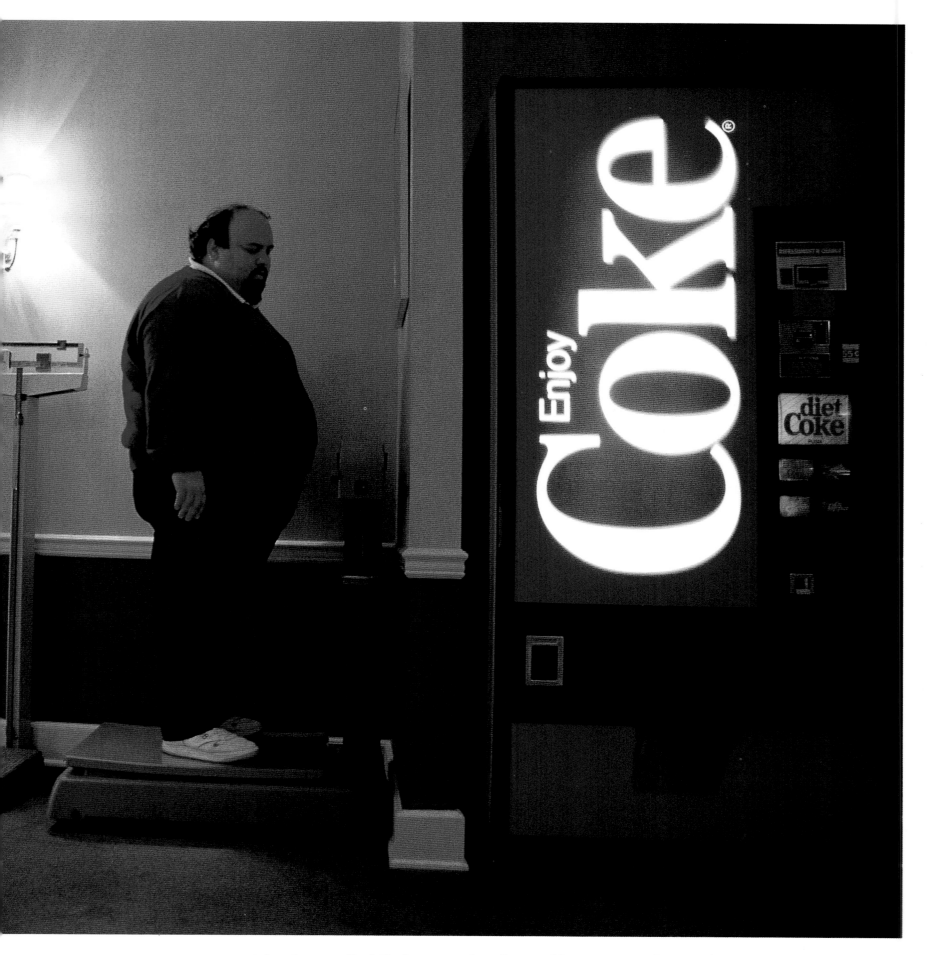

▲ **Americans are the fattest people in the world,** with twenty-two percent of adult men and twenty-seven percent of adult women officially categorized as clinically obese. Jack Margareten of Forest Hills, New York, weighs himself after two weeks at Structure House, one of many residential weight-loss facilities in Durham, North Carolina. Margareten, who stands five feet, five inches tall, topped out at 372 pounds and says that his six-week stay at Structure House — full of aerobic walking, visits with doctors and nurses, seminars on stress management, classes on nutrition and menu planning, and group and individual therapy sessions — has inspired him to believe he can cut his weight in half.
Photo by Annie Griffiths Belt

range of devices, from miniature biosensors, implanted under the skin, that dispense drugs with astonishing accuracy, to futuristic nanomachines, themselves hardly larger than red blood cells, that course through our blood-stream, scrubbing the insides of our arteries.

Even more fundamental will be gene replacement therapy, in which missing or defective genes are supplied by the physician. Such procedures are being developed to treat serious illness, but they will eventually be used to boost enzyme levels and hormone production, to retard aging, and to increase vigor.

Accompanying the use of more refined technology to prevent and treat illness, psychoimmunology, the science that deals with the mind's role in helping the immune system to fight disease, will become a vitally important clinical field in the years to come—perhaps the most important medical field in the twenty-first century, supplanting our present emphasis on oncology and cardiology. The encouragement of healthy thinking may eventually become an integral aspect of treatment for everything from allergies to liver transplants.

What all this means is that our present concept of medicine will disappear. Pressed both by patients and its own advancing technology, medicine will change its focus from treatment to enhancement, from repair to improvement, from diminished sickness to increased performance. That transformation has already begun. And it will reach its logical conclusion when the first sixty-five-year-old stands atop Mount Everest, and the relationship of humanity and medicine enters a new and extraordinary era.

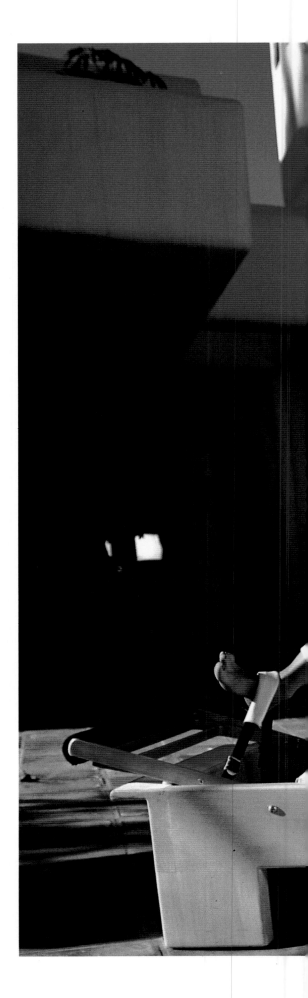

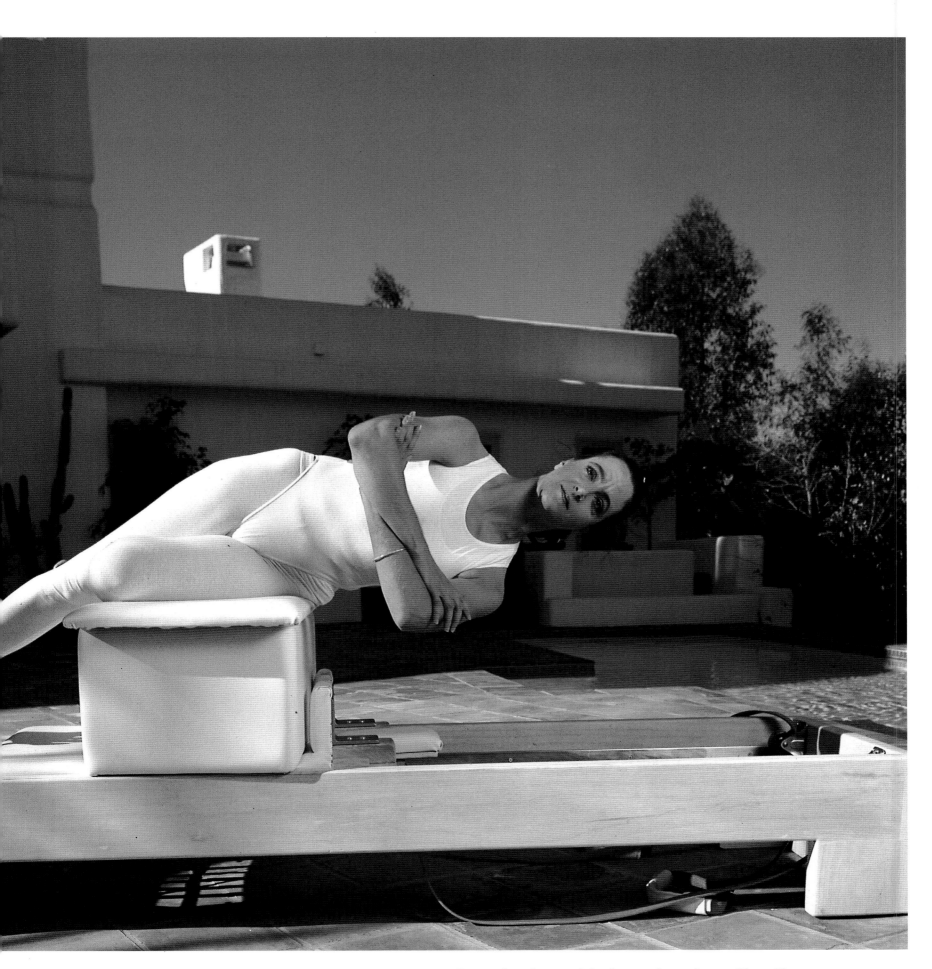

▲ **The exercise machine of the 1990s?** Siri Galliano, a physical trainer to the stars, works out on a Pilates machine, named after the German boxer and nurse who invented it and brought it to the United States in the 1920s.

Dancers have long used the device as an exercise aid, but its recent spread into other circles may catapult it into must-have status. "It can be used for back injury rehabilitation, posture problems, or cosmetically," says Galliano, whose clients include

Jessica Lange, Glenn Close, Danny DeVito, Sidney Poitier, and Shelley Long. "There are over 100 exercises on it, and they're all no-impact." *Photo by Alon Reininger*

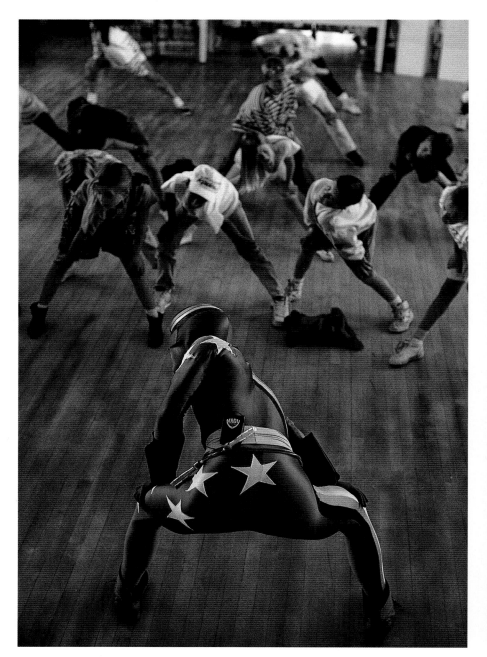

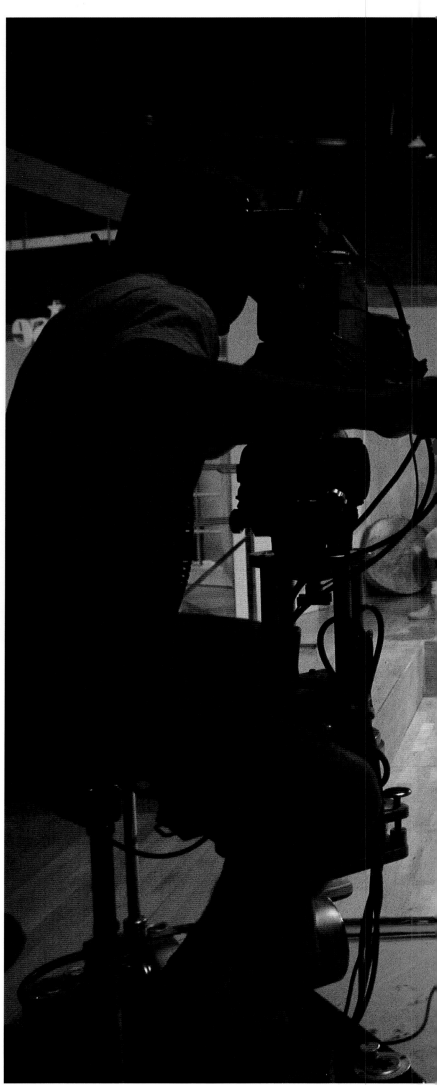

▲ **Four out of every ten kids in America between the ages of five and eight show at least one heart disease risk factor** (obesity, elevated cholesterol, high blood pressure, or physical inactivity), and one out of every six is considered physically underdeveloped. Thirty-three-year-old Kirk Lawrence, alias FitKid, takes his exercise message to schools throughout California, saying he wants children to "think about fitness, not fatness." But it may take more than one lone superhero to improve the woeful physical condition of the country's youth: only one state, Illinois, requires daily physical education classes for every student from kindergarten through twelfth grade. As a result, only one-third of the nation's children are enrolled in daily phys ed classes.
Photo by Matthew Naythons, M.D.

▶ **A pioneer in the aerobics craze,** exercise entrepreneur Judi Sheppard Missett, forty-four, videotapes her latest batch of Jazzercise routines. The tape will be sent to owners of the 4,100 Jazzercise franchises in the United States and several foreign countries, including Canada, Australia, and Japan; franchise instructors are then expected to work the new routines into their classes. Missett founded Jazzercise — "a total body conditioning program based on jazz dance, in which artistic creativity is paramount" — in 1969, but the boom years for her business didn't begin until 1976. Today, some twenty-four million Americans participate in aerobics classes.
Photo by Karen Kasmauski

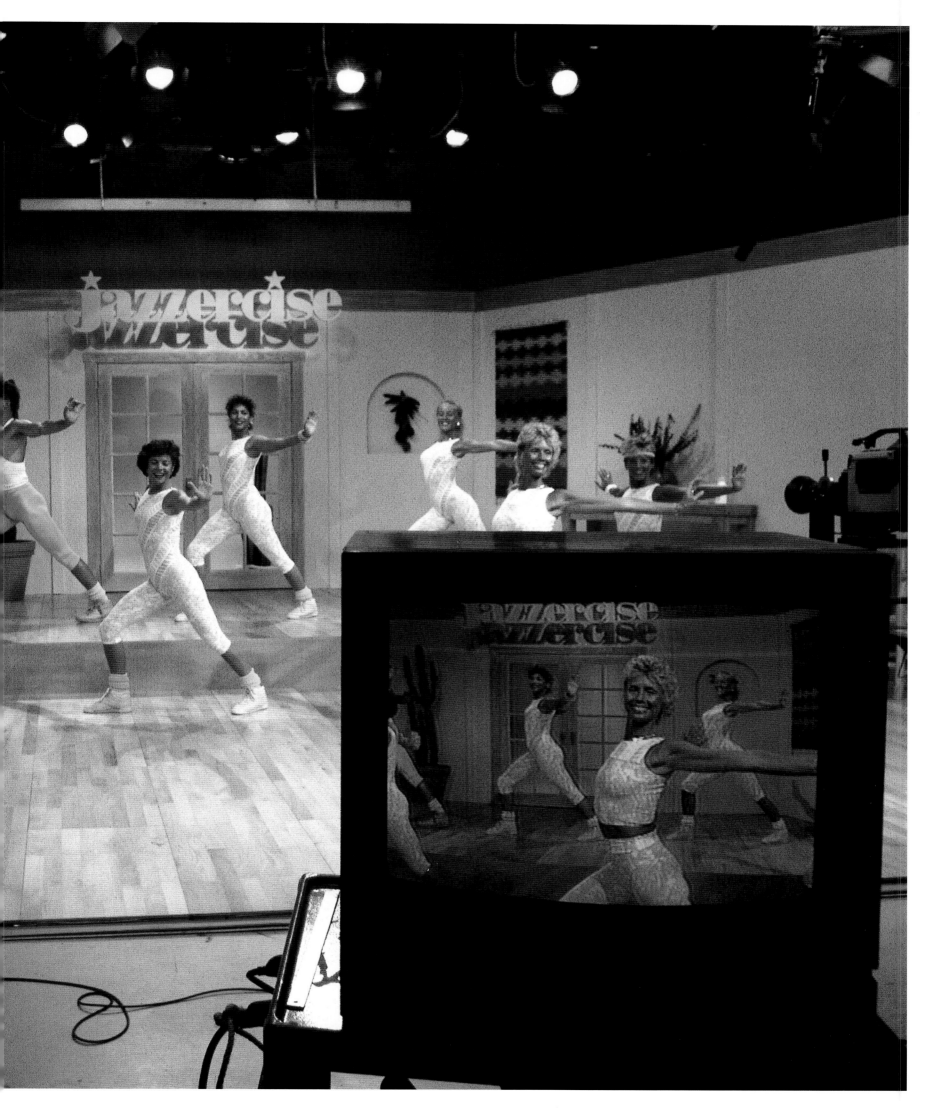

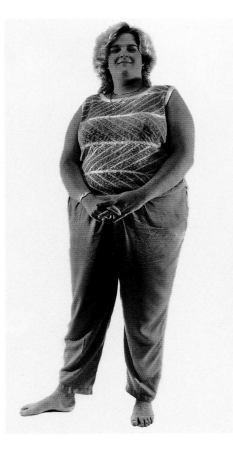

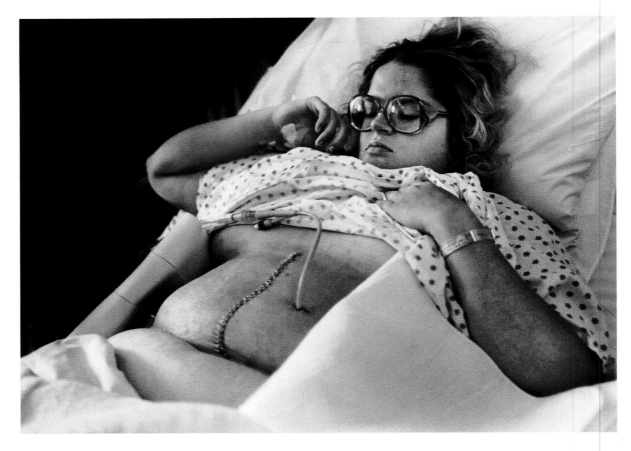

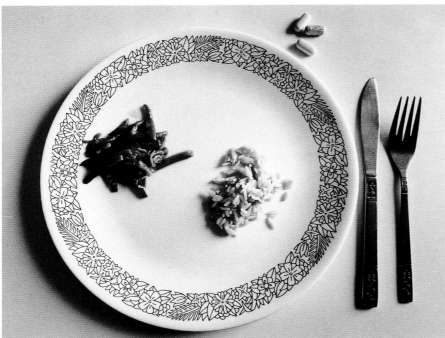

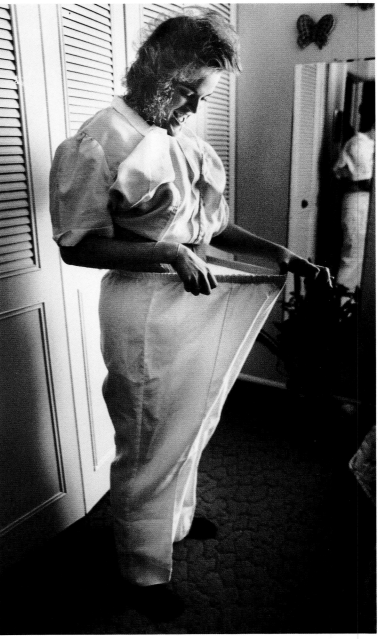

▲ **At the age of twenty-one, registered nurse Wendy Fraser** (*above left*) entered a Pittsburgh hospital to radically shrink her stomach with the permanent insertion of seventy steel staples. "It was an act of desperation," says Fraser, who weighed nearly 270 pounds. A temporary tube near the surgical incision relieves gas as Fraser recovers from the operation (*above right*). With her stomach's food-storage capacity reduced to about one ounce from the normal human capacity of forty-eight ounces, Fraser's first meals after the operation were spartan (*above*). "Now I'm able to eat a normal meal," she says, "but I don't go back for seconds or thirds." Within a year Fraser had lost more than 100 pounds (*right*). Says Tom Fraser of his daughter, playing ball with her nephew Jared (*far right*): "There's been a 100 percent turnaround in her mood since the operation." *Photos by Melissa Farlow*

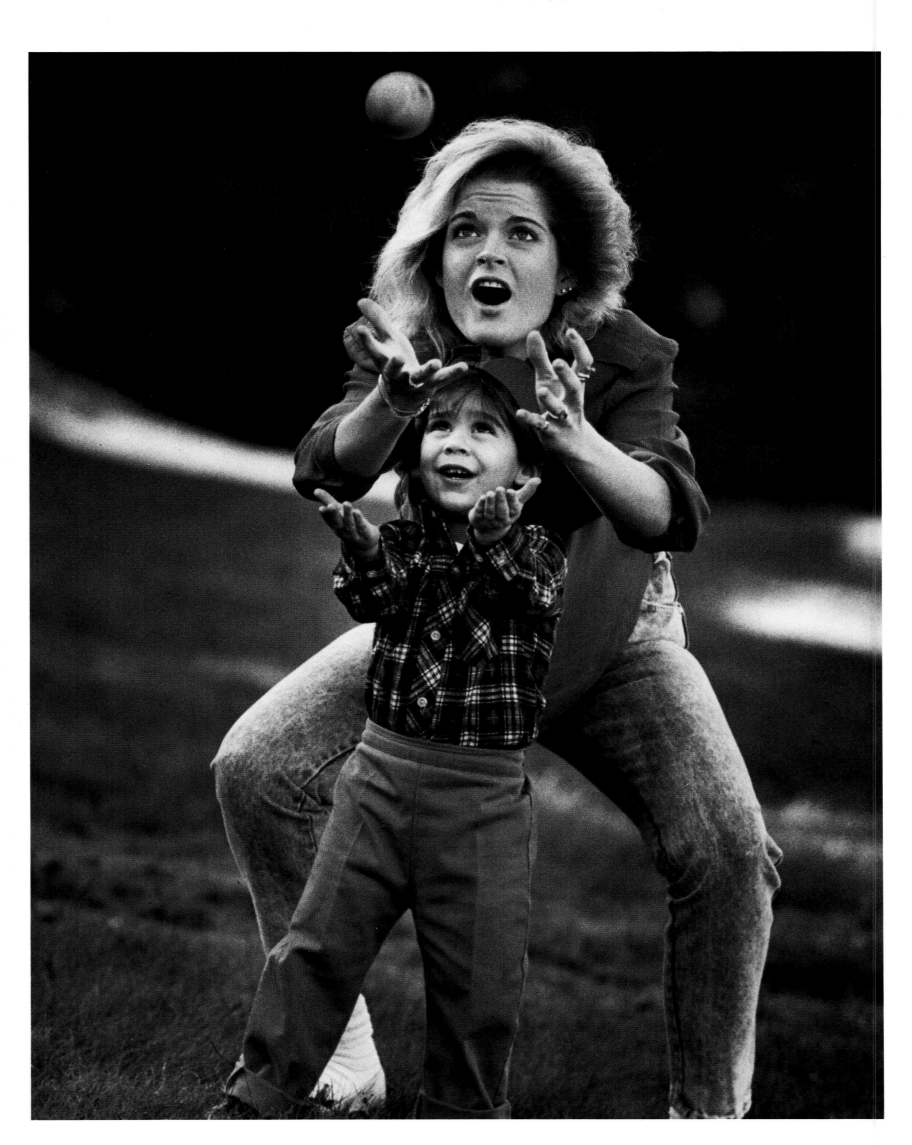

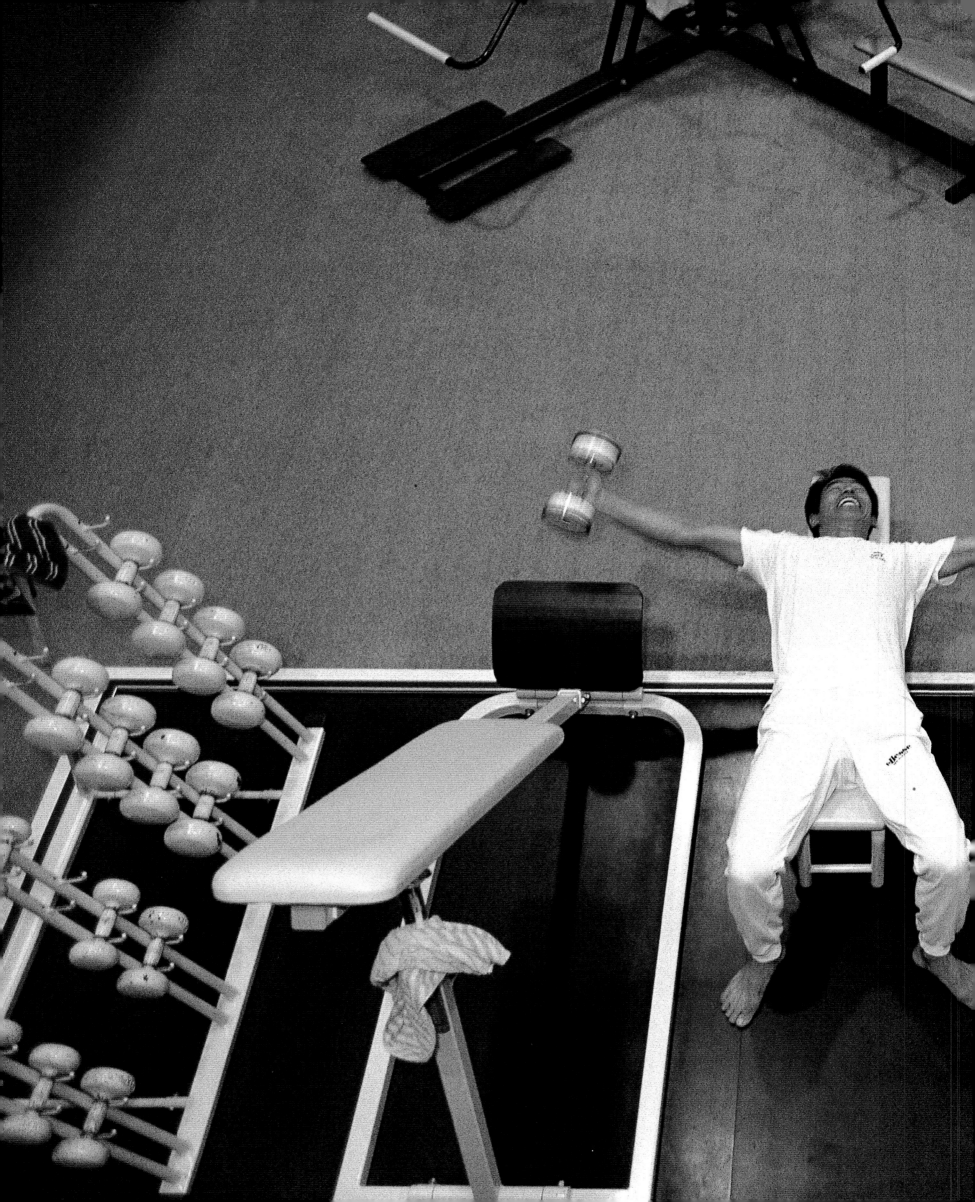

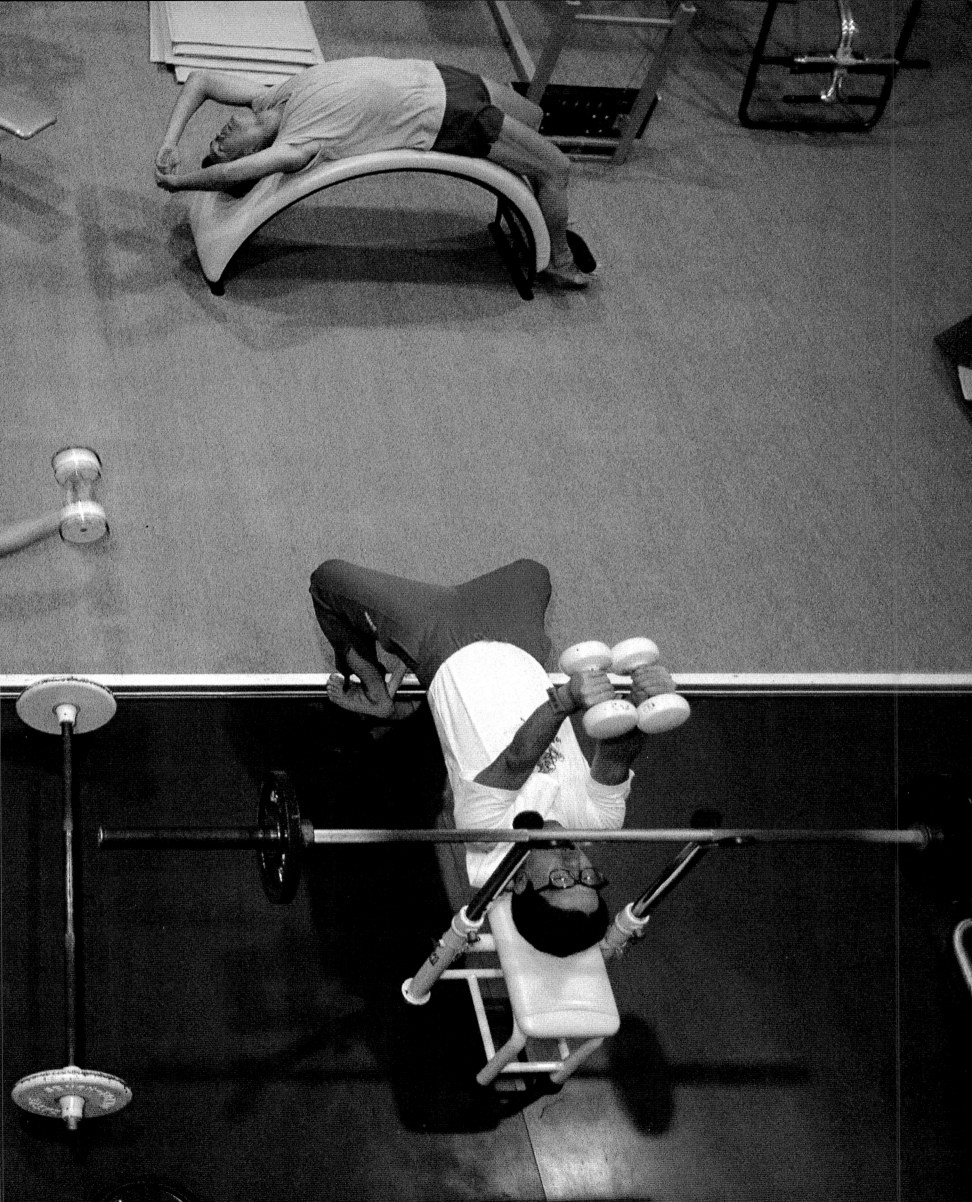

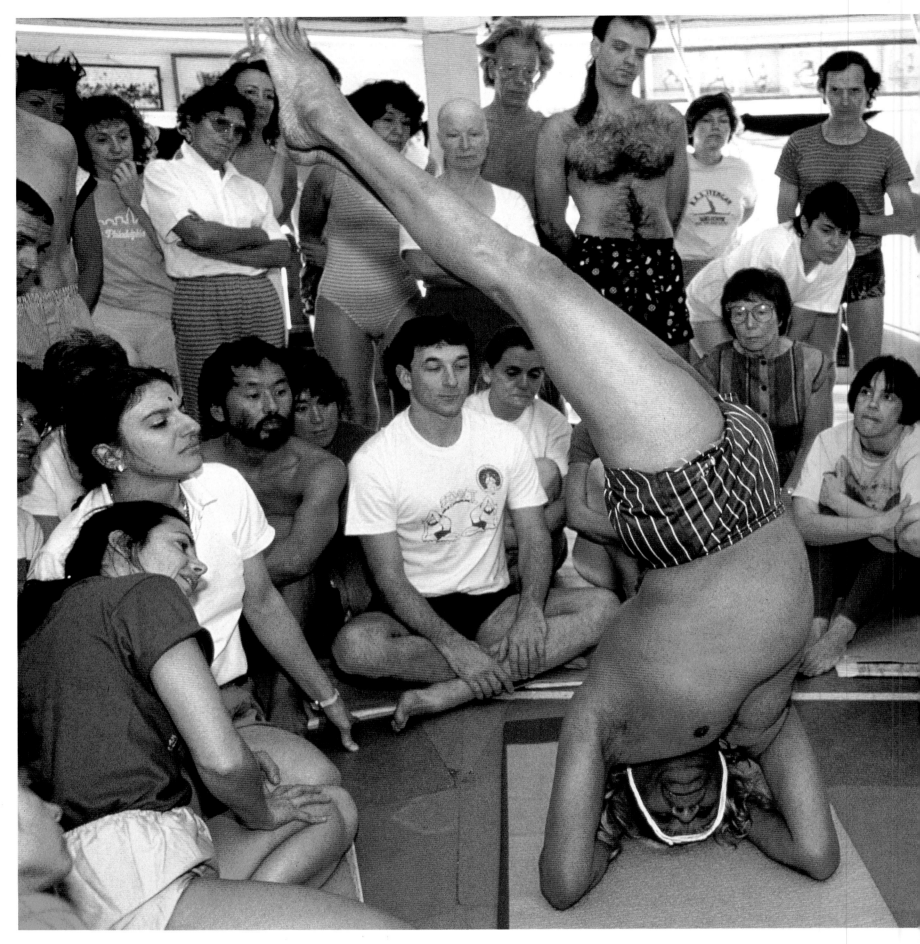

◀ A sound body and a sound mind mean good workers: that's the philosophy at the Nissan Corporation in Tokyo, where employees grunt and groan in the company-sponsored Nissan Sports Plaza. The eleven-story sports center was built in 1983 to help reduce stress and improve the health of Nissan's Japanese workers and their families — important goals in a country where the six-day workweek is still prevalent, and where reserving a public tennis court must be done by lottery two months in advance. But the Sports Plaza isn't just for locals: any of Nissan's 53,000 employees around the world may use the facility free of charge when in Tokyo on business. *Photo by Torin Boyd*

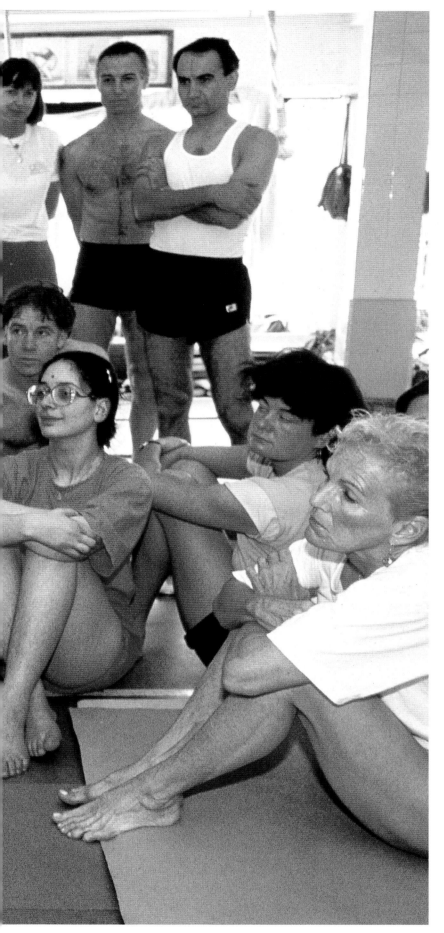

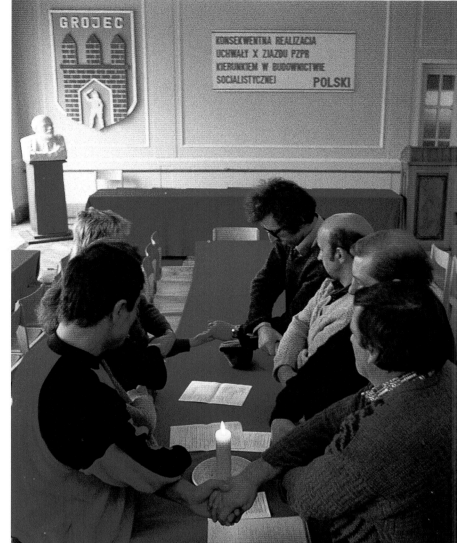

◄ **Seventy-one-year-old yogi B.K.S. Iyengar,** whose method has inspired the creation of more than 125 yoga centers in North America, twists into the *parsva sirsasana* position at his home base in Pune, India. Practitioners of Iyengar yoga use benches, ropes, sandbags, mats, chairs, and other devices to adopt poses designed to develop strength, endurance, and correct body alignment. "Yoga," says Iyengar, "aims for complete awareness in everything you do." *Photo by Alon Reininger*

▲ **Using the twelve-step program to fight alcoholism is a growing trend in Poland,** where some 6,000 people attend meetings of Alcoholics Anonymous. The message of AA — the self-help group founded in Akron, Ohio, by a doctor and a stockbroker in 1935 — has now spread to more than 140 countries; in the United States, there are nearly a million members. Because AA's twelve simple principles, or steps, are easily adapted to fighting other types of addiction, the 1980s saw an explosion of AA-like support groups. A sampler of twelve-step programs now includes Gamblers Anonymous, Overeaters Anonymous, Debtors Anonymous, and Sexaholics Anonymous. *Photo by Tomasz Tomaszewski*

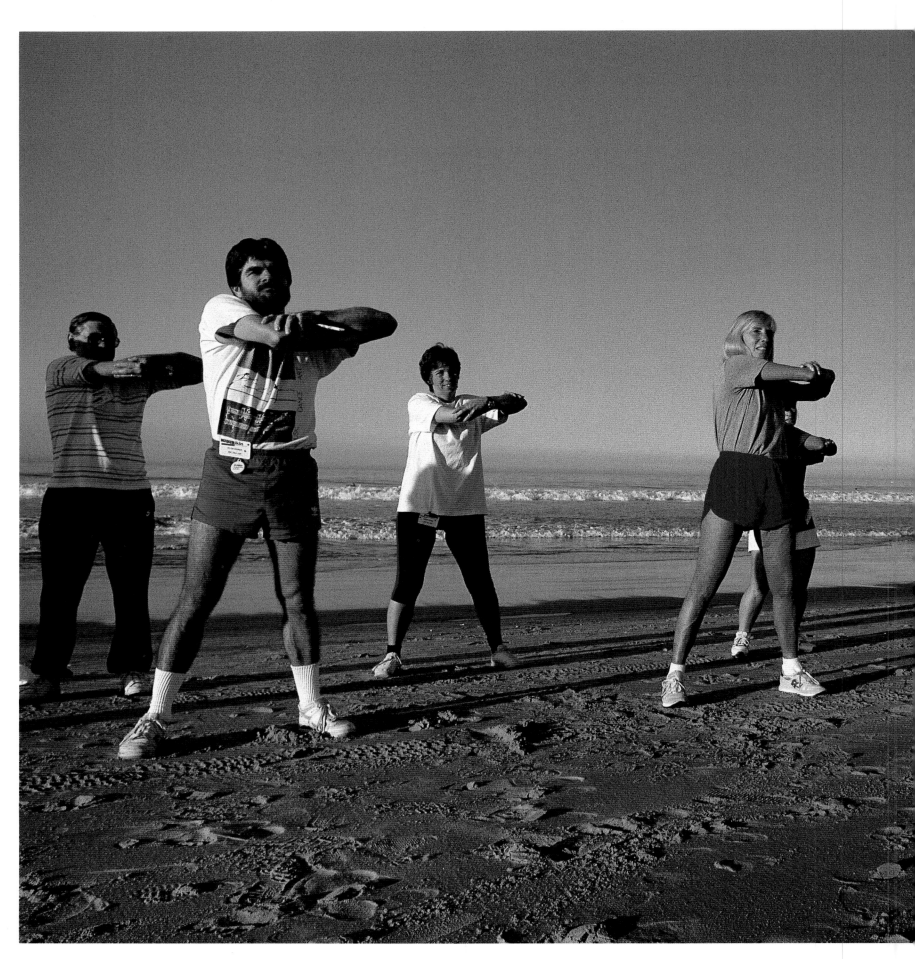

▲ **New morning, new lives: 7:30 is stretching and toning time on a Santa Monica beach** for participants in a short-term residential program at the Pritikin Longevity Center in California. On a typical day, the morning stretch will be followed by two health lectures, two exercise classes, a doctor's appointment, a cooking class, an outdoor jog, a stress-management lecture, and evening entertainment. While the three Pritikin Centers in the United States claim impressive results in lowering cholesterol, weight, and high blood pressure, the solutions don't come cheap: the thirteen-day program costs $5,500, and the twenty-six-day program close to $10,000.
Photo by Rick Smolan

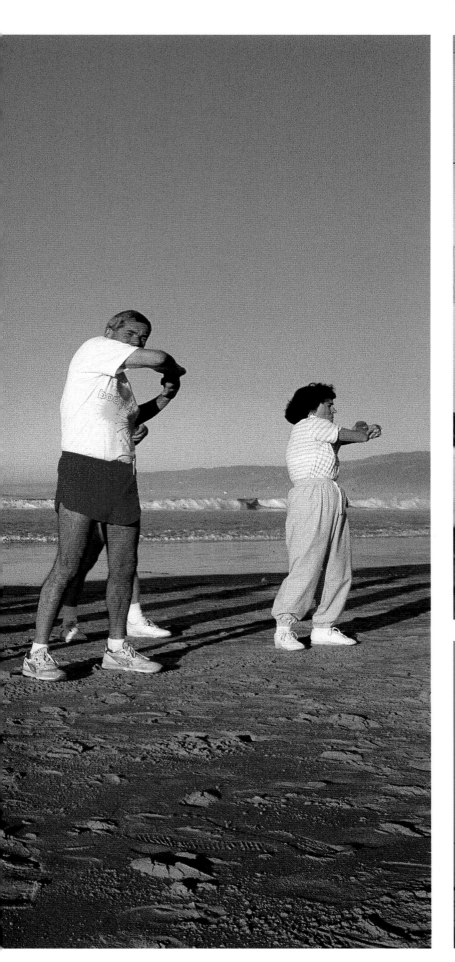

▲▲ Developing new eating habits is a key part of the Pritikin program, so Susan Massaron uses her daily cooking classes to teach participants how to make tasty meals with only ten percent fat — as opposed to the forty or fifty percent fat that graces most American dinner tables. Here, she shares her recipes for spicy raspberry chicken, fish in lime sauce, brown-and-wild-rice vegetable salad with dill dressing, and banana cake.
Photo by Rick Smolan

▲ The electronic death count changes nearly every minute on this Los Angeles billboard, which tracks the toll of America's deadliest drug. The billboard looms over the heavily traveled Little Santa Monica Boulevard, and was commissioned and donated by a local businessman in 1987. Although cigarette smoking in the United States has declined every year since 1981, tobacco-related diseases still kill nearly 400,000 Americans per year, far more than all other narcotics-related fatalities combined.
Photo by Torin Boyd

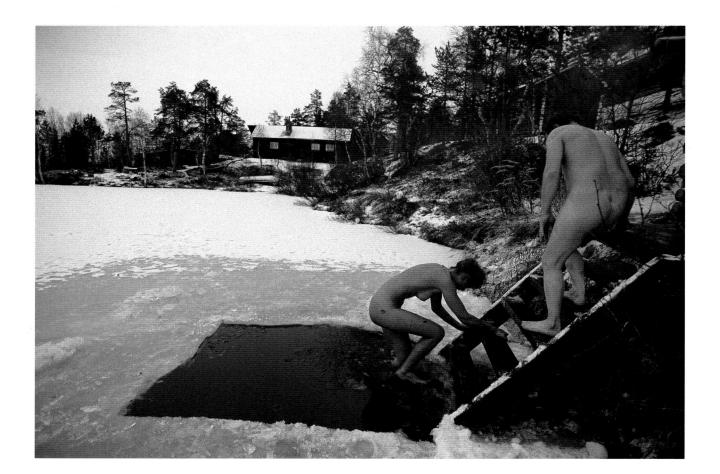

▲ **At thirty-four degrees Fahrenheit,** the water is the perfect temperature for the dip that refreshes after a sauna in Ivalo, Finland. Doctors are not sure the hot-to-cold dash has any long-term health benefits; in fact, some caution that it might be dangerous. But the sauna-loving Finns are undeterred. Insisting that a cold jolt to the system after several minutes of dry heat improves circulation, they take an average of two saunas per week.
Photo by Stephanie Maze

▶ **An ornate holdover from the Turkish occupation,** the sixteenth-century Kiraly Baths in Budapest are a magnet for visitors seeking relief from the hurly-burly of modern life. Some form of water treatment, or hydrotherapy, is a part of many of the world's cultures. Here in the Hungarian capital, dozens of thermal bathhouses also include medical clinics that treat rheumatism, degenerative joint and spinal problems, respiratory diseases, and even infertility.
Photo by Péter Korniss

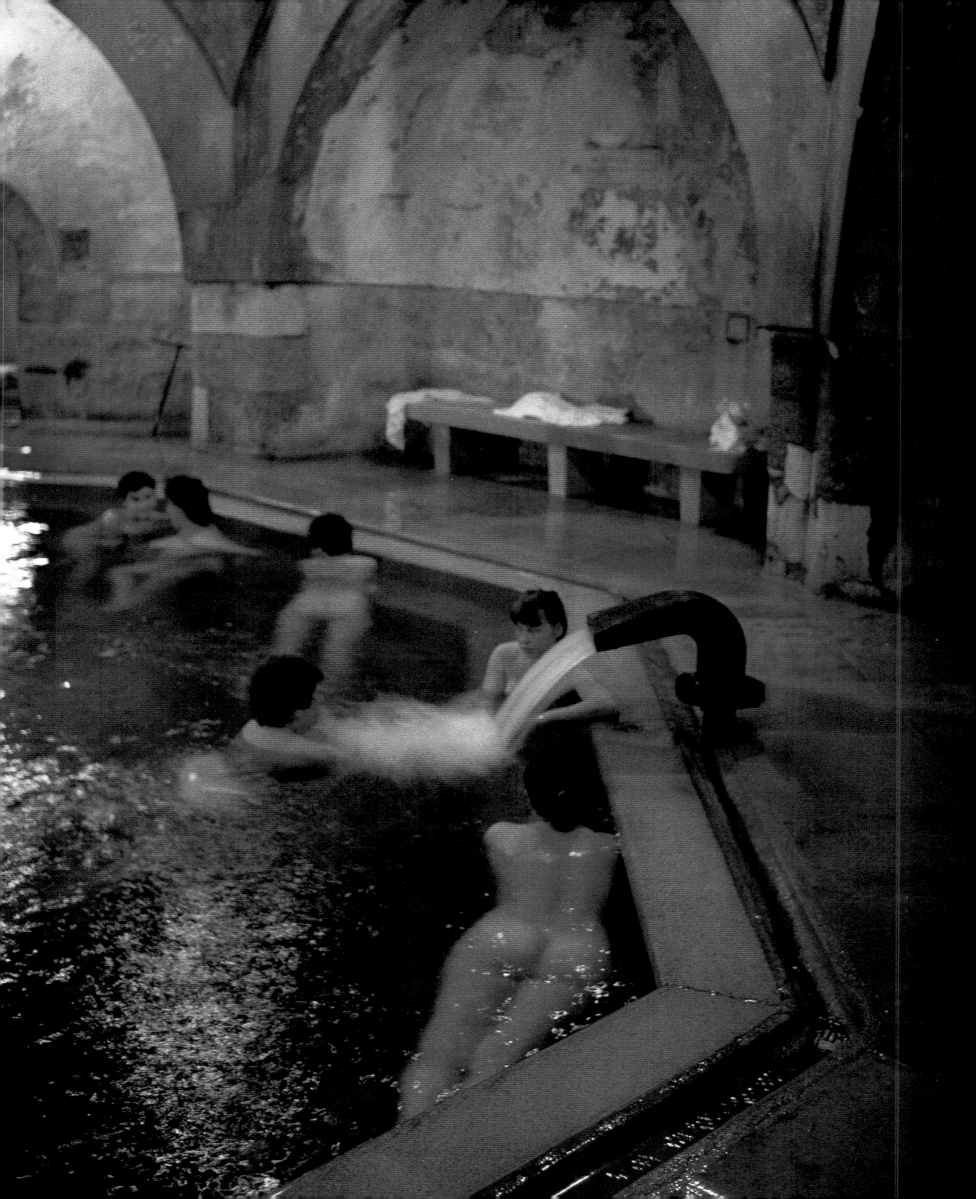

What is your secret to long life?

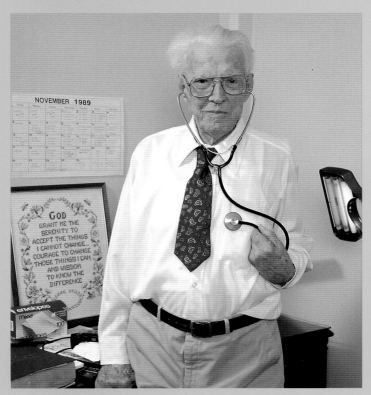

"I am a Christian. Jesus Christ is my savior." Dr. Willis Butler, Hermitage, TN. 101 years old. *Photo by J.P. Laffont*

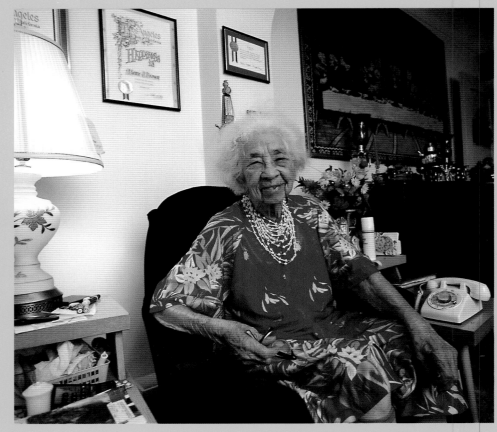

"I have a highball every day at 4 o'clock. It's my medicine." Mattie Brown, Los Angeles, CA. 104 years old. *Photo by Dana Fineman*

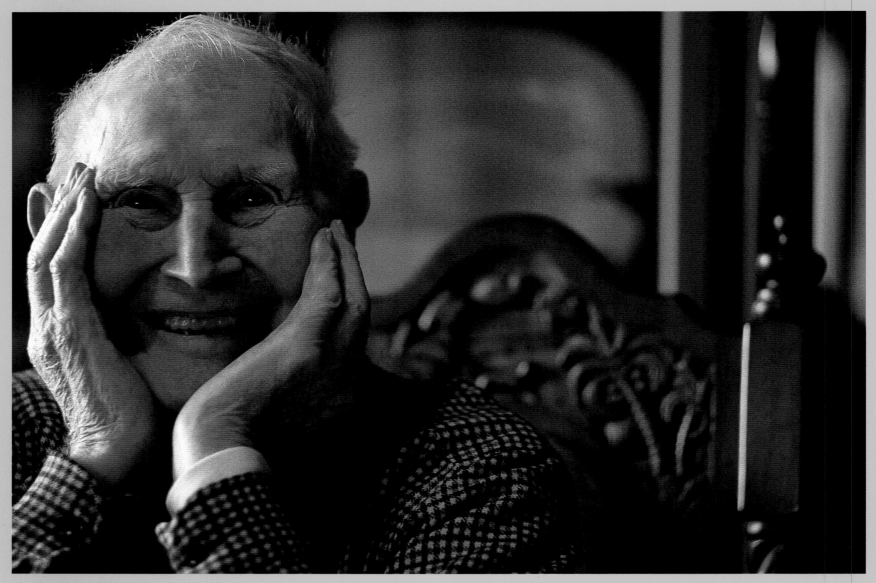

"I worked hard. If hard work killed I'd have been dead long ago." Bill Schilperoort, Olympia, WA. 100 years old. *Photo by Alan Berner*

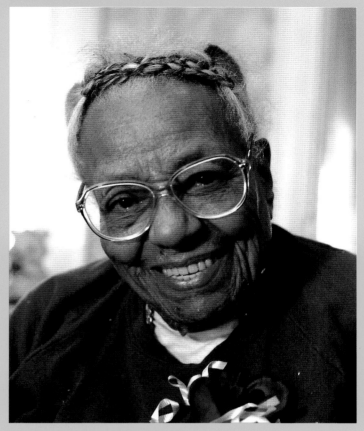

"I eat onions. Lots of them, even on ice cream." Minerva Bedford, Paris, KY. 103 years old. *Photo by Henry Clay Owen III*

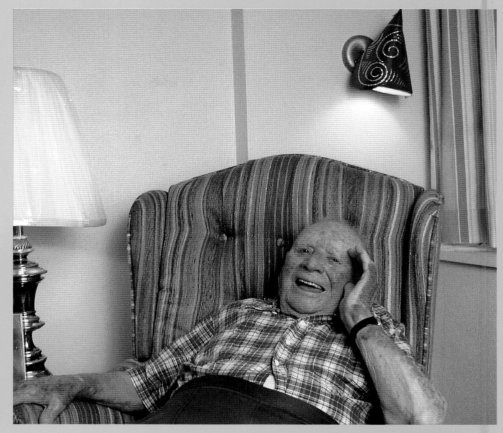

"I worked hard and I like beer." Samuel Low, Dallas, TX. 105 years old. *Photo by J.W. Fry*

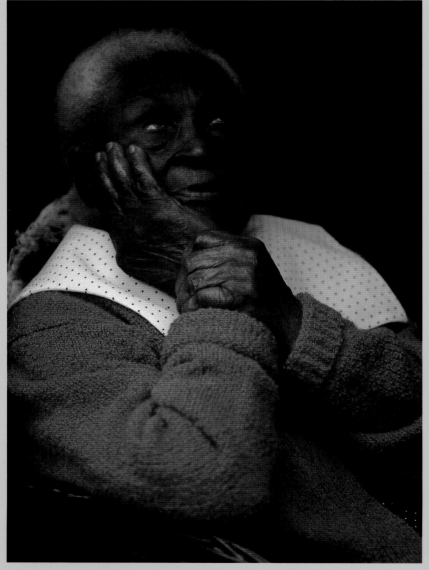

"God is my secret." Susie Brunson, Wilmington, NC. 118 years old. *Photo by Annie Griffiths Belt*

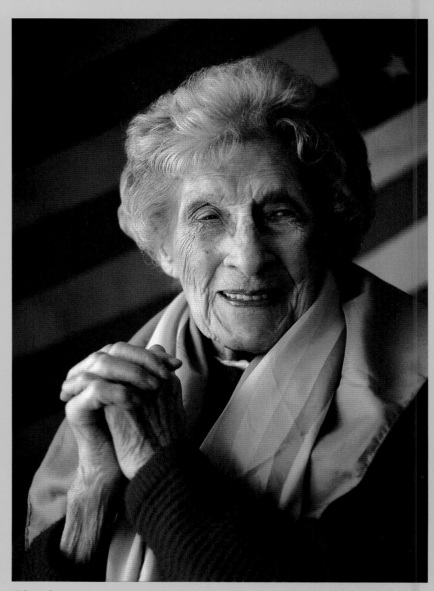

"I loved my parents a lot. And I loved to dance." Wilhelmina Pier, South Bend, IN. 109 years old. *Photo by Gary S. Chapman*

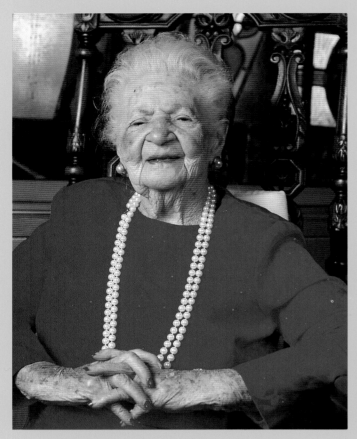

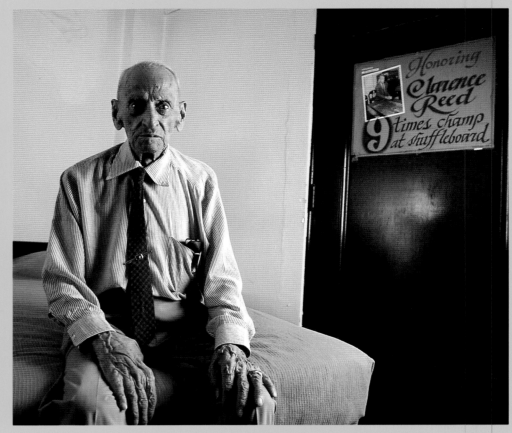

"I never hurt anyone. I was honest and helped charities."
Mollie Silberman, Dallas, TX. 104 years old. *Photo by J.W. Fry*

"I'm too far gone to give advice, kiddo. I drink a lot of water." Clarence Reed, Bedford, VA.
101 years old. *Photo by Cindy Pinkston*

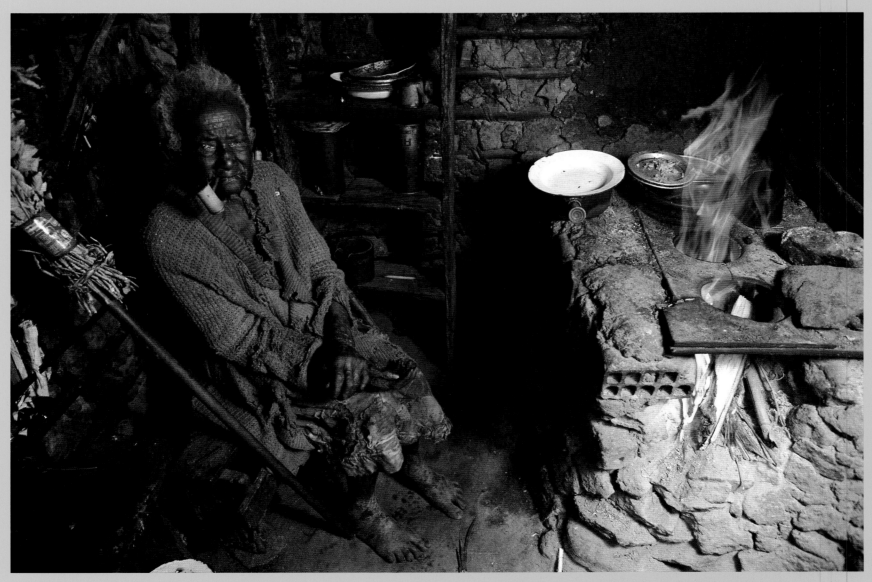

"I smoke my pipe every day, and until recently I drank sugar cane liquor every day." Maria Madalena Venanca Da Silva, Belmiro Braga, Brazil. 103 years old.
Photo by Claus C. Meyer

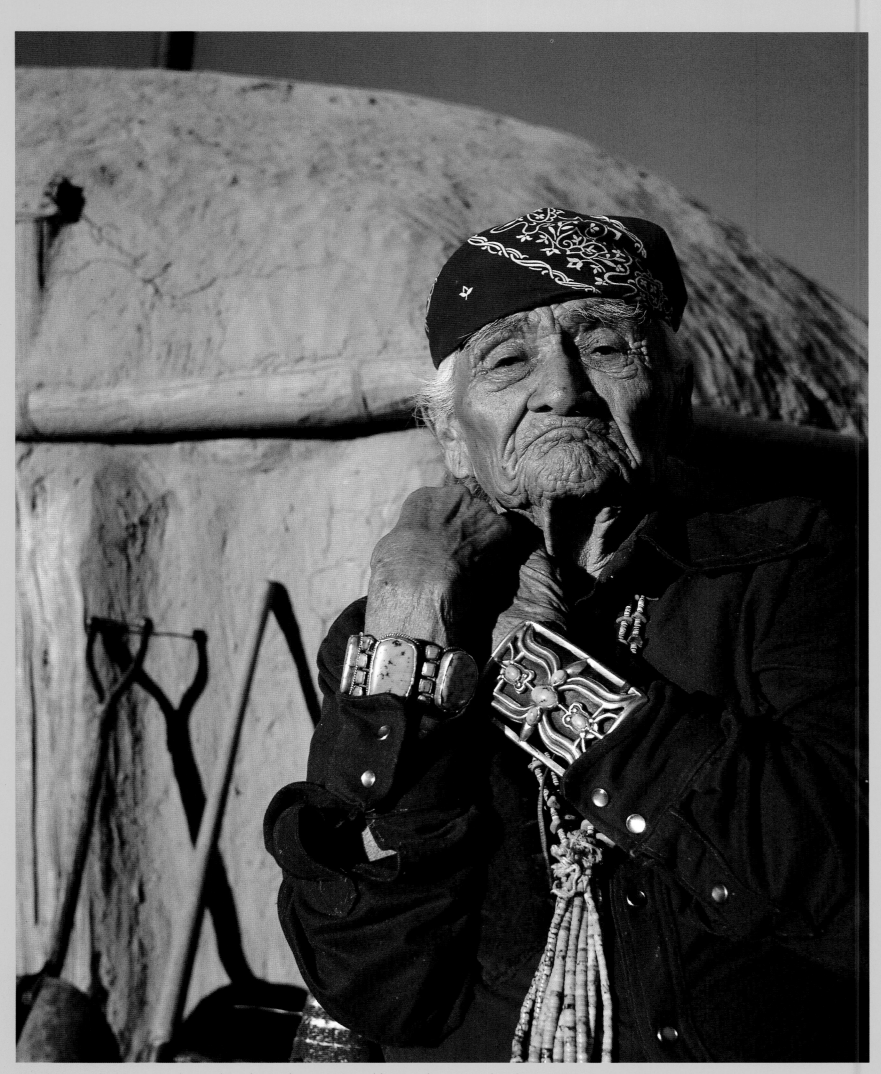

"Until I was eighty-four I ran three miles a day. In the winter I would run in the snow with only my underwear on." John Parrish, medicine man, Monument Valley, AZ. 104 years old. *Photo by Ethan Hoffman*

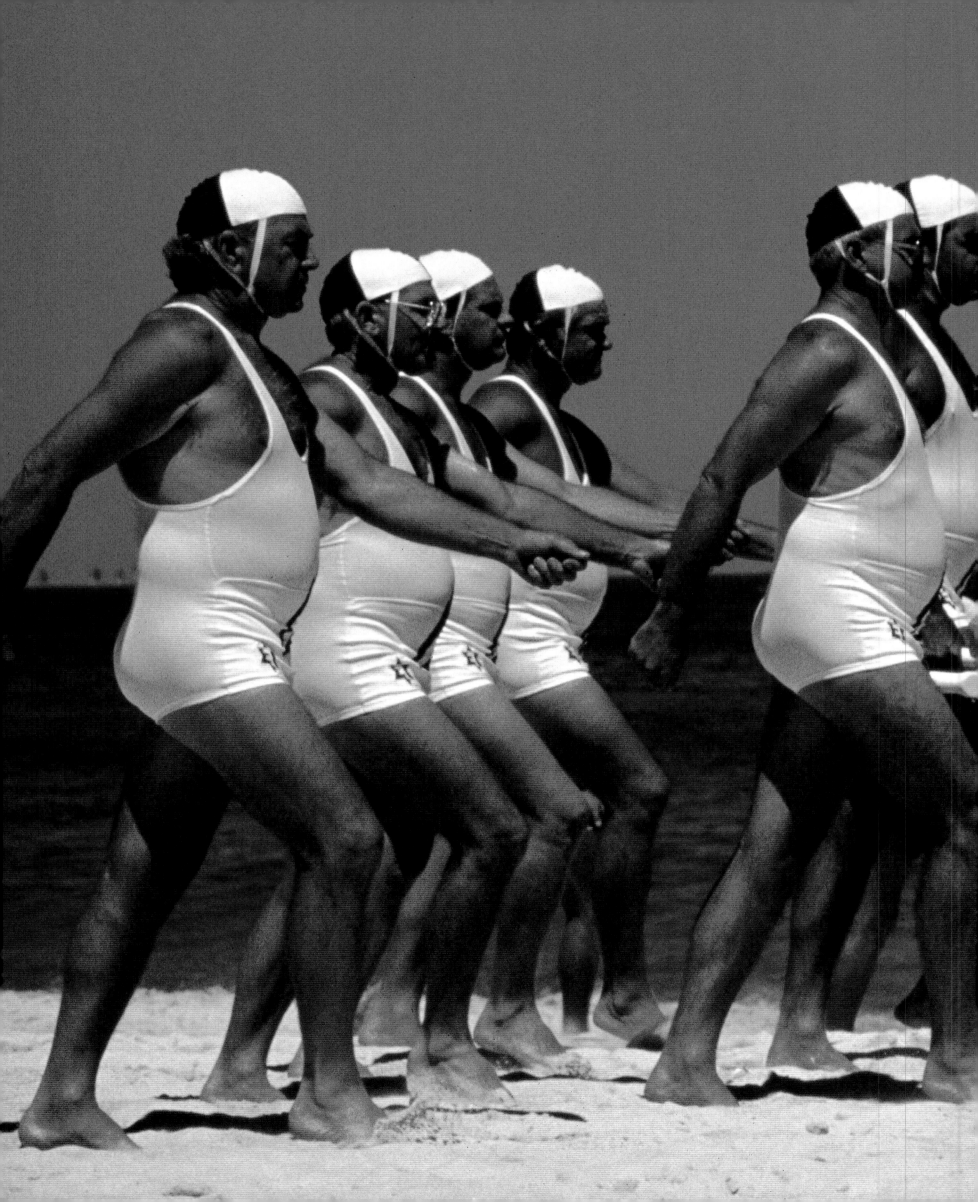

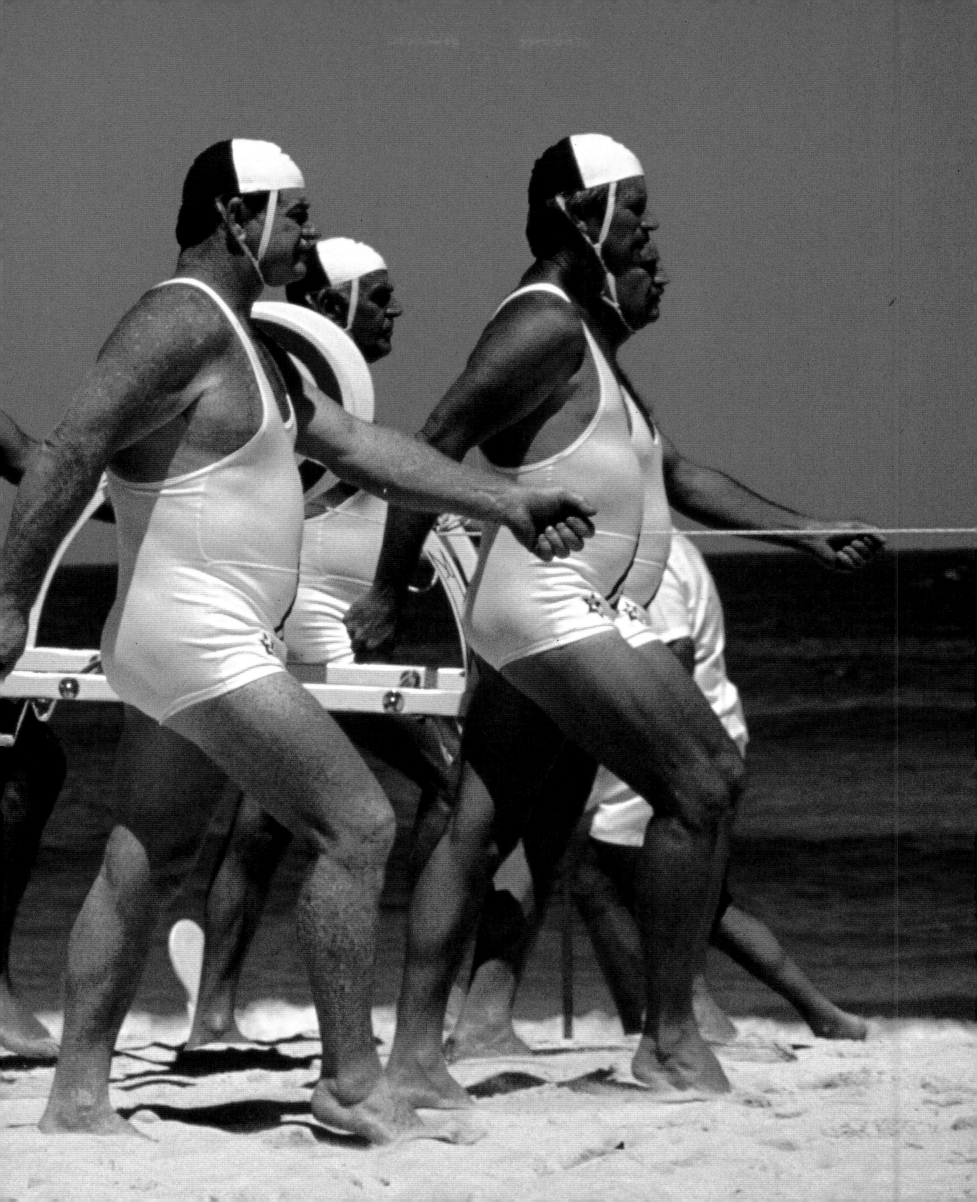

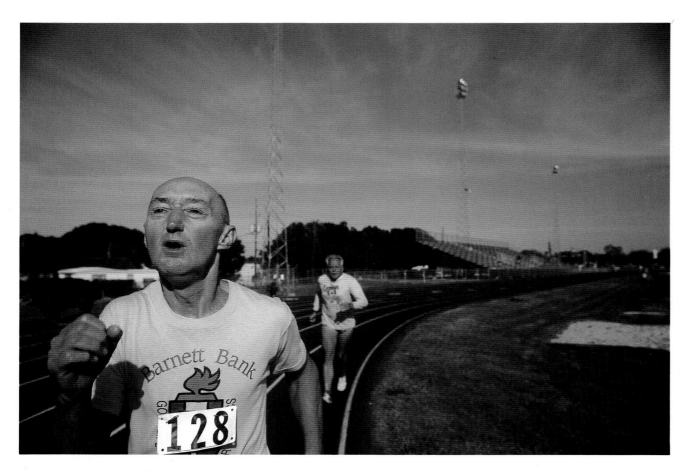

◄ **Saving lives at the Australian seashore isn't just for the young:** volunteer lifeguards in Sydney, their ages ranging from thirty-six to fifty-nine, walk smartly on the beach in preparation for the Surf Life Saving Club Association carnival — a televised, twenty-two-event competition among the country's more than 250 lifeguard clubs. These men, from the Freshwater club, train four hours a week for the March Past event, which is judged on precision, style, and coordination.
Photo by Klaus Bossemeyer

▲ **Pacemaker and all,** sixty-two-year-old Bob Moore spurts to victory in the 1500-meter race at the Good Life Games in Clearwater, Florida. More than 2,000 seniors from Pinellas County compete each year in eighteen events, which some participants use as a springboard to the Senior National Olympics. Moore, whose winning time here was 9:09, says he would have won the gold at the National Olympics last year "if I hadn't had to replace my pacemaker a few months before the race. That slowed me down."
Photo by Jerry Valente

► **Still supple at seventy-five,** Foofie Harlan of the Sun City Poms credits much of her shapeliness to her pantyhose — "heavy, shiny pairs that hold me in real good." Harlan moved to the Arizona retirement community sixteen years ago and has no formal training in acrobatics. She and the other Poms, average age seventy-four, strut their stuff each year in parades across the country.
Photo by Alon Reininger

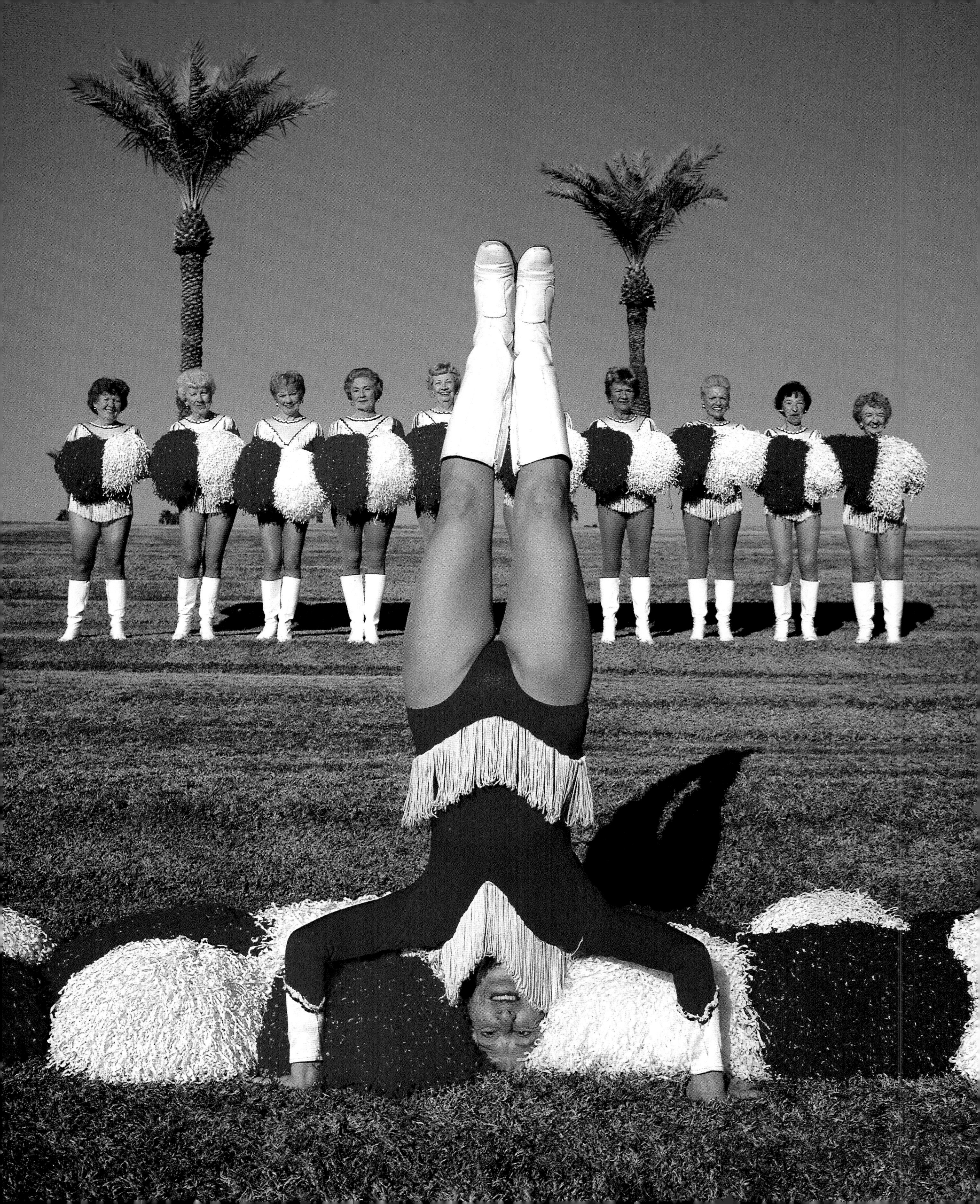

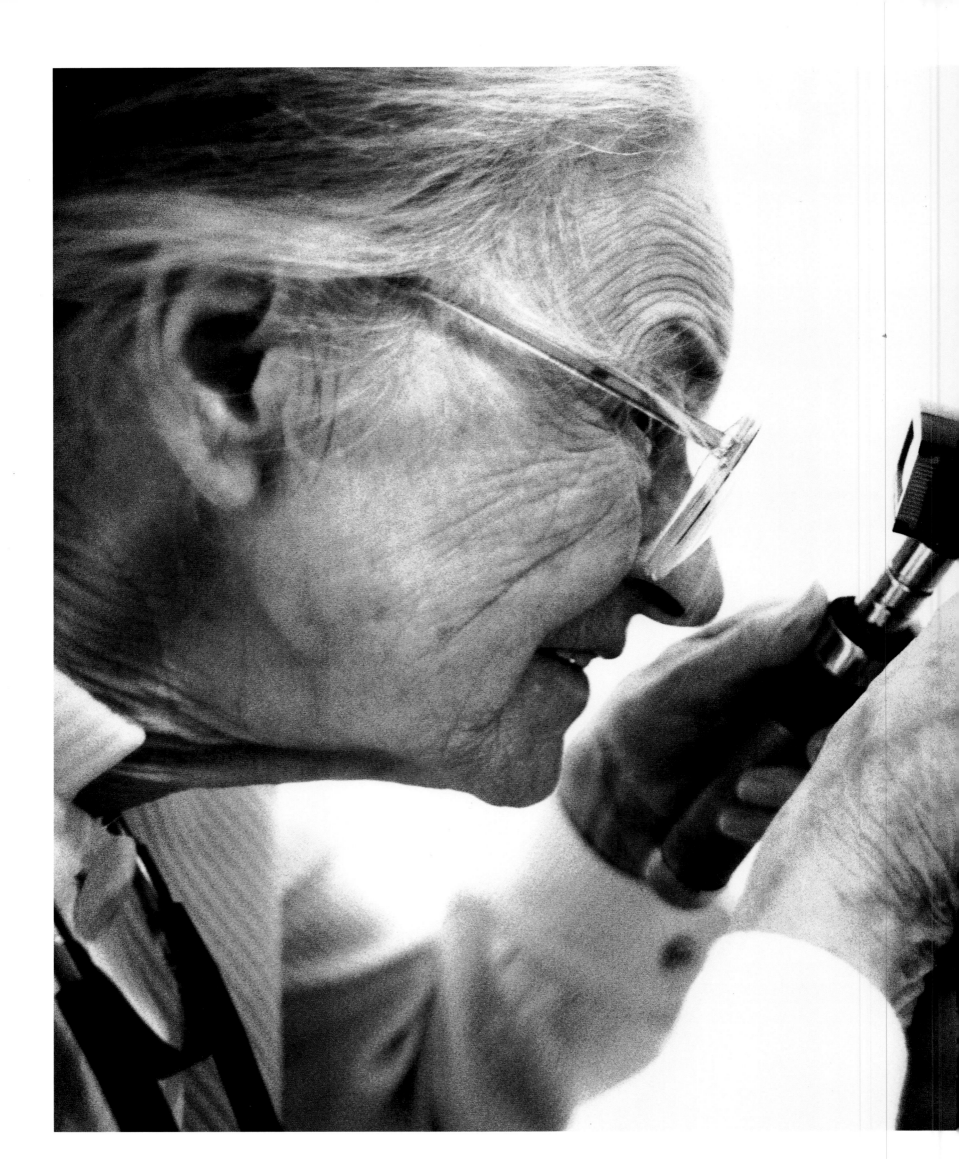

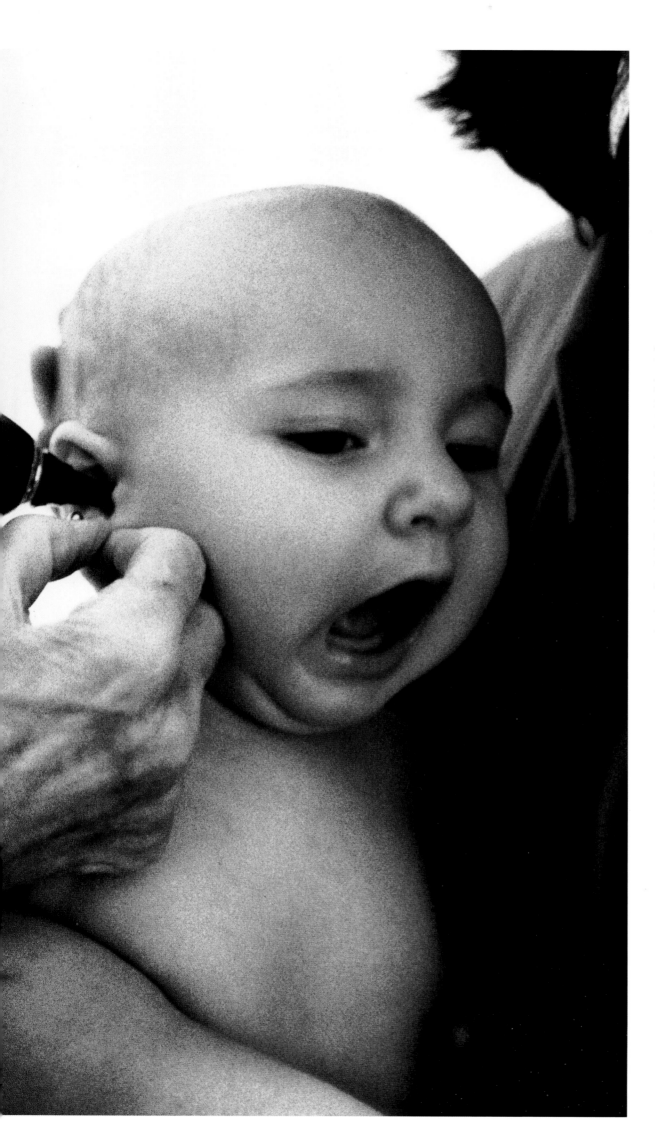

◄ **Using medicine's human touch to bridge several generations,** Dr. Leila Denmark, born in 1898, peers into the ear of her patient Rebekah De Avila, born in 1989. Denmark, who says she'll continue to practice medicine "as long as I'm able," was the third woman ever to graduate from the Medical College of Georgia in Augusta. She has practiced in Georgia ever since her 1928 graduation; besides her own practice four days a week, she also saw patients one day a week for fifty-six years in a charity clinic. "But I've never worked," says the grandmother of two, one of whom is a medical student. "If you love what you're doing, it's not work." *Photo by Jerry Valente*

A Century of Progress

The twentieth century has been an astonishing time in humanity's quest to gain power over illness and disease. The first nine decades of this century of progress in science, medicine, and public health policy have featured:

A victory over bacteria. The most significant medical achievement of the century's first half was the 1928 discovery of penicillin, which was first used to treat a human patient in 1941. With penicillin and the other antibiotics that followed, most infectious bacterial diseases, such as scarlet fever, rheumatic fever, gonorrhea, and meningitis, can be cured.

The end of smallpox. In 1980 the World Health Organization announced the eradication of smallpox. As recently as 1967, there were ten million new sufferers of smallpox in the world annually, two million of whom died. Never before in recorded history had an infectious disease been wiped off the earth.

Hope for cancer patients. Four of every ten Americans diagnosed with cancer today will be alive five years from now. In 1930, fewer than two Americans in ten survived at least five years after being diagnosed.

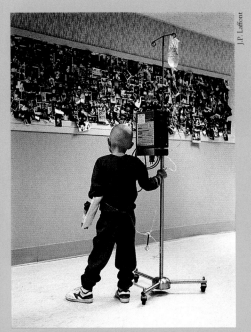

J.P. Laffont

Understanding genetics. The 1951 discovery of the DNA molecule's double helix structure may be the most remarkable medical breakthrough of the twentieth century. It opened up an entirely new field of medicine, which has led to bioengineered drugs such as blood-clot-dissolving agents and a more reliable and plentiful vaccine for hepatitis B, a sometimes fatal viral disease. What's more, gene defects can now be correlated with specific diseases. Researchers are looking forward to the day when new genes can be inserted into diseased bodies to effect cures for hundreds of diseases and maladies.

Healthier hearts. With Americans smoking less, exercising more, and watching what they eat — and with the innovations over the past twenty years of coronary bypass surgery, clot busters, and angioplasty — the coronary heart disease death rate has dropped almost in half since its 1963 peak.

Insights into the mind. In 1900 Sigmund Freud published *The Interpretation of Dreams*, which began to focus scientific attention on his theories of the workings of the human psyche. Later in the century, Carl Gustav Jung and others built on Freud's work by providing diagnostic tools and standard treatments for mental and emotional disorders.

New kidneys, hearts, and livers. In 1967 Dr. Christiaan Barnard drew on research by doctors around the world to perform the first heart transplant. Some 1,500 heart transplants have been performed since. Other transplantable organs include the heart and lungs together, the kidneys, the liver, and the pancreas.

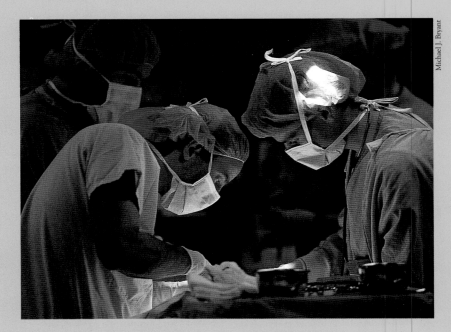

Michael J. Bryant

Control of diabetes. In 1920 life expectancy for many diabetics was just a handful of years after the disease's onset. Insulin, discovered in 1921, is now the key to survival for nearly two million of the twelve million American diabetics.

Radiation as a life force. In 1904 Pierre and Marie Curie proved that radium kills diseased cells preferentially, leading to its use in fighting cancer. Radioactive substances are now also used to treat a host of disorders, including thyroid disease and an overabundance of red blood cells.

The decline of polio. Health officials hope to announce the worldwide elimination of polio by the year 2000, less than fifty years after the development of the Salk vaccine.

Dentistry without pain. Novocaine was introduced in 1910.

Immunization against childhood killers. In 1901 German doctor Emil von Behring won the first Nobel Prize in Medicine for his development of an antitoxin for diphtheria, which was killing as many as 20,000 American children annually. Immunization for diphtheria, whooping cough, and tetanus is now a routine event in an American child's first year.

Computers as diagnostic aids. The 1973 introduction of computerized axial tomography, or CAT scans, and the 1984 introduction of magnetic resonance imaging, or MRI, have greatly aided doctors in their ability to diagnose disorders of the brain and nervous system. In 1980 only ten percent of victims of severe head trauma were expected to live. By 1990, thanks in part to the diagnostic abilities of CAT scans and MRI, that figure had jumped to nearly ninety percent.

The Challenges That Remain

Despite the impressive medical accomplishments in this century, we still face imposing health problems — many of which are questions of public policy or human neglect as much as questions of scientific research. Here are but a few of the health challenges of coming years:

The killer virus. The human immunodeficiency virus, which causes AIDS, infects about 10,000 people in the world monthly.

The killer microorganism. Malaria strikes 150 million people worldwide each year, causing some 2 million deaths. Half the world's people live in areas where the disease is common.

Death by influenza. Despite the development of flu vaccines in the early 1940s, the rapidly mutating flu virus continues to outwit scientists. More than 40,000 Americans are killed by the flu in a typical epidemic year.

Dying young in America. The U.S. infant mortality rate ranks twenty-first in the world.

The ravages of tobacco. Tobacco kills more Americans each year, nearly 400,000, than died in World War II. Around the world, smoking kills about 2.5 million people annually — not even counting deaths in the Third World from smoking-induced heart disease.

Access to health care. One of every eight Americans is without health insurance.

Sickle-cell anemia, Tay-Sachs, and cystic fibrosis. These genetically transmitted — and so far incurable — diseases strike primarily young people whose ancestors came from equatorial Africa, eastern Europe, and northern Europe, respectively. Sickle-cell patients can live past the age of forty, and cystic fibrosis sufferers often live into their mid-twenties, but children born with Tay-Sachs die before the age of five.

Heart disease: still the big killer. Almost as many Americans die each year of cardiovascular disease — about a million — as from all other causes of death combined.

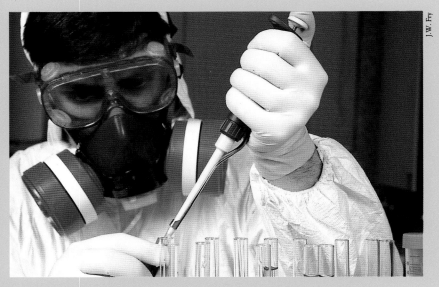

The cost of health. The average American hospital stay in 1984 cost $4,657. By 1990, that cost had doubled.

The world toll of tuberculosis, syphilis, and measles. These three treatable diseases — which are experiencing mild comebacks in the United States — each kill about two million people around the world annually.

More cancer than ever. About one in 275 Americans is diagnosed with cancer annually, a fourteen percent increase since 1973. Seventy million Americans will develop cancer in their lifetime.

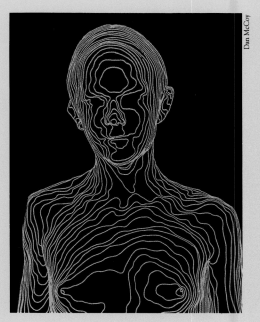

Disenfranchised in America. African-American men in Harlem are less likely to reach age sixty-five than are men in Bangladesh.

Cocaine's grip. While overall cocaine use in the United States decreased in the 1980s, the number of Americans who use the drug at least once a week rose to nearly 900,000.

Hunger and illness. One of every five people in the world goes to bed sick or malnourished.

Preventable blindness. Around twenty million people in the world are blind from cataracts. The cost of effective and routine cataract surgery remains beyond the means of most cataract sufferers in the developing world.

Deathly spirits. About 105,000 Americans die each year from injuries or diseases linked to alcohol, and some 8,000 alcohol-damaged babies are born in the United States each year.

The lack of minority doctors. Hispanic-Americans make up about five percent of all doctors in the United States, and African-Americans account for about three percent.

Unchecked tropical diseases. About half a billion people in the world suffer from tropical diseases such as malaria, leprosy, and African sleeping sickness.

A place for the aged. About 600,000 Americans over the age of eighty-five now require nursing home care. In fifty years, that number is expected to be around four million.

Still no cure. Hundreds of diseases remain incurable, among them arthritis, multiple sclerosis, cerebral palsy, Alzheimer's disease, muscular dystrophy, amyotrophic lateral sclerosis (Lou Gehrig's disease), lupus, and the common cold.

Biographies

Joseph Chaikin
For nearly a decade Chaikin directed one of the most influential experimental theater groups in the United States, the Open Theatre, which he founded in 1963 after working as an actor with the Living Theatre. He has received three Obie Awards for his directing and acting, and his work with the Open Theatre earned him the first Lifetime Achievement Obie Award in 1977. In 1984 Chaikin suffered a stroke, which left him with aphasia. Despite his language impairment, he has continued to act and direct, and in 1987 he received the Edwin Booth Award for his contribution to New York theater.

Norman Cousins
Cousins's long history of journalism and public service includes thirty-five years as editor of *Saturday Review*, diplomatic missions abroad for three presidents, numerous awards (including the United Nations Peace Medal), and an honorary degree in medicine from Yale University. His twenty-five books include *Anatomy of an Illness* and *Head First: The Biology of Hope*. Cousins currently teaches at the UCLA School of Medicine.

Michael Crichton, M.D.
Educated at Harvard Medical School, Crichton has since turned his hand to more literary pursuits. He has authored several novels, including *The Andromeda Strain*, *The Terminal Man*, and *The Great Train Robbery*. His four works of nonfiction include *Five Patients*, a book about American hospital medicine. He has directed six feature films, including *Coma*, *The Great Train Robbery*, and most recently, *Physical Evidence* in 1989. Crichton also collects modern art and creates computer games.

Wade Davis, Ph.D.
Davis, educated in ethnobotany at Harvard University, has done extensive field work in Haiti and in the Amazon region of South America, resulting in two books: *The Serpent and the Rainbow* and *Passage of Darkness*. Davis's articles and photographs have been published in dozens of periodicals as diverse as *People* and the *Journal of Ethnopharmacology*, and he has led workshops on folk healing. A native of Canada, he now divides his time between homes in Washington, D.C., and West Vancouver, British Columbia.

Barbara Ehrenreich, Ph.D.
Feminist writer and lecturer Ehrenreich is the co-author of *For Her Own Good: 150 Years of the Experts' Advice to Women*, *The American Health Empire: Power, Profits and Politics*, and *Witches, Midwives and Nurses: A History of Women Healers*. She has written for numerous publications, ranging from *Vogue* to the *Wall Street Journal* to *Mother Jones*, and was the recipient of the 1980 National Magazine Award for Excellence in Reporting. She holds a Ph.D. in biology from Rockefeller University. Ehrenreich's latest book, *Fear of Falling: The Inner Life of the Middle Class*, was nominated for a National Book Critics Circle Award in 1989.

Maxine Hong Kingston
Born in Stockton, California, Kingston is the author of three books that chronicle and comment on the Chinese-American experience — *The Woman Warrior*, winner of the National Book Critics Circle Award in 1976, *China Men*, for which she received the 1981 American Book Award, and *Tripmaster Monkey, His Fake Book*. She lives in Oakland, California, with her husband, the actor Earll Kingston.

Elisabeth Kübler-Ross, M.D.
Kübler-Ross's 1969 book, *On Death and Dying*, was a landmark study of human emotional response and methods of coping with loss. The book's profound influence led to the author's selection by *Ladies' Home Journal* as Woman of the Decade ten years later. A native of Switzerland, Kübler-Ross emigrated to the United States in 1958 and has taught at the University of Chicago and the University of Colorado. She currently serves on the faculty of the University of Virginia. Her latest book is *AIDS: The Ultimate Challenge*.

George Leonard
Leonard was a senior editor at *Look* magazine from 1953 to 1970, and has won thirteen national awards for education reporting. His many books include *Education & Ecstasy*, *The Ultimate Athlete*, and *Silent Pulse*. He has written articles for a wide range of magazines, including *Esquire*, for which he is a contributing editor and produces the annual "Ultimate Health and Fitness" issue. He is also the co-owner of an aikido school and holds a third-degree black belt.

Phillip Moffitt
Moffitt, co-creator of *The Power to Heal*, was editor in chief of *Esquire* magazine and chief executive officer of the Esquire Magazine Group from 1979 to 1986. Prior to his years at *Esquire*, Moffitt co-founded the 13-30 Corporation (now Whittle Communications), serving as both editor in chief and president. He is a co-founder of Light Source, a computer graphics software publishing company; a director of the C.G. Jung Foundation; and a founding member of the Social Venture Network, a group of entrepreneurs working for socially responsible values in business practices. In 1989 *Inc.* magazine named Moffitt one of the top entrepreneurs of the decade.

John Poppy
Born in Prague, Czechoslovakia, Poppy has co-written and edited six books, including *Minamata* with W. Eugene Smith and Aileen Smith, which was nominated for a National Book Award in 1975. He served as a senior editor at *Look* and is currently a contributing editor for *In Health*. Believing that "prudent attention to health is better than obsession," Poppy jogs two miles three times a week. His column, "Active Health," appears monthly in *Esquire*.

Richard Restak, M.D.
Restak, one of the world's foremost neuropsychiatrists, is the author of five books concerning the human brain. He has served as a consultant for West German television, the Smithsonian Institution, and the U.S. Congress. His extensive publishing credits include the *World Book Encyclopedia*, *Newsday*, the *Washington Post*, *Vogue*, *Science Digest*, and *Publisher's Weekly*, and his commentary has been broadcast on National Public Radio.

Judith Thurman
Born in New York and educated at Brandeis University, Thurman is the author of *Isak Dinesen: The Life of a Storyteller*, which won the 1983 National Book Award for Biography and has been translated into eleven languages. The book was the basis for the motion picture *Out of Africa*, for which Thurman was an associate producer. She is a frequent contributor to the *New Yorker* and is at work on a biography of Colette, which Knopf will publish in 1994.

Jean-Claude van Itallie
Van Itallie was born in Brussels, raised in Long Island, and educated at Harvard University. His trilogy of one-act plays, *America Hurrah*, was hailed as the landmark off-Broadway show of the 1960s. He has received Vernon Rice, Obie, and Drama Desk awards as well as numerous grants and fellowships. He has taught playwriting and theater at Princeton University, the University of Colorado, New York University, and the Naropa Institute.

Rick Weiss
Weiss, a licensed medical technologist, is life sciences and biomedicine editor at *Science News* magazine in Washington, D.C. His work has appeared in the *Washington Post*, the *Los Angeles Times*, the *San Jose Mercury-News*, and the *Tribune* of Oakland, California. He received a B.A. in biology from Cornell University and a master's degree in journalism from the University of California at Berkeley.

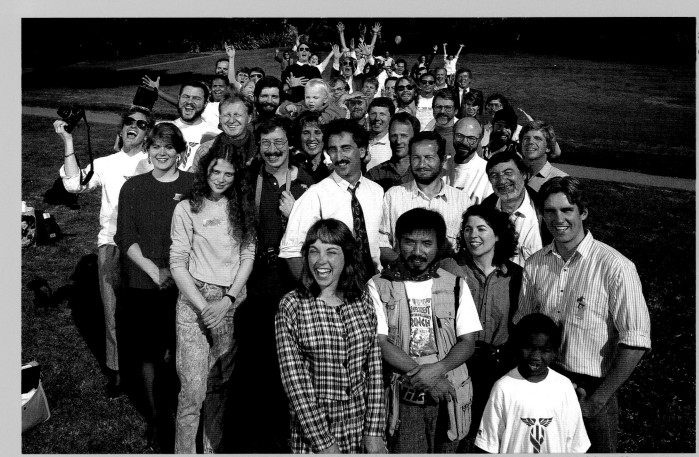

The staff of The Power to Heal *and many of the project's photographers gather in San Francisco before scattering to their assignments around the world.*

Photographers

Monica Almeida, American
Almeida began her career at the *Los Angeles Times* as part of the team of journalists awarded the 1984 Pulitzer Prize for coverage of California's Hispanic community. Since 1986 she has been a staff photographer for the *New York Daily News*.

Shlomo Arad, Israeli
Born in Austria, Arad escaped Nazi Germany as a child. Best known for his combat and war photography, he has been on contract with *Newsweek* for the last twelve years. He regularly publishes work in *Life, Bunte*, and the *New York Times Magazine*.

José Azel, American
Cuban-born Azel is a regular contributor to *National Geographic*. His work also appears in *Smithsonian* and *Time*, and his coverage of the 1988 Summer Olympics earned him a World Press Photo Foundation award.

Eric Lars Bakke, American
During his seventeen-year career, Bakke has covered events ranging from the World Series and the Super Bowl to insect infestation in Utah and fire storms in Yellowstone National Park. His work has been published in *Time, Sports Illustrated, Business Week*, and *National Geographic*.

Nina Barnett, American
Barnett is a New York-based freelance photographer whose work appears in *Fortune, Forbes, New York Woman*, and *Money*. In 1989 *American Photographer* nominated her as a "New Face" in American photojournalism.

Annie Griffiths Belt, American
Belt began assignment work for *National Geographic* in 1978, and has worked since on more than two dozen magazine and book projects. Her work has also appeared in *Newsweek, Geo*, and *Stern*, and she has exhibited in New York, Washington, D.C., Moscow, and Tokyo.

Nicole Bengiveno, American
In 1986 Bengiveno joined the staff of the *New York Daily News* after eight years with the *San Francisco Examiner*, where she was named Bay Area Press Photographer of the Year in 1979. In 1987 and 1989 she won first-place honors in feature photography from the New York Associated Press for her work from the Soviet Union.

P.F. Bentley, American
Bentley is a *Time* magazine photographer based in Stinson Beach, California. His awards include first-place honors in the

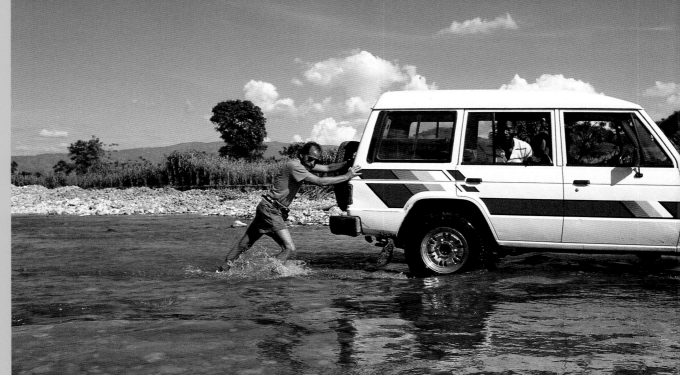

Photographer P.F. Bentley on the road in the central highlands of Haiti.

National Press Photographers Association Pictures of the Year competitions in 1984 and 1988 for his coverage of the United States presidential campaigns.

Alan Berner, American
Berner worked for five newspapers before joining the *Seattle Times*. He has twice been named a National Press Photographers Association Regional Photographer of the Year, and he won the Robert F. Kennedy Journalism Award for Outstanding Coverage of the Disadvantaged.

Klaus Bossemeyer, German
Since 1979 Bossemeyer has been a freelance photographer, working primarily for German publications such as *Stern, Geo*, and *Merian*.

Torin Boyd, American
A veteran of many *Day in the Life* projects, Boyd began his career as a surfing photographer at the age of seventeen in Florida. Now based in Tokyo, he contributes to *Fortune, Newsweek, Time, U.S. News & World Report*, and several Japanese magazines.

Michael J. Bryant, American
A staff photographer at the *Philadelphia Inquirer*, Bryant has won Photographer of the Year honors in Pennsylvania (1988), California (1980), and Michigan (1979).

George Y.F. Chan, Chinese
Chan has written and photographed in two dozen countries as a staff photographer for the *Earth Chinese Geographic Monthly*. His work has been exhibited in Hong Kong, Taipei, and Tokyo.

Gary S. Chapman, American
A staff photographer for the Sunday magazine of the *Louisville*

Courier-Journal, Chapman has also participated in seven *Day in the Life* projects, as well as freelancing for the National Geographic Society, *Time, Newsweek, Sports Illustrated*, and *Forbes*.

Paul Chesley, American
As a freelancer with the National Geographic Society since 1975, Chesley has traveled regularly to Europe and Asia. Solo exhibitions of his work have appeared in museums in London, Tokyo, and New York. He has participated in eight *Day in the Life* projects.

Bradley E. Clift, American
Clift, now a staff photographer for the *Hartford Courant*, won the National Press Photographers Association Photographer of the Year Award and a World Press Photo Foundation award in 1986, and he won the Robert F. Kennedy Award for Photojournalism in 1987. The cover of *A Day in the Life of California* features a picture taken by Clift.

Jay Dickman, American
A 1983 Pulitzer Prize winner and gold medalist in the World Press Photo Foundation competition, Dickman is a freelancer based in Denver. His work appears in *Time, Life, Geo, Bunte*, and *Stern*.

Don Doll, S.J., American
Doll recently completed an eight-month study of the Athabascan Indians along the Yukon River in Alaska that appeared in *National Geographic*. In the 1989 Pictures of the Year competition, sponsored by the National Press Photographers Association, he won first place in the magazine feature photograph category.

Dan Dry, American
Dry has received more than 300 awards, including National Newspaper Photographer of the Year in 1981 for his work while on staff at the *Louisville Courier-Journal* and the *Louisville Times*. In 1984 one of his photos appeared on the cover of *A Day in the Life of Hawaii*.

Misha Erwitt, American
Erwitt has been taking pictures since he was eleven years old and is now on the staff of the *New York Daily News*. His work has been published in *Esquire, People*, and *Manhattan, inc.*, and he has participated in six *Day in the Life* projects.

Jürgen Escher, West German
Escher began his study of photography while attending a design high school in Bielefeld, West Germany. Since 1983 he has been member of the photo agency Present/Essen, working as a freelance photographer.

David Eulitt, American
Eulitt was twice named College Photographer of the Year by the National Press Photographers Association. Before joining the staff of the *San Bernardino Sun* in 1988, he interned with the *Indianapolis News* and the *Flint Journal*. He was a student at the 1989 Eddie Adams Workshop.

Melissa Farlow, American
In 1975 Farlow was a member of the *Louisville Courier-Journal* and *Louisville Times* photography staff that received a Pulitzer Prize for its coverage of desegregation of the public schools. Now a staff photographer for the *Pittsburgh Press*, she is a two-time Pittsburgh Photographer of the Year.

Enrico Ferorelli, Italian
A freelance photographer for twenty-four years, Ferorelli travels widely on assignment, and his pictures have appeared in *National Geographic, Time, Newsweek, Life, Smithsonian, Sports Illustrated*, and the *London Sunday Times*.

Dana Fineman, American
A member of the Sygma photo agency, Fineman studied at the Art Center College of Design in Pasadena, California. Her work appears regularly in *New York Magazine, People, Time, Newsweek*, and *Stern*.

Joachim Fischer, M.D., West German
Now a pediatrician at Herdecke University Hospital, Fischer worked in New Zealand for several years as both a doctor and a photographer. His photos have appeared in *Geo* and *Die Zeit*.

Victor Fisher, Canadian
Fisher is a Toronto-based freelance photographer who shoots regularly for *Newsweek, People*, the *New York Times, Canadian Living*, and *Maclean's*.

Sam Forenich, American
Forencich was a staff photographer for the *Peninsula (Palo Alto) Times Tribune* for five years before starting his freelance career in 1988. He works for *USA Today*, the *Christian Science Monitor*, the *San Jose Mercury News*, and the *San Francisco Examiner*.

Peter Freed, American
Freed started his photojournalism career as a freelancer for the *New York Times*, logging more than 1,000 assignments in his first three years. His work appears regularly in *Newsweek, Forbes, Business*

Gene Kunz

Week, the *New York Times*, and *New York Magazine*.

J.W. Fry, American
After receiving his degree in photography from East Texas State University, Fry worked as a freelance photographer in Dallas. In 1989 he was accepted to the Eddie Adams Workshop, where he won a one-year fellowship with the Professional Photography Division of Eastman Kodak.

Raphaël Gaillarde, French
Gaillarde is associated with Gamma Presse Images, and his pictures of world events have appeared in many European magazines. He has participated in several *Day in the Life* projects.

Sam Garcia, American
Garcia is on staff with Nikon Professional Services. In his fourteen years with Nikon he has covered most major sporting events, including four Olympic Games, and he has trained America's space shuttle astronauts to use 35mm still equipment. A participant in six *Day in the Life* projects, Garcia is also on the faculty of the Eddie Adams Workshop.

William F. Gentile, American
Gentile is *Newsweek*'s Latin America and Caribbean photographer, and has lived in Nicaragua since 1983. His book, *Nicaragua*, was published in 1989 by W.W. Norton.

Diego Goldberg, Argentine
After beginning his career in Latin America, Goldberg moved to Paris in 1977 as a Sygma staff photographer. In 1985 he returned to his native Argentina. His work has been featured in the world's major magazines, and in 1984 he won a World Press Photo Foundation award.

George Grall, American
Grall is on the staff of the National Aquarium in Baltimore, and exhibits his work throughout the aquatic facility. A photojournalist for nineteen years, he has published work in *Life*, *National Geographic World*, and *Science*.

Peter S. Greenberg, American
Greenberg, a freelance photographer for more than twenty years, is the former west coast correspondent for *Newsweek*. He also writes for several magazines, including *Rolling Stone* and *Playboy*.

Judy Griesedieck, American
As a staff photographer for the *San Jose Mercury News*, Griesedieck has covered the 1984 Democratic Convention, the Calgary Winter Olympics, and the Super Bowl. She was California Photographer of the Year in 1986. While a staff

photographer for the *Hartford Courant*, she was named Connecticut Photographer of the Year in 1983.

Skeeter Hagler, American
During his fifteen years with the *Dallas Times Herald*, Hagler won numerous state and national awards, including the Pulitzer Prize for feature photography in 1980 for his series on the Texas cowboy. Recently President George Bush requested a set of the series to be displayed in the White House.

Henry Hilliard, American
Hilliard has traveled the world on assignment for a variety of editorial and corporate clients. His recent assignments have taken him to the Soviet republics of Uzbekistan and Armenia, the rainforests of Central America, and the Swiss Alps.

Volker Hinz, West German
For the last sixteen years, Hinz has been a staff photographer for *Stern* magazine. His pictures also appear in many other publications, including *Vanity Fair*, *Time*, *Newsweek*, *Life*, and *Paris Match*.

Ethan Hoffman, American
Hoffman's work has appeared in a wide variety of publications including *Life*, *Stern*, *Geo*, and *Fortune*. He was nominated for a National Book Award in 1981 for *Concrete Mama: Prison Profiles from Walla Walla*. His last book was *Butoh: Dance of the Dark Soul*. Hoffman was killed while on assignment in June, 1990, at the age of 40.

Doug Hulcher, American
Hulcher lives in Bangkok, Thailand, where he is executive director of the Refugee Family Reunification Project. He has published work in *National Geographic*, *Geo*, and the *Minneapolis Star Tribune*.

Lynn Johnson, American
After working for seven years for the *Pittsburgh Press*, Johnson joined Black Star photo agency in 1984. She has shot on assignment for *Time*, *Fortune*, *Forbes*, *National Geographic*, and the *New York Times Magazine*, and her work is represented in the permanent collection of the Carnegie Museum of Art. She is a 1988 World Press Photo Foundation award winner.

Karen Kasmauski, American
Kasmauski spent five years with the *Virginian Pilot/Ledger-Star* before becoming a freelancer. Her awards include special recognition in the 1983 Robert F. Kennedy

Torin Boyd prepares to begin shooting at Toyota Memorial Hospital in Tokyo.

Journalism Awards for Outstanding Coverage of the Disadvantaged.

Nick Kelsh, American
Kelsh's photos have appeared in *Time*, *Life*, *Newsweek*, *National Geographic*, *Forbes*, *Fortune*, and *Business Week*. In 1986 he co-founded Kelsh Marr Studios, a company that specializes in the design of and photography for annual reports and other corporate publications. A picture taken by Kelsh is featured on the cover of *A Day in the Life of China*.

Robb Kendrick, American
Kendrick has published work in *Time*, *Life*, *Sports Illustrated*, *National Geographic*, *Geo*, *Merian*, *Fortune*, and the *New York Times*. A recent solo exhibition at the FotoFest in Houston featured his work on Texas ranching.

Kim Komenich, American
Since 1982 Komenich has been a staff photographer for the *San Francisco Examiner*, and in 1987 he received the Pulitzer Prize for his coverage of the revolution in the Philippines. In addition, he freelances for *Time*, *Newsweek*, *U.S. News & World Report*, and other magazines.

Péter Korniss, Hungarian
Korniss has worked as a photographer since 1958, including a thirteen-year project photographing folk culture in Hungary and other Eastern European countries. He is a three-time juror for the World Press Photo Foundation competition and a member of the W. Eugene Smith Memorial Fund advisory board.

J.P. Laffont, French
Laffont was a founding member of the Gamma and Sygma photo agencies. He has won awards from the New York Newspaper Guild and the Overseas Press Club of America, and has received the

World Press General Picture Award and the Nikon World Understanding Award. His work appears regularly in the world's leading newsmagazines.

Frans Lanting, Dutch
Lanting is a freelancer whose work has been honored by the World Press Photo Foundation and the American Society of Magazine Photographers. One of his photos graces the cover of the best-selling *A Day in the Life of America*.

Frederic Larson, American
Larson is a staff photographer for the *San Francisco Chronicle*, and in 1989 he was named Photographer of the Year by the California Press Photographers Association. He was also recently elected to the Football Photography Hall of Fame in Canton, Ohio.

Sarah Leen, American
A freelancer based in Philadelphia, Leen works primarily for *National Geographic* and is associated with Matrix International. In 1986 she received honorable mention in the Robert F. Kennedy Journalism Awards for her work on Alzheimer's disease.

Leong Ka Tai, Chinese
Leong has traveled extensively for editorial and corporate clients. He is a founding member of the Hong Kong Institute of Professional Photographers.

Andy Levin, American
A seven-time *Day in the Life* participant, Levin has covered a wide variety of medical subjects for magazines. In 1985 he received top honors in the National Press Photographers Association Pictures of the Year competition for his essay on a Nebraska

farm family. In 1986 his essay on the Statue of Liberty won similar honors.

Barry Lewis, British
Lewis was a founding member of the Network agency. He works for *Life*, *Geo*, the *London Sunday Times*, and the *Observer*, and has photos on display in several U.S. and British museums.

Douglas Lewis, M.D., American
Lewis divides his time between photography and medicine. A graduate of Yale Medical School, he completed his residency and fellowship training at Harvard University. He has exhibited work in San Diego, San Francisco, New Haven, and Tahiti.

Vickie Lewis, American
Currently based in Washington, D.C., Lewis has contributed pictures to *Stern*, *People*, *National Geographic World*, and *Sport*.

Gerd Ludwig, West German
A founding member of the Visum photo agency in Hamburg, Ludwig is a regular contributor to *Geo*, *Life*, *Stern*, *Fortune*, and *Zeit Magazin*. He is an honorary member of the Deutsche Gesellschaft für Fotografie.

Mary Ellen Mark, American
Winner of numerous grants and awards, including the George W. Polk, Robert F. Kennedy, and Philippe Halsman awards for photojournalism, Mark has exhibited her work throughout the world. She currently contributes to *Life*, *Stern*, *Vanity Fair*, and the *New York Times*.

John Marmaras, Australian
Now based in Sydney, Marmaras spent eight years in London and thirteen years in New York. He has worked on assignment for major magazines including *Time*,

Newsweek, the London Daily Telegraph, Esquire, and Sports Illustrated.

Richard Marshall, American
A three-time regional National Press Photographers Association Photographer of the Year, Marshall currently works for the St. Paul Pioneer Press Dispatch. In 1985 he was Gannett Group Photographer of the Year for his black and white photography.

Stephanie Maze, American
Since 1979 Maze has been a freelance photographer for National Geographic. She has covered three Olympic Games and won a first-place award from the White House Press Photographers Association in 1985.

James McGoon, American
McGoon specializes in editorial portraiture and reportage. He began his career in 1982, and has since published work in Fortune, Esquire, Manhattan, inc., New York Magazine, and Texas Monthly. He has contributed to exhibitions in the United States and Europe.

Wally McNamee, American
For more than twenty years, McNamee has been a staff photographer for Newsweek, to which he has contributed more than 100 cover pictures. He is a four-time winner of the White House News Photographers Association's Photographer of the Year Award.

Dilip Mehta, Canadian
An original member of Contact Press Images, Mehta is a regular contributor to Time, Fortune, Geo, Paris Match, and the London Sunday Times. He frequently returns to his native India to cover news events. His images of the chemical disaster in Bhopal and the aftermath of the assassination of Indira Gandhi earned him two World Press Photo Foundation awards in 1985.

Jim Mendenhall, American
Mendenhall, a former Orange County Register staff photographer who now works for the Los Angeles Times, has been published in more than seventy magazines, including National Geographic, Life, Sports Illustrated, and Geo.

Doug Menuez, American
Menuez works on assignment around the world for Time, Newsweek, Fortune and other newsmagazines. In 1987 he established Reportage, an agency specializing in the design and production of annual reports, brochures, and photo essays. In 1989 Menuez co-directed 15 Seconds: The Great California Earthquake of 1989, a book project

that sold 50,000 copies and raised more than $500,000 for earthquake relief.

Claus C. Meyer, West German
Meyer was selected in 1985 by Communications World as one of the top annual-report photographers in the world. His color photography has been recognized by Kodak and Nikon, and in 1981 he won a Nikon International Grand Prize. He has published several books on Brazil.

Robin Moyer, American
Now based in Hong Kong as a staff photographer for Time, Moyer has won many awards for his photography of Asia and the Middle East, including Photo of the Year in the World Press Photo Foundation competition and the Robert Capa Gold Medal Citation from the Overseas Press Club of America. His work is represented in the Masters of Photography Collection of the Library of Congress in Washington, D.C.

Matthew Naythons, M.D., American
Co-creator of The Power to Heal, Naythons previously led parallel lives, practicing emergency-room medicine in California and traveling the world as an award-winning Time magazine photojournalist. In response to the horrors he witnessed while covering the 1979 Cambodian refugee exodus, he formed International Medical

Teams, a relief organization that brought medical care to refugees on the Thai-Cambodian border. His most recent assignment was a two-year photo essay for National Geographic on the Centers for Disease Control.

Roland Neveu, French
Neveu began his career in 1973 at the age of twenty-three, working on assignment for Time and various European magazines. While continuing to shoot for newsmagazines, he has worked since 1986 as a special and still photographer for movie productions, including Platoon and Born on the Fourth of July. He divides his time between Los Angeles and Paris.

Seny Norasingh, Laotian
Twice named North Carolina Photographer of the Year, Norasingh moved to the United States from Laos when he was seventeen. His newspaper career has included positions with the Raleigh News and Observer and the Raleigh Times. Norasingh is now a freelancer, and his work has appeared in National Geographic, Time, Newsweek, U.S. News & World Report, the Washington Post, and the Time-Life book series.

Randy Olson, American
Olson worked for the San Jose Mercury News, the Charleston (West Virginia) Gazette, and the Palm Beach Post before joining the

staff of the Pittsburgh Press. In addition to his newspaper work, he freelances for National Geographic, Fortune, and Time, and participates in Day in the Life projects. While teaching photojournalism at the University of Missouri, he received a National Archives grant for work with the Pictures of the Year Archives.

Graeme Outerbridge, Bermudian
Named the 1985 Outstanding Young Person of the Year in Bermuda, Outerbridge has exhibited work in New York, Washington, D.C., Boston, London, and Helsinki. He has published two books, the most recent of which — finished in 1989 — is on bridges of the world.

Henry Clay Owen III, American
Owen interned at the Los Angeles Times before beginning a freelance career with the Lexington Herald-Leader. In 1989 he was one of 99 young photographers chosen from more than 800 applicants to participate in the Eddie Adams Workshop, which led to his being selected to contribute to The Power to Heal.

Mark Peters, Zimbabwean
A one-time South African Press Photographer of the Year, Peters has covered all the African countries as a contract photographer for Newsweek and for newspapers around the world. His work also appears in Time and Life.

Bill Pierce, American
A contract photographer for U.S. News & World Report, Pierce played back-up guitar for Jimi Hendrix before choosing photojournalism as a career. His photos of Beirut and Belfast won him the Overseas Press Club's Oliver Rebbot Award for international photo-reportage.

Cindy Pinkston, American
Pinkston joined the staff of the Roanoke Times & World-News after interning at the Florida Times-Union and the Jacksonville Journal. Her participation in the 1989 Eddie Adams Workshop led to her being selected to shoot for The Power to Heal.

Larry C. Price, American
Price, a two-time Pulitzer Prize winner, received the honor in 1981 for his coverage of the Liberian coup and in 1985 for pictures taken in Angola and El Salvador. He is currently a staff photographer for the Philadelphia Inquirer, and his work has been honored by the Overseas Press Club, the World Press Photo Foundation, the Pan American Press Association, and the National Press Photographers Association.

Louie Psihoyos, American
In 1980 Psihoyos became a full-time contract photographer with National Geographic. Now a freelance photographer, he is

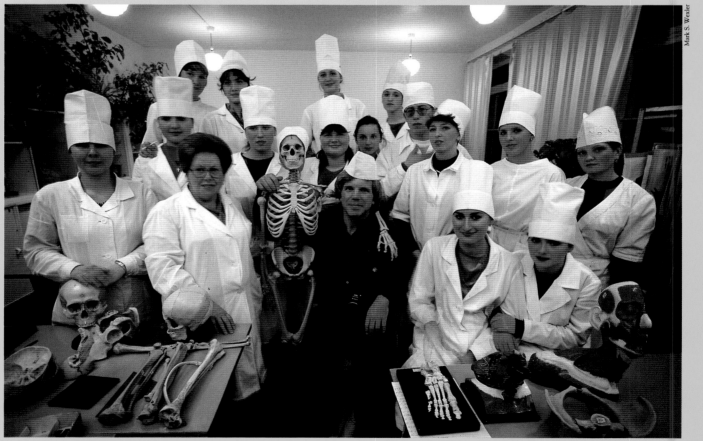

Photographer Mark S. Wexler and friends at the Magadan Nursing Institute in Siberia.

affiliated with Matrix International and shoots regularly for *Fortune*, *U.S. News & World Report*, and *Sports Illustrated*.

Alon Reininger, American/Israeli
One of the original members of Contact Press Images, Reininger's coverage of AIDS won him Press Photo of the Year from the World Press Photo Foundation in 1986 and the Philippe Halsman Award for Photojournalism in 1987. He is a regular contributor to *Time*, *Life*, *Fortune*, and the *London Sunday Times*.

Geneviève Renson, French
Renson is a self-taught photographer who has been a freelancer specializing in animal and nature photography since her first trip to Africa in 1969. Her work has appeared in *Geo*, *Marie Claire*, *Le Figaro*, and *Playboy*.

Eugene Richards, American
A member of Magnum Photos since 1981, Richards has published work in *Life*, *Stern*, the *New York Times Magazine*, *Geo*, and *Smithsonian*, and has taught at M.I.T., Harvard University, Yale University, and the International Center of Photography. His awards include a Guggenheim Fellowship in 1980, and the Canon Photo Essay Award in 1989.

Jim Richardson, American
Richardson is a freelancer whose images appear in *Time*, *Fortune*,

and *National Geographic*. His photos of the American Midwest have been honored at the World Understanding Contest with three Special Recognition awards.

Rick Rickman, American
During the five years he worked for the *Des Moines Register*, Rickman was named Iowa Photographer of the Year three times. In 1985 he brought a Pulitzer Prize to the *Orange County Register* for coverage of the 1984 Summer Olympics, and was chosen California Photographer of the Year.

Steve Ringman, American
Twice honored as Photographer of the Year by the National Press Photographers Association, and a four-time Bay Area Newspaper Photographer of the Year, Ringman has been on staff at the *San Francisco Chronicle* for ten years. Known for his compassionate work, he shot one of the first photo essays on AIDS patients.

Galen Rowell, American
The 1984 recipient of the Ansel Adams Award, Rowell has exhibited his work at Nikon House, the International Center of Photography, and the Smithsonian Institution. He has nine large-format books to his credit, including *The Yosemite*, published by Sierra Club Books, and *The Art of Adventure*, published by Collins Publishers.

April Saul, American
Saul joined the staff of the *Philadelphia Inquirer* in 1981, and since then has won numerous awards, including the Robert F. Kennedy Journalism Award in 1983 and special recognition in the Canon Photo Essayist Award in 1985. She was a finalist for the Pulitzer Prize in 1987.

Michael A. Schwarz, American
Schwarz worked for the *Baltimore News American*, the *Texarkana Gazette*, and the Associated Press before joining the staff of the *Atlanta Journal Constitution* in 1987. The same year, *Life* magazine honored him as one of the outstanding young photographers in North America.

Stephen Shames, American
Shames has published work in several newsmagazines, including *Time*, *Newsweek*, *New York Magazine*, *Stern*, and *People*. He received honors from the Robert F. Kennedy Journalism Foundation in 1983, 1986, and 1987, and was awarded the Leica Medal of Excellence in Photojournalism in 1983 and 1984.

Bhawan Singh, Indian
A self-taught photographer, Singh is a picture editor for *India Today*, the largest-circulation Indian newsmagazine. His honors include awards from the Nikon Photo Contest and the World Press Photo Foundation.

Leif Skoogfors, Swedish
Skoogfors has published work in thirty-seven countries. He started the photography department at Moore College of Art in Philadelphia and has also taught at Philadelphia College of Art and at Temple University. His pictures are represented in the permanent collections of the Philadelphia Museum of Art and the Corcoran Gallery of Art.

Karel Sláma, Czechoslovakian
Sláma, a retired engineer whose hobby is photojournalism, was a finalist in the 1988 World Health Organization Health for All — All for Health international photo contest.

Rodney Smith, American
Smith has exhibited his work in New York, New Haven, Boston, and New Orleans. He has also taught photography at Yale University, Duke University, and the Maine Photographic Workshops.

Rick Smolan, American
Co-creator of *The Power to Heal*, Smolan is also the creator of the award-winning *Day in the Life* series. A founding member of Contact Press Images, he was one of *Time* magazine's chief photographers in Asia and Australia. His work has appeared in *National Geographic*, *Newsweek*, *Life*, *Fortune*, the *New York Times*, the *London Sunday Times*, *Stern*, and *Paris Match*.

Feliks Solovyov, Soviet
Solovyov has been taking pictures professionally since 1959. A freelancer who works in all genres, he has published work in many Soviet publications and in *Stern*, *Der Spiegel*, and *Quick*.

George Steinmetz, American
Before graduating from Stanford University with a degree in geophysics, Steinmetz took two-and-a-half years to hitchhike through more than twenty African countries. His work currently appears in *Time*, *Fortune*, *Life*, *Geo*, and *National Geographic*.

Thomas Stephan, German
Since 1982 Stephan has worked as a freelance photographer. In 1988 he won top honors in the science and technology category of the World Press Photo Foundation contest for his essay on prematurely born quintuplets.

Mišo Suchý, Czechoslovakian
A photographer and documentary filmmaker, Suchý divides his time between Washington, D.C. and Bratislava, Czechoslovakia. His recent projects include photo-

graphing family life in the United States, military training, and Gypsies.

Patrick Tehan, American
A photographer for the *Orange County Register*, Tehan won top honors in the magazine division of the National Press Photographers Association's Pictures of the Year competition in 1986. He has been a regular participant in *Day in the Life* projects.

Tomasz Tomaszewski, Polish
Tomaszewski's pictures have appeared in *Stern*, *Geo*, and *National Geographic*. In 1985 his exhibition "Remnants —The Last Jews of Poland" received the underground Solidarity Award for best cultural event. Since then, the exhibit has traveled to the International Center of Photography in New York, the National Press Club in Washington, D.C., and the Museum of the Jewish Diaspora in Tel Aviv.

David Turnley, American
The Paris-based Turnley, a correspondent for the *Detroit Free Press* who is affiliated with Black Star photo agency, won the 1990 Pulitzer Prize for his photos of the tumultuous world political events of 1989. His work has appeared in *Time*, *Newsweek*, *Life*, and *National Geographic*. In 1988 he won Picture of the Year from the World Press Photo Foundation.

Jerry Valente, American
A participant in several *Day in the Life* projects, Valente pursues corporate and industrial work. When not taking pictures, he helps run a New York food bank.

David H. Wells, American
Wells has received fellowships from the Pennsylvania Arts Council, Columbia University, and the National Press Foundation. He has published work in *Geo*, *Life*, *National Geographic*, *Time*, *Newsweek*, and the *New York Times Magazine*.

Mark S. Wexler, American
Wexler travels the world as a photographer for a variety of clients, including *Time*, *Life*, *National Geographic*, *Smithsonian*, and *Geo*. He won three World Press Photo Foundation awards for his work on *A Day in the Life of Japan*.

Michael S. Yamashita, American
A regular contributor to *National Geographic* since 1979, Yamashita has also published in *Portfolio*, *Vis à Vis*, and *Travel & Leisure*. He has exhibited his work at the Smithsonian Institution, at Kodak's Professional Photographer's Showcase at Epcot Center, and at the National Gallery in Japan.

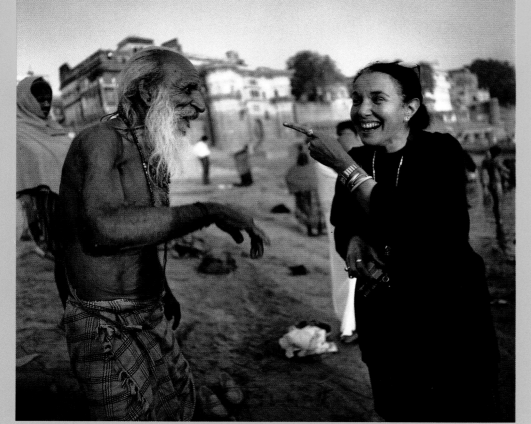
Mary Ellen Mark on assignment in Varanasi, India.

Sponsors, Contributors, and Friends

Major Sponsors
Eastman Kodak Company
Parke-Davis
United States Surgical Company
Empire Blue Cross & Blue Shield
Pan American World Airways
Apple Computer Inc.
Nikon Inc.
San Francisco Marriott

Specialty Group Sponsors
Abbott Laboratories
G.D. Searle and Company
Lederle Laboratories
Miles Inc., Pharmaceutical Division
Schering-Plough Corporation
Syva Company
The Upjohn Company

Major Contributors
Aldus Corporation
Articulate Systems
Barneyscan
Iomega Corporation
Federal Express
Longly Communications
MACsetra
National Instruments
Outbound Systems
Pallas Photo
QMS Inc.
Sausalito Hotel
Shiva Networks
Silicon Beach Software
Sunventure Travel
SuperMac Technology
The Bonnier Group
The New Lab
United Airlines

Software Contributors
Adobe Systems
CE Software
Claris
Connect Inc.
Emerald City Software
Farallon Computing
Intuit
Lundeen & Associates
Microsoft Corporation
Portfolio Systems
Software Ventures
Symantec Corporation

Contributors
ABC News Interactive
Aga Khan Foundation USA
AIDSCOM/Academy of Educational Development
Alaska Airlines
Alfieri & Griffiths
American College of Traditional Chinese Medicine
American Express Publishing
American Fertility Society
American Medical Association
American Medical News
American Red Cross
Associated Press
Astra Research Corporation
Bering Air Inc.
Beyond Words Press
Black Star Publishing
Bowling Green State University
Brigham and Women's Hospital
C.G. Jung Foundation
Camillus Health Concern
Celestial Productions
Center for Investigative Reporting
Centers for Disease Control
Collins San Francisco
Colorado Outward Bound
Cone Communications
Contact Press Images
Creative Artists Agency
Crested Butte Ski Area
Criswell Communications

Duke University Medical Center
DynaMac
Eastern Health Center
Embassy of Finland
Embassy of Zimbabwe
Environmental Traveling Companions
Esquire Magazine
Finnish Tourist Board
FPG International
Friends of Hibakusha
Friends of Photography
Hahnemann University
Handicap International
Hanover Hospital
Hearst Magazines Division
Herbert Birch Services
Howard University
Institute for Circumpolar Health
Institute for Health Policy Studies
Institute for the Future
International Center of Photography
International Committee of the Red Cross
Interplast
Iowa City Free Medical Clinic
Japan External Trade Organization
Japanese American Library, San Francisco
Jordan High School, Los Angeles
Joslin Diabetes Center
Kayenta Health Center
Kelton Labs
King Drew Medical Magnet High School, Los Angeles
Kodalux
KUSA-TV Channel 9, Denver
La Leche League International
Lecture Literary Management
Light Source
Lotus West
MacWeek
Magna
Maine Photographic Workshops
McClean Public Relations
Metro Dade Fire Rescue
Mocrophor, Inc.
Mütter Museum
NASA
National Association of Childbearing Centers
National Geographic Society
National Women's Health Network
New Orleans Planned Parenthood
New York Hospital-Cornell Medical Center
New York University Medical Center
Newsweek Magazine
Novosti Press Agency
Pacific Presbyterian Medical Center
Pairs Software, Inc,
Perth/Aboriginal Medical Service
Pharmaceutical Manufacturers Association
Planetree Health Resource Center
Primal Screen
Professional Photographic Services
Project Concern
Rainforest Action Network
Royal Flying Doctor Service of Australia
Samy's Cameras
San Francisco AIDS Foundation
Sausalito Medical and Surgical Clinic
Scripps Clinic and Research Foundation
Sirpa Sante
Sony Corporation of America
South Carolina Medical Association

South Mississippi Home Health, Inc.
Southwest Foundation for Biomedical Research
St. Luke's-Roosevelt Hospital
Stanford Medical Center
Stern Magazine
TechArt
The Jordan Group, Inc.
The MDS/PRA Group
The Mudd Creek Clinic
The Wellness Community
Time Magazine
Tokyo Hilton International
United States Air Force
University of California San Francisco Medical School
University of Iowa
University of Papua New Guinea
Urban Health Study
USA Today
Victoria Anti-Cancer Campaign
Villa Ki-Yi Dance and Theater Troupe
West Alabama Health Services
West Suburban Hospital Medical Center
Woodfin Camp & Associates
World Health Organization
Yale University
Yerkes Primate Research Center
Ziff Davis Publishing

Friends and Advisors
Mary Abboud
Frederick Able
Alyssa & Eddie Adams
Katherine Adler
Deborah Agre
Mariann Alcorn
Bill Allen
Dr. Brian Allen
Tomoko Amano
Diana Anderson
Lisa Anderson
Dr. Paul Andrews
Mary Lou Aquino
Harry Arader
Dr. Jorge Arias
Rachael Arvallo
Bill Atkinson
Cecilia Atkinson
Dr. William Atkinson
Karen Bakke
Anna Maria Bambara
Jill Bamberg
Martin Bander
John Barch
Debra Bard
Howard Barney
Lori Barra
Terry Bartlett
Dr. Artie Ann Bates
Ben Bauermeister
Andy Bechtolsheim
Ross Beck
Dr. Sergei Belenky
Dr. Harold Benjamin
Mark Benninghoff
Dr. Herbert Benson
Dr. Margaret Bentley
Larry Berkin
Michele Bernard
George & Keetje Berndt
Bill Berry
Jeffrey Bertsch
David Bethune
Vince Bielski
Lionel Bird
Dr. James Birrell
Cindy Black
Gerald Blake
Britt Blaser
Chris Bleck
Gene Blumberg
Nicola Blundell-Brown
Janice Boardley
Richard Boardley
Urs Boegli
David Bohrman
Mike Boich
Roger Boissoneault
Tony Bonelli

Amy Bonetti
Alberto Bonvicini
Mark Booth
Susan Bowldy
Dr. Jim Boyle
Jessica Brackman
Patricia Bradbury
Paul Brainerd
Kandes Bregman
Elizabeth Broughton
Dr. Jeff Brown
Russell Brown
Barbara Browning
Karen Bruck
Cecilia Brunazzi
Laurie Bryant
Diane Burns
James Busby
Thomas Bvuma
Victor Byrd
JoAnn Cabello
Bill Calhoun
Sean Callahan
Woody Camp
Bill Campbell
Dr. Henrique Moisés Canter
Cornell Capa
Albert A. Cardone
Paige Carlin
Perry Carson
Richard Cartiere
Michael Castleman
Gina & Mike Cerre
Nancy Chambers
Howard Chapnick
Sarah Charf
Brad Chase
Dr. Edward Chaum
Hen Sen Chin
Judy Ann Christensen
Maria Christidou
Albert Chu
Dr. Da Tong Chu
John Clark
Dr. Margaret Clark
Paul Clark
Dr. Harris Clearfield
Dr. Alwyn Cohall
Dr. Herbert Cohen
Richard Cohn
Jennifer Coley
Christie Collins
Vicky Comiskey
Maggie Condon
Carol Cone
Dave Conklin
Donald Conklin
Alex Conn
Sheila M. Conn
Rob Cook
Scott Cook
Edward Corboy
Mary Core
Sonia Corea
Helen & Jack Corn
Tracey Cosgrove
Lisa Court
Kelly Courtney
Brad Coyle
George Craig
Kim Criswell
Sue Crowdis
Steve Crowe
Jim Cullen
Joe D'Arco
Bill Dalton
Rob Daniels
Peter Danos
Jennifer Daves
Paula David
Liz Davila
Sashka T. Dawg
Laura De Young
Dr. Enrico Deaglio
Cliff Deeds
François DeLorme
Jim DeMain
Wayne Dickerson
Joe Dilger
Chickie Diogardi
Carol Squire Diomande
Jim Domke
Sheila Donnelly

Annette Doornbos
Clifford Douglas
Mark Dowie
Michael Downey
Arnold & Elaine Drapkin
Gayle & Gene Driskell
Natasha Driskell
John David Dupree
John Durniak
Esther Dyson
Oscar Dystell
Mary Dawn Early
Fred Ebrahimi
Steve Edelman
Lisa Edmondson
Dr. Peter Eisenberg
Sean Elder
Gloria Emerson
Robert Engle
Dr. David Epstein
Ellen Erwitt
Elliott Erwitt
Jeanette Erwitt
Gordon Eubanks
Dr. Michael Evans
Valerie Fahey
Lisa Falco
Beth Churchill Fantz
Daniel Farber
Tibor Farkas
Jason Farrow
Elizabeth Faulkner
Dr. Shotsy Faust
Diane Feldman
Harlan Felt
Roy Fidler
Bill Finelli
Phyllis Fischer
Dr. Susan Fitzpatrick
Mary Fleming
Dorothy Flippo
Iris J. Fluellen
Connie Folleth
Paulette & Lazlo Fono
Tony Fontaine
Hazel Foster
Cindy Fox-Aisen
Fred Francis
Richard Frankel
Sara Frankel
Bruce Fraser
Dr. Charles Fraser
Janice Fraser
Eleanor Freedman
Henry Freedman
Ed Fritzky
John Frook
Chuck Fry
Dr. Robert Gale
Leslie & Marvin Gans
Jenni Gant
Rebecca Gardner
J.P. Garnier
Wilbur E. Garrett
Lucy Garrick
Silvio Gasbarrino
Joe Gasparrini
Jean Louis Gassée
Bill Gates
Charlotte Gay
Rich Gazer
Seth Geiger
Noreen Geistle
Marge Gibbons
Mark Gielecki
Candy Gilar
Peg &Tom Gildersleeve
Sheldon Gilgore
Catherine Gilmore
Laura Gilpin
Dr. Martin Gittleman
Tom Gliatto
Robbie Gluckson
Vicky Godbey
Kate Godfrey
Cathy Golden
Nate Goldhaber
Dr. Jeff Goldhagen
Marc Gombeaud
Christine Gomez
Dr. Charles Good
Danny Goodman
Jim Gordon

Joel Gottler
Henry Gougelman
Brian Grazer
Harry Greene
Dr. Joe Greer
Mark Greyson
Lisa Griffins
Tom & Rusty Grimaldi
Bonnie Grimes
Jane Gross
Sheila Groves
Claire Gruppo
Nellie Gupta
Susan Gurley
Steve Guttman
Don & Lily Guy
Dr. Penn Handwerker
Karen Hansen
Dr. Karen Hardy
Dr. Maria Hari
Nick Harris
Ginni Hassrick
Steve Haugan
Barry Haynes
Richard Heckler
Vince Heidenreich
Steve Heiner
Ruth-Inge Heinze
Hugh Helm
Diana Hembree
Dr. William Hendee
Dr. Joseph Henderson
Lori Henderson
Stuart Henigson
Holly S. Herman
Amy Herndon
José Herrera
Brad Herrmann
Lenore Hershey
Andy Hertzfeld
Steve Higgins
Bill Hinchberger
David Hindawi
William Hindmarch
Dr. Harry Hirsch
Leon Hirsch
Art Hoffman
Mike Hoffman
Ulla Hoikkala
Mike Holm
Carol Holmelund
Marc Honig
Elena Hortado
Maureen Houlihan
John Howard
Ron Howard
Shay Huffman
Dr. Sandral Hullett
Lynn Hutto
Dora Hyde
Dr. John Ireland
Vern Iuppa
Charlie Jackson
Tom Jackson
Ken Jacobs
Rita D. Jacobs
Dr. Mark Jacobs
Janice James
Peter Jarrett
Dr. David Jensen
Kathy and Phillip Jiang
Steve Jobs
Ken Jones
Dr. Brigitte Jordan
Judy Jorgensen
Turey Josefsen
Mike Joseph
Bill Joy
Linda S. Jue
Karen Kai
Susan Kare
George Kaufmann
S. Kawasaki
Dr. Daniel Kelly
Kevin Kelly
Kim Kelly
Nathalie Kelly
Susan Kelly
Alison Kennedy
Robert Kennedy
Tom Kennedy
Dr. Robert Kerlan
Mel Kerner

223

Brad Kibbel
Tina King
Dr. William Knaus
Kent Kobersteen
Maritta Koch-Weser
Melanie Kohn
Jerome Kossoff
Tony Krantz
Susan Krattiger
Susan Krenn
Jeff Kriendler
Andrew Kruger
Chris Kuebler
Kambowa Kukyuwa
Miki Kurosu
Jim Kurshuk
Eliane Laffont
Jim Lamb
Linda Lamb
Rupta & Vishuas Lambley
Sonia Land
Sandra Lane
Dr. Douglas Lanes
Steve Langer
Leo Laporte
George Larrieu
Denise & Jim Larsen
Dr. Allen Lavee
Steve Lawrence
Pat Layton
Polly Leach-Lychee
Billie Geanne Lebda
Dr. Aleksei Lebedev
Richard Leclair
John Leddy
Frankie Lee
Klaus Lempke
James & Susan Lenfestey
Sharon Levandovich
Martin Levin
Howard Levine
Jim & Lynn Levinson
Thad Lewallen
Lisa Lewis
Shirley Lewis
Maureen Liberti
Katherine Lindstrom
Wayne Llano
Dunbar Lockwood
Dail Lodge
John Loengard
Richard LoPinto
Bill Lord
Barbara Lubin
Tim Lundeen
Donna Lundsford
David Lyman
Thomas Lytle
Jenny Macdonnell
Maria Tereza Machado-Menuez
Dr. Robert Mack
Mark E. Mackbee
Karen MacMaster
Dr. Julie Madorsky
Judi Magann
Linda Maita
Dr. Ted Mala
Alfred Mandel
Elisa Mantel
Katherine Mann
Sophia Marchand
Thom Marchionna
Kevin Mardorf
David Markus
Peter Marshall
Ikuo Masaki
Greg Mason
Dr. Edward Mason
Susan Massaron
Dixie Matthews
Lucienne & Richard Matthews
Gil Maurer
Fred Mayer
Elizabeth McAllister
Dan McCammon
Laurie McClean
Theresa McCormick
Mary McDaniels
Nancy McDonald
Carro McFadyen
Kathleen McKenna
Dr. Howard McKinney, Jr.
Christy McLaren

Charlotte "Arkie" Meisner
Dorothy Mendolson
Karen Meredith
James Merker
Kathi Merritt
Tripp Mikich
Ron Millender
Jill Miller
Ivan Mimica
Bob Minnis
Marlene Mitrovich
Brenda Moffitt
Robert Moore
Tom Moore
Dana Morgan
Dr. Bernard Moriniere
Harriet & Michael Moritz
Naheed Morrill
Rev. Scott Morris
Ann Moscicki
Karen Mullarkey
Mary Munly
Dr. Stanley Music
Dr. Jane Mutambirwa
Mahesh Naithani
Susanna Napierala
Jean Jacques Naudet
Benjamin Naythons
William Naythons
Sherry Neff
Harry Nelson
Nick Nishida
Joe Noel
Rod Nordland
Peggy Northrop
Peter Nosco
Dr. Mark Novitch
Boxer & Yvonne Nthabu
Jonas Nyren
Elizabeth & Michael O'Brien
Maeve O'Connor
Kathleen O'Donnell
John O'Neal
Wendy Oakes
Harry Oberkfell
T. Ogasawara
Tetsu Okumoto
Karen Olcott
Kathryn Olney
Dan Oshima
Gene Ostroff
John Owen
Melville Owen
Carrie Padilla
Bill Pakela
Dr. Jorge Palacios
Rusty Pallas
Beverly Palmer
Paula Palmer
Wendy Palmer
Rick Pappas
Dr. John Parascandola
Dr. K.J. Pataki-Schweizer
Jim Patchen
Daniel Paul
Sylvia Paull
Micha X. Peled
Carl Pelzel
Holly Peppe
Tyler Peppel
Gabe Perle
Dave Pernock
Brent Peterson
Donna Pfeiffer
David Pfieffer
Pamela Pfiffner
Christine Phillip
Mike Phillips
David Phinney
Sandy Pickup
Joe Pieroni
Robert Pledge
Sue Pondrom
Jane Popolizio
Ginny Power
Christine Preble
Robert Pritikin
Darcy Provo
Douglas Putnam
Cathy Quealy
Mamiki & Sonny Ramithibela
Michael Rand
Hilary Raskin

Barry Reder
Dorothy Redfield
Dr. Irwin Redlener
Pamela Reed
Sharon Reed
Dr. Bill Reger
Sidney Regnier
Carl Reichel
Dr. Quentin Reilly
Marta Remenius
Helen Ressini
Sister Agnes Reynolds
David Rice
Rich Richardson
Thomas P. Rielly
Dennis Ring
Ken Ritvo
Jack Robbins
Jerry Roberts
Ty Roberts
Joan Robertson
Rick Rocamora
Monty Roessell
Michael Rooks
Leslie Rosen
Bob & Joan Rosenberg
Dr. John Rosenberg
Gerald Rosenberg
Marilyn Rosenthal
Dr. Jane Ross
John Ross
Dr. Barry Rostek
Jim Rowe
Tom Rowe
Joann Rubeck
Ann Rubin
Robin Ruse-Rinehart
Cornelia Rutledge
Tom Ryder
Mark Rykoff
Dana Sachs
Paul Saffo
Nola Safro
Myron Sailer
Janet & Sanjay Sakhuja
Akihiko Sakuda
Louis Saliba
Marianne Samenko
Ismail Samji
Bob Sanders
Dr. Joseph Santana
Jenny & Murray Sayle
Cynthia Schartzer
Steve Scheier
Eric Schlesinger
Paul Schmidman
Sue Schmidt
Steve Schneider
Dr. Larry Schonberger
Kaiulani Schuler
Dr. Debra Schumann
Paul Seaton
Steve Seekins
Dr. Milton Seifert
Tom Sellars
Karen Seriguchi
Ann Jennings Shackelford
Bill Shapiro
Audrey Shehyn
Ron Shelton
Joanne Sherer
Stephanie Sherman
Bob Shimek
Rimi Shiraishi
Wayne Silby
Andrew Singer
Laura Singer
Bob Siroka
Susan Skand
Richard Skeie
Brian Smiga
Dr. Betsy Smith
Karen Smith
Polly Smith
Rick Smith
Gloria Smolan
Leslie Smolan
Sandy Smolan
Michael Snowden
Nancy Sobin-Dryer
Joy & Marty Solomon
Lou Sosa
Dr. Melanie Sovine

Barbara Sparks
Roger Spottiswoode
Douglas Squires
Mary Stainton
Don Stang
Mike Stark
Shirley Starke
Mark Stephens
Michele Stephenson
Suzanne Stewart
John Stimson
John Clay Stites
Julie Stock
Jim Stockton
Wendy Storch
David Stout
Lew Stowbunenko
Marilee Strong
Charles Stroupe
Jill Sullivan
Daryl Summers
Barry Sundermeier
Phyllis Susser
Peter Sutch
Doug Swartz
Norma Swenson
Martin Swig
Gayle Tagliatera
Dr. Sinezio Talhari
Kathy Tallone
Shingo Tanaka
Ron Taniwaki
David Taylor
Rebecca Taylor
Michael Tchao
Dr. John Templer
Bob Terifay
Bill Thompson
Jim Thylin
Stephen Tiger
Laura Toland
Doug Tompkins
Vivian Tourlis
Patricia Townsend
Mario Trivizas
Andy Trohanis
Linda Troller
Vivian Tsu
Karen Tucker
David Valdez
Dan Valerio
Willem Van Buren
Della Van Heyst
Vea Van Kessel
Nick van Praag
Vicki Vance
Chuck Vaughn
Doug Vennell
Ryan P. Ver Berkmoes
Dr. Jacques & Larry Vidal
Alicia Villanueva
Marjorie Vinnedge
Joyce Volk
T. Wada
Loretta Wagner
George Walker
Robert Walker
Robert T. Walker
Susan Walker
Jeannette Walker
Vickie Walter
Bill Warner
John Warnock
Drs. Linda & Roger Warren
John Watters
Dr. Andrew Weil
Irwin Weiner
Leonora Wiener
Nan Wiener
Kevin Weldon
Dr. Charles Wells
David White
Terry Whitman
Gregory Wilker
Frederick D. Wilkinson Jr.
Dr. George Wilkinson
Mary Joan Willard
Barbara Williams
Russell Willier
Janice Wilson
Joan Winch
Dave Winer
Fred Winninger

Jim Witous
Dan Wohlfeiler
Robin Wolaner
Mary Celio Wolf
Jimmy Woods
Amy Woodworth
Gretchen Worden
Simon Worrin
John Woychcik
Tanner Wray
Richard Saul Wurman

Kitty Yancy
René Yañez
Junichi Yano
Stan Yoder
Dr. David Young
Kate Yuschenkoff
Joyce Zeitz
Mel & Pat Ziegler
Dr. Philip Ziring
Peter Zogas

About this book...

Despite the complex logistics involved in researching and coordinating assignments for 100 photographers around the world, editing their nearly 300,000 photographs down to the 200 or so in the finished book, designing and organizing the presentation of the photos, and researching and writing captions and essays, The Power to Heal was produced, start to finish, in seven months — less than half the time most publishers take to produce a book.

The key to this project was our use of Apple's Macintosh computers, with their desktop-publishing and related technologies. Each of our seventeen full-time staff members used a Macintosh SE and a SuperMac DataFrame hard disk. Our computers were part of a local area network connected through Farallon Computing's PhoneNet Plus and CE Software's QuickMail electronic mail system. Detailed research was facilitated with Dialog's online database using Farallon's 9600-baud modem. Farallon's Timbuktu program allowed editors to consult online with researchers at their workstations. Traveling staff communicated back to the office with Connect's MacNet online service.

Assignment ideas were organized and logged in with Symantec's More outlining program. The database and word processing modules of Microsoft Works were combined with Lundeen & Associates' WorksPlus Spell to keep track of photographers and create mail-merged letters for their global photo shoots.

The design and production were done on three Macintosh IIcx computers using SuperMac Trinitron monitors with Spectrum/24 series 111 color cards. The images were digitized on both a Barneyscan Imagescanner and an Apple flatbed scanner and then saved onto 44-megabyte cartridges on a dual Bernoulli drive. Image scanning was done with technical assistance from Light Source. Layout was done using Aldus PageMaker, with final assembly and linkage of the layouts stored on Macsetra's Genesis 6000 erasable optical drive. We proofed the book on a QMS model 100 color printer, which allowed us to preview the entire book in color and show it to bookstore representatives many months ahead of publication.

Final output was generated on a Linotronic 300 printer at Digital Prepress International in San Francisco. Traditional color separations and printing were done at Dai Nippon Printing Co., Ltd. in Tokyo.

Other software used in producing The Power to Heal included: Claris' MacWrite II and Filemaker II, Adobe Systems' Adobe Type Manager and Photoshop, Emerald City's TypeAlign, Software Ventures' MicroPhone II, Intuit's Quicken, Portfolio Systems' DynoDex, CE Software's CalendarMaker and Articulate Systems' Voice Navigator.

We gratefully acknowledge these companies for their generous support of The Power to Heal.